SIXTH EDITION

Controlling Stress and Tension

Daniel A. Girdano

George S. Everly Jr.

Dorothy E. Dusek

Allyn and Bacon

Boston • London • Toronto • Sydney • Tokyo • Singapore

Vice President: *Paul A. Smith*
Publisher: *Joseph E. Burns*
Series Editorial Assistant: *Annemarie Kennedy*
Composition and Prepress Buyer: *Linda Cox*
Manufacturing Buyer: *Julie McNeill*
Cover Administrator: *Linda Knowles*
Editorial-Production Service: *Shepherd, Inc.*

Library of Congress Cataloging-in-Publication Data

Girdano, Daniel A.
  Controlling stress and tension / Daniel A. Girdano, Dorothy E. Dusek, George S.
Everly.—6th ed.
    p. cm.
  Includes bibilographical references and index.
  ISBN 0–205–31724–3
  1. Stress management. 2. Stress (Psychology) I. Dusek, Dorothy. II. Everly, George S.,
1950- III. Title

RA785.G57 2001
155.9'042—dc21

                                                                          00-044764

Printed in the United States of America

10 9 8 7 6 5 4 3 2 1   04 03 02 01 00

CONTENTS

Preface   xiii

1 Stress, Stressors, and Stress Management   1

Stressors in Life   1
Frequency, Intensity, Duration, and Valence   2

Stress and Disease   4
Disorders of Arousal   5

Stress Management   9
Intervention Points   9
Free Will and Mindfulness   9
Choices   11

Sources Cited   14

2 Systems That Control Stress Arousal   15

The Purpose of the Stress Response   15

The Basic Systems of Control   16
The Autonomic Nervous System (ANS)   16
Autonomic Control of the Stress Response   25

The Endocrine System   25
The Pituitary: The Master Gland   26
The Adrenal Glands   26

Sources Cited   28

3 The Body's Response to Stress   29

The Stress Response Pathway   29
The Muscles' Response   35
The Gastrointestinal Response   36
The Brain's Response   39
The Cardiovascular Response   40
The Skin's Response   43

The Immune System's Response   44
Structure and Function of the Immune System   44
Stress and the Immune System   46

The Prevention and Treatment of Diseases of Arousal   47

Sources Cited   49

4   Stressful Emotions, Thoughts, and Beliefs   50

The Development of Human Emotion   51
Self-Assessment Exercise 1   55
Pain and Pleasure   56

Emotional Energy   56
Stressful Emotional Patterns   58
Emotion Recall Exercise   59
Breaking Unhealthy Emotional Cycles   60

Thoughts and Beliefs   61
Thoughts   61
Beliefs   62

Exercises to Decrease Emotional Stress   64
Learn Anger Management   64
Examine Beliefs Regarding Anger   65
Explore Your Fear History   65
Take Action   65
Give Away Fear   66
Examine Beliefs Regarding Fear   66

Sources Cited   66

5   The Human Spirit   68

Living the Spiritual Life   69

Stress in Seeking Spirit   71

Two Insights from Science   72

Personality and Individuality   73

The Forces   75

Steps toward Enlightenment   75

Exercises   77
   Honor Code   77
   Lies I Have Told   78
   The Four Major Questions   78
   Mysteries and Miracles   78

Sources Cited and Recommended Readings   79

6 Patterns of Behavior   80

Self-Perception   80
   Self-Assessment Exercise 2   81
   Components of Self-Concept   82
   Effects on Behavior   83
   Effects on Disease   84

Enhancing Self-Concept   84
   List Your Resources   85
   List Subpersonalities   85
   Affirmations   85
   Compliments   86
   Assertiveness   86
   The Assertiveness Ladder   87
   Interpersonal Effectiveness Training   89
   Recognition   89
   Analysis   90
   Action   90
   Avoid Negative Self-Talk   90
   Examine Negative Beliefs   91
   "Go Fever"   91
   Self-Assessment Exercise 3   94

Exercises   95
   Practice Concentration   95
   Planning   95
   Examine Attachment Involvement   96
   Anxiety   96
   Self-Assessment Exercise 4   98

Exercises   100
   Thought Stopping   100
   Stress and the Need for Control   100
   Self-Assessment Exercise 5   101

Exercises 103

    Keep a Journal 103
    Calm Yourself 104
    Reality Check 104
    Let Go of Judgments 104
    Cognitive Restructuring 104
    Examine Beliefs 106

Sources Cited 106

7 Demands and Expectations 108

Change 108

    Self-Assessment Exercise 6 110
    Control 113
    Challenge 113
    Commitment 113

Exercises 114

    Establish Routines 114
    Avoid Change 114
    Plan for Change 115
    Action Plan 115
    Frustration 116
    Overcrowding 116
    Self-Assessment Exercise 7 117
    Discrimination 118
    Socioeconomic Factors 118
    Bureaucracy 119

Exercises 121

    Express Your Frustration 121
    Determine Your Real Outcomes 121
    Choose Alternatives 122
    Examine Beliefs 124
    Question 125
    Answers 125
    Turning Beliefs Around 125
    Take Action 126
    Behavioral Skills 126

Overload 126

    Urban Overload 126
    Self-Assessment Exercise 8 127
    Occupational Overload 128
    Academic Overload 129
    Domestic Overload 129

Exercises   130

Expressing Your Feelings   130
Negotiate   130
Manage Time   131
Say What You Want   132
Delegate   132
Expectation History   132
Examine Beliefs   133

Decision Making and Problem Solving   133

Exercise   135
Boredom and Loneliness   136
Self-Assessment Exercise 9   137

Exercises   138

Keep a Journal   138
Physical Activity   138
Join a Social Group   138
Ask for Human Contact   138
Examine Beliefs   139

Sources Cited   138

8   Stress and the Human Environment Interaction   141

Time and Body Rhythms   141

Self-Assessment Exercise 10   143

Eating and Drinking Habits   144

Sympathomimetic Agents   144
Hypoglycemic Stress   145
Sodium Intake and Fluid Retention   146
Eating Guidelines   148
Drugs, Alcohol, and Tobacco   150
Noise Pollution   154
Music Therapy   156

Climate and Altitude   157

Sources Cited   158

9   Stress in Relationships   159

Love   159

Relationships   161

Making a Relationship Work   164
Living Together   165

Communication   166
Fighting Fair   168
Areas of Stressful Conflict   169
Sexual Relations   169
Recall Exercise   170
Money   172
Personal Habits   172
Jealousy   172
In-laws   173

Separation   173

Loneliness   174

Sources Cited   177

10   Crisis, Violence, and Posttraumatic Stress   178

Historical Background   178

Posttraumatic Stress Disorder   180
Consequences   181
The Nature of Posttraumatic Stress   181
Traumatic Events   184
Coping with Traumatic Stress   185

Violence: A Special Form of Crisis   187

Sources Cited   188

11   Stress in the Workplace   189

Job Stress   189

Occupational Stressors   191

Self-Assessment Exercise 11   192

Organizational Stressors   193
Lack of Financial Rewards   193
Lack of Career Guidance   193
Overspecialization   194
Work Overload   194
Decision Making   196

Individual Stressors   198
Occupational Frustration   198
Job Ambiguity and Role Conflict   198
Stifled Communication   199

Discrimination   199
Bureaucracy   200
Inactivity and Boredom   200

Environmental Stressors   201
Change and Adaptation   202
Violence in the Workplace   203
Retirement   204

Biological Factors in the Workplace   205
Time Change   205
Noise   205
Lighting   206
Computers and Eye Strain   206
Carpal Tunnel Syndrome   207
Temperature   208
Physical Posture   208
Compassion Fatigue: The Stress
    of Caring Too Much   208
Occupational Stress Management   209
Sources Cited   210

12   Breathing and Relaxation   213

Breathing Correctly   213
Upper Costal Breathing   215
Middle Costal Breathing   215
Diaphragmatic Breathing   215
Very Deep Breathing   215

Breathing Exercises   216
Breathing Down   216
Controlled Tempo Breathing   217
Breath Counting   218
Aromatherapy   218

Sources Cited   221

13   Muscle Relaxation   222

Neuromuscular Exercises   223
The Learning Phase   224
Preparation   224
Lower Extremities   225
Hips and Knees   226
Trunk   227

Upper Extremities   228
Head, Neck, and Face   230

Biofeedback   232

Massage and Bodywork   234
Traditional Massage   234
Structural/Functional/Movement Integration   235

Sources Cited   238

14   Autogenics and Visual Imagery   239

Autogenic Relaxation Training: Relaxation Recall   239

Legs Heavy and Warm   241
Center of Warmth   241
Arms Heavy and Warm   242
Freedom Posturing   242
Situation 1   243
Situation 2   243
Your Special Place   244

Visual Imagery   245

Sources Cited   246

15   Yoga and Stretch-Relaxation   247

Yoga   247

Stretch-Relaxation Exercises   247

Toe Raise, Knee Stretch, Toe Touch   248
Back Stretch Forward and Reverse, Standing
    Trunk Bend   250
Wall Reach, Sky Reach, Shoulder Roll, Back Reach,
Shoulder Elevation   253

Sources Cited   260

16   Meditation   261

Brainwaves   262

Types of Meditation   263

Concentration   264

Contemplation   265

Meditation and the Reduction of Stress Arousal   266

How to Meditate   267

Mindfulness and Insight Meditation   271
The Need for Practice   272

Sources Cited   273

17   Stress Reduction through Physical Activity   274

Physical Activity as Treatment   275

Physical Activity in the Prevention of Disease   276

Exercise for Well-Being and Tranquility   277

Beyond Competition   278

High-Risk Activity   279

Exercise Assessment   279

Exercise Program Benefits and Guidelines   282

Stronger Heart and Better "Tuning"
of the Heartbeat   282
Increased Muscle Strength and Endurance   282
Increased Lung Capacity   282
Stronger Bones   282
Improved Serum-Cholesterol Level
and HDL/LDL Ratio   283
Improved Body Composition   283
Increased Range of Motion   283
Greater Efficiency, Attention, and Economy
of Movement   283
Greater Alertness   283
Diminished Effects of Aging   283

Preprogram Guidelines and Principles   284

Regularity   284
Variety   284
The Overload Principle   284
Aerobics Program   285
Heart Rate   285
Intensity and Duration   286
Flexibility Program   287
Muscular Strength and Endurance Programs   287

Sources Cited   288

18   **Your Personal Stress-Management Plan**   **289**

Developing the Plan   290

Step 1. What Do You Want to Accomplish?   290
Step 2. How Will Things Be Different or Better
    in Your Life?   293

Outcome Visualization   294

Step 3. How Do You Know When You Have
    Achieved an Outcome?   294
Step 4. What Are Your Useful Resources?   295
    Finding a Resource State   295
Step 5. What are Your Blocks to Success?   298
    Fear of Failure   298
    Fear of Success   298
Step 6. Devise an Action Plan   299
Step 7. Devise a Revised Plan   300

A Sample Practice Plan   301

Sources Cited   305

Appendix: Personal Stressor Profile Summary   306

Index   309

PREFACE

A major factor in the maintenance of health is the ability to live in harmony within society while keeping to a minimum the detrimental effects of one pervasive by-product of modern society—excess stress and tension.

Stress is a multidimensional phenomenon. Reducing its detrimental effects is best accomplished by modifying many varied aspects of your lifestyle. This modification involves reducing the stressfulness of interactions with other people and the environment. An often unspoken, yet very important aspect of stress is that it is a by-product of your belief system, which is an outgrowth of your personal philosophy. Aligning your behavior with your philosophy may be the ultimate stress-reduction technique. Behavior is dependent upon becoming aware of your emotional response system and learning how to balance your feelings with appropriate social behaviors. Finally, becoming aware of the connection between mind and body as it applies to both arousal and relaxation and mastering techniques of relaxation provide a healthy means of perceiving the inner and outer world. Incorporating nutritional and exercise patterns completes the stress-management package.

This book teaches a multifaceted and holistic approach to the control of stress and tension. This approach operates on many levels, encompassing both self and environment and incorporating the physical, emotional, mental, social, and spiritual facets of life. The first part of the book discusses the stress problem and our potential for achieving a solution, examining the relationship between mind and body, the nature of stress and the stress response, the mind-body theory of disease, and the psychoneuroimmunological mechanisms that link stress and illness. An in-depth look at emotions, thoughts, and beliefs is followed by a thought-provoking look at stress and the human spirit.

The next several chapters examine a number of specific categories of potential stress-producing elements in everyday life. Examples of these categories are patterns of behavior; demands and expectations; environmental relationships; human relationships; crisis, violence, and trauma; and job stress. Through self-assessment exercises in each category, readers have the opportunity to determine the stressful factors in their own lives. The self-assessment techniques culminate in the construction of a personal stress profile. Stress-management techniques and many original and other popular time-tested relaxation methods and exercises are presented for each stress problem and combined into a complete stress-management system.

The remainder of the book consists of techniques used to alleviate stress and tension. Some are specific to the causes of stress mentioned previously, while others are general techniques for reducing stress reactions, such as deep breathing and meditation. Detailed instructions are provided along with discussion of the basic mechanism underlying each technique.

In the final chapter, readers participate in a step-by-step procedure to build their own holistic stress-management programs based on their personal insights, needs, and abilities.

Acknowledgments

We would like to thank the following reviewers: Barbara Brehm-Curtis, Smith College; Allen Kelley, Essex Community College; Frances McGrath-Kovank, San Francisco State University; Kathy Pignatelli, Bergen Community College; Glen Richardson, University of Utah; Andrew Ryan Jr., USC at Columbia; Walter Schneider, St. Thomas Aquinas College; Jon Swanson, Benedictine University; and Bill Thompson, Belmont University.

CHAPTER

1

Stress, Stressors, and Stress Management

Stress is a mind-body arousal that can, on the one hand, save our lives and, on the other, fatigue body systems to the point of malfunction and disease. Stress is both a physical response that protects us and a natural defense mechanism that has allowed our species to survive. We need stress and would not want to eradicate our capacity for the stress response even if this were possible. Stress can be motivating, energizing, exciting, and fun; it can challenge us to greater endeavor. At the same time, it is known to be implicated in at least 80 percent of the illnesses that plague modern society.

Stressors in Life

A stressor is any condition or event that causes a stress response. Stressors can be physical, emotional, intellectual, social, economic, or spiritual. A stressor may be real or imagined; however, the response to the stressor (i.e., the human stress response), is always real.

Look at your surroundings, your situation, and your life in general. Opportunities to be stressed are everywhere, from minor annoyances, such as not being able to find a parking spot, to major fears, such as getting fired or failing to get into grad school.

Interestingly enough, the greatest challenge to your serenity is not next week's test or finding the right employment—it is human relationships: intimate partners, friends, children, parents, employers, co-workers, teachers, siblings, even campus cops and store clerks. Imagine a circus juggler tossing knives up in the air and fretfully managing to keep them safely in motion. Such is the stress of relationships—trying to balance your needs with those of others and still be loved, cared for, admired, and rewarded. The stress of relationships may be summed up in one word: expectations. Stress in human relationships comes from a combination of failure to meet the expectations of others and failure to get your needs met. On the positive side, relationships pressure us to grow and change, and they ground us when they are loving.

Intimate relationships bring up issues such as loyalty, values, morals, defending lifestyle choices, competition, rivalry, compatibility, jealousy, and control. These same issues follow us into the workplace: trying to please, get noticed, get promoted, and get a raise. The workplace has great potential for satisfaction, yet it also has potential for disappointment, frustration, and discrimination, what some call *occupational stress*.

1

Personal safety is becoming a greater concern for everyone. Terrible incidents such as the Columbine High School shootings make us wonder whether any place is safe. Conflict is a universal stressor with profound implications for health and well-being. Fear, worry, anger, and revenge are emotions that are directly related to stress. Posttraumatic stress and its treatment have become a given for those who have survived (or for many who have even observed) traumatic experiences such as rape, murder, bombings, and natural disasters.

Underlying all of our short- and long-term stressors is the inner conflict of matching our behaviors with our personal code of ethics. Most of us struggle with an inner conflict, a clash of values, a war waged on a philosophical/spiritual level for control of our behavior. We struggle between what we know is right and what is convenient or economical or feels good at the moment. We practice self-deception with rationalization, denial, and other psychological defense mechanisms. "Everyone else is doing it." "I'll suck it up now, make big money, and straighten out my life after I'm at the top." How many are brave enough to follow their personal code of ethics? How many even know what their personal code of ethics is?

Much of this book is about psychology, that is, what we think and how we think. All stress relates to how we think or we perceive the world—in other words, our philosophy of life, our ideals, and our beliefs. Philosophy has many aspects, and one is the belief that there is order to the universe and our place in it. This order dictates that a right way and a wrong way, a loving way and a fearful way all exist. Inner peace, which comes from a more joyful and less stressed life, is the result of living closer to what we believe is right and loving. Both Eastern and Western philosophers agree that our spiritual path transforms our consciousness and that the forces that create suffering and stress in ourselves and in the world, such as greed, hatred, ignorance, fear, envy, and jealousy, originate in our hearts.

Frequency, Intensity, Duration, and Valence

In physical terms, stress means strain, pressure, or force on a system. In the context of the human experience, it is the body's reacting to the environment through the buildup of internal pressure and the strain of muscles tensing for action. If prolonged, this physical pressure and strain can fatigue or damage the body. W. B. Cannon (1939) first defined stress as the fight-or-flight syndrome: When one becomes stressed, the proper use of that stress is either to fight off the threat or to run from it. To do either, the body prepares itself through the psychological mechanisms of coping and cognition and the motor act (behavior) that alleviates the stressor. The goal is to manage stress by diminishing the excess stress in our lives, the stress that is inappropriate for accomplishing our objectives.

Three aspects that help frame an understanding of stress are frequency, intensity, and duration. The most important of these is the duration of the stress response. Even stress that is not particularly severe can, if prolonged, fatigue and damage the body to the point of malfunction and disease. Disease is not the only focus. A more immediate consequence is that excess stress robs us of joy in our lives. If we are worried about money, success, or image, if we are pressured by expectations and work demands, if we are angry and looking for ways to get revenge, we eventually lose our ability to feel the happiness, joy, and love that represent the core of the human experience. When we are under stress, our attention focuses on survival, and we retreat to escapist daydreams of a better tomorrow instead of finding ways to live each moment with joy and enthusiasm. Most philosophers and religious leaders teach that the purpose of life is to increase our enlightenment and to perfect our spirit. This becomes difficult to accomplish when our stressed lives do not allow for the silence so necessary for introspection. Stress can be a thief that robs us of not only our health but also our happiness.

The stress response of modern man and woman is often inappropriate both to the situation and in its level of intensity. Although physical stressors still exist, most of the stressors of modern society are primarily social or ego related. When a stressor is ego related or is a response to a social situation, it cannot be solved by a physical response. In addition, it may not be alleviated for a long period. If the threat is imagined and the stress response is stimulated, we cannot physically run from it. Pressure builds up, and part of us wants to strike out while the other part strains to hold back. Externally, nothing happens. Internally, the body is trapped in the tension.

Stressors occur daily; they are part of life. However, we must examine the valence of the stressor when we talk about its effect on health. Stress is negative when it exceeds our ability to cope, fatigues body systems, and causes behavioral or physical problems. Stress is positive when it forces us to adapt and thus to increase the strength of our adaptation mechanisms. Stress is also positive when it warns us that we are not coping well and that a lifestyle change is warranted if we are to maintain optimal health. When the body tolerates stress and uses it to overcome lethargy or enhance performance, the stress is positive, healthy, and challenging. Hans Selye, one of the pioneers of the modern study of stress, termed this *eustress*. This action-enhancing stress gives the athlete the competitive edge and the public speaker the enthusiasm to project optimally. Selye termed negative, debilitating, or harmful stress *distress*. Distress produces overreaction, confusion, poor concentration, and performance anxiety and usually results in subpar performance. An individual in distress cannot cope competently. Prolonged distress moves the organism into the health danger zone. Somewhere between eustress and distress is a level of optimal stress. Figure 1.1 illustrates this concept.

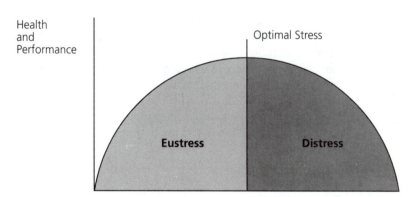

FIGURE 1.1   **Point of Optimal Stress**

The best way to find and use our optimal stress level is to develop the ability to recognize the signs and symptoms of distress. That sounds simple enough, but in actuality is not, because the body's sensitivity to the awareness of stress arousal tends to wane. The human organism characteristically becomes accustomed to its level of arousal, which often becomes the body's normal state. In other words, people become conditioned to their level of stress arousal if it lasts for a few weeks.

Stress and Disease

Stress may be thought of as a response that links a stressor stimulus to any stress-related disease, symptom, or dysfunction (see Figure 1.2).

All too often our interest in health begins when it deteriorates and when pain and dysfunction begin to dictate a lifestyle of diminished capacity. Virtually everyone knows disease. It is a condition of the body that presents symptoms peculiar to it. Disease or the fear of diminished capacity has prompted the study of stress, now a well-documented cause of illness. The primary vehicle and unifying thread in this research is the mind-body concept that simply means the mind and the body working in harmony and with mutual influence and effect.

The mind-body concept of illness explains how our environment and social interactions, our perception of our environment, and our personal choices and emotional states produce a physical stress response. Moreover, it explains how stress arousal can eventually lead to illness and reveals a map of the interrelations among our mind, body, and social environment.

The mind-body influence on illness is not a new concept, as written accounts appeared in earliest Greek literature and reemerged in relation to modern medicine around 1927 with the teachings of Felix Deutsch (later published in 1959) and with the writings of Helen Dunbar (1935). Mind-body disease refers to any condition thought to be the result of excess emotional arousal, maladaptive coping, and chronic distress. The basis for this concept is that emotional disturbances such as anxiety, anger, fear, and frustration can increase the body's susceptibility to organic diseases.

In 1965 René Dubos noted that even infectious organic diseases do not commonly occur simply from pathogenic (disease-causing) microbes entering the body. Dubos studied the role of what we are calling the mind-body phenomenon. The sciences concerned with microbial diseases, he explained, developed almost exclusively from the study of acute or semiacute infections caused by virulent microorganisms acquired through exposure to an external agent.

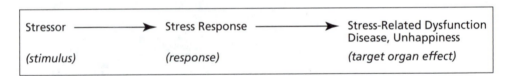

FIGURE 1.2   Stress and Disease

In contrast, the microbial diseases most common in our communities today arise from microorganisms that are always present in the environment. These organisms remain in the body and under normal conditions do not cause obvious harm; they have pathological effects only when a person is under conditions of stress. In this type of microbial disease, the event of infection is less important than the hidden manifestation of the smoldering infectious process. The stressful disturbance that converts latent infection into overt pathology is all-important. Stress appears to lower the body's resistance or immunity to disease. Dubos pointed out that being infected or having some organ system begin to degenerate is not the critical factor in the course of the illness. The critical factor is the body's ability to defend itself against these common infectious and degenerative processes, which are part of everyday life. We now know that distress impedes the body's ability to defend itself against all diseases.

Thus, stress may act as a catalyst for an organic disease already present by (1) allowing the disease to establish a foothold in the body from which to spread destruction or (2) accelerating the spread of the disease throughout the body. In short, almost any organic disease may have a psychosomatic component, depending, of course, on an individual's psychological makeup.

Disorders of Arousal

Research has substantially increased our understanding of how stress arousal can be precipitated by a wide variety of environmental stimuli. In addition, stress arousal can result in an equally wide variety of disorders whose only common characteristic is that they occur in response to the arousal. Therefore, diseases caused or characterized by excessive stress arousal are commonly called disorders of arousal. They can be psychological disorders, such as those caused by anxiety, or very definable stress-related syndromes, such as cardiovascular or gastrointestinal diseases.

Research on the physiology of arousal is centered in the areas of the brain below the thinking cortex within the limbic, hypothalamic, and reticular activation centers (these areas are illustrated in Chapter 2). These "hardwired" centers communicate with the cells of the entire body through informational substances that interact with receptor sites throughout the various systems, especially the gut, spinal column, endocrine glands, and the immune system (Pert 1999). In the latter half of the the twentieth century, these centers of the brain have continued to be the focal point of research into emotional arousal. Involved in sensory stimulation and emotional expression, these brain structures are also responsible for integration of the nerve stimuli sent from the brain to the body and thus have a profound impact on physical and mental health.

These same brain structures contribute to states of hyperalertness, hypersensitivity, and nervous-system hyperactivity in association with worry, threat, and the avoidance behavior of flight. Limbic-system arousal and sensitization have been implicated in a variety of anxiety disorders, personality disorders, posttraumatic reactions, addictive disorders, and withdrawal syndromes (Pert 1995).

One of the most substantial advances in the study of mind-body interaction is the theory that various disorders of the informational substance network that includes neurohormones, steroid hormones, peptides, growth factors, and polypeptides (what Pert calls the "molecules of emotion") are involved in disease. This theory implicates stress in the development of diseases ranging from the common cold to cancer. There is little doubt that information received from the environment, the way it is perceived and evaluated, and its influence on thought processes and muscle activity contribute to disease. The pathway from the social environment to ill health is a complex one that involves the interaction of mind and body (Figure 1.3). Even positive events can produce stress when they demand change and adaptation, but most stress begins with the negative, painful, and unpleasant events of our lives. An inseparable aspect of environmental stress is our varied and complex social interaction, fraught with feelings, expectations, and often frustration.

Different pathways, two of which are represented in Figure 1.3, process the information from the environment. One pathway is thought to be largely subconscious and is thus named the subconscious-appraisal pathway. If this pathway is stimulated, coping action may eventually be required, in which case the pathway's innate

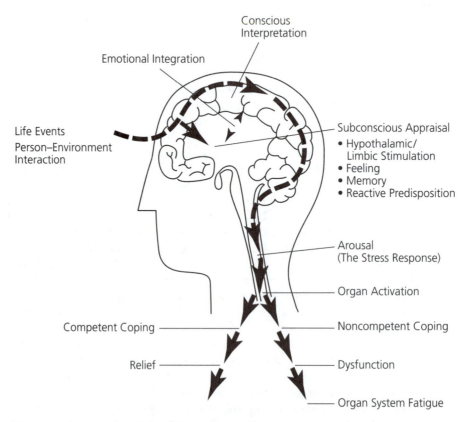

FIGURE 1.3 Mind/Body Pathways to Illness

physical and emotional reflexes prepare the body for action. It is important to note that this system only prepares the body for action and that this preparation is independent of the final action. It is the second, or voluntary, pathway that determines whether this arousal is necessary and used.

The voluntary pathway controls perception, evaluation, and decision making and is responsible for voluntary action. How you perceive an event largely depends on your concept of self, ego strengths, value system, mood, temperament, and even heredity. The emotions aroused are tempered by your psychological defenses, which are gained from experience, especially childhood responses. These lead to physical arousal, and you feel a need to act. Action itself is also complex; as a result of the consequences of a possible action, the reaction to a stressor is often no action at all. (For example, you may hold back a harsh comment after you realize it may hurt someone's feelings.)

Background action is very important here—it is arousal that is not conscious or noticed by the individual. It supports any potential action that may follow. The idea of background action is intriguing because it probably developed from the superior intelligence of humans and their capacity to perform several activities simultaneously. Sport offers a good example. Novice basketball players must concentrate very intensely when learning to dribble, just as novice ice skaters must work very hard to remain balanced in an upright position on their skates. As people learn a sport, they establish the neural pathways that allow the most efficient transmission of messages between the brain and the muscles. They develop the necessary muscles and build the confidence to perform the activity. Day by day the activity becomes more automatic until the accomplished basketball player can dribble the length of the court while remembering the coach's selection of plays in any situation. Now apply this example to stress behaviors. If we live stressful lives, the body learns how to position itself for action very efficiently. Imagine a boxer having to think about tensing his muscles or concentrate on getting his heart to pump more blood to his muscles while he tries to defend himself.

When we are frightened by a situation or hurt because of the way people talked or looked at us, our bodies are affected by stress responses that have become automatic. We can be (and usually are) stressed. We behave in a stressful or defensive manner without knowing it because we respond to the stressful situation on that automatic or subconscious level that allows us to do two or more things at once. Pert (1999) believes that the subconscious is the body and that body cells hold a memory pattern. A person who has a low threshold for frustration and is quick to become defensive might have developed a predisposition to be reactive. This predisposition is referred to as "tone." The person who is highly toned is conditioned to react in a stressful manner when any number of situational triggers are present. Often the triggers are unknown on a conscious level or are forgotten if a certain memory is too painful to think about. Victims of childhood physical, emotional, and/or sexual abuses often bury the memory of the actual abuse. However, the body remembers the feeling and responds to triggers in a stressful manner even when no conscious appraisal is apparent. Thus our emotions exert an all-important measure of background control over our thoughts and behaviors.

To summarize, we become very efficient at being aroused even when we are not conscious of the arousal (the triggering situation). We often feel stressed and do not know why. Not until we consciously interpret the stress arousal can we begin to deal with the stress, for at this point our emotions are integrated with our thoughts, and we interpret the experience in light of our knowledge and the situation. If we appraise the threat and no solution is forthcoming, our stress arousal is compounded by stress arising from fear of failure or harm. If a solution is forthcoming and involves an angry attack on the stressor, then the stress is likewise compounded. If a solution is planned and then inhibited, stress arousal is again compounded. If a solution is forthcoming, stress arousal can begin to dissipate; however, the physiological resolution may take as long as twenty-four hours.

As Figure 1.3 illustrates, both the subconscious and voluntary pathways can lead to physical arousal; arousal is not totally dependent upon voluntary action. If the body prepares for action (for example, by bracing itself in a defensive posture) but then finds the action thwarted, the person is often left with chronic low-to-moderate tension. Prolonged physical arousal can go unheeded when its symptoms are not overt and do not produce noticeable pain or discomfort. However, if fatigue of an organ system ensues or if the system malfunctions, noticeable symptoms will appear.

The signs and symptoms of stress arousal appear when a body system is excessively stimulated. The signs usually include feelings such as moodiness, irritability, depression, and anxiety and behavior such as withdrawal, drug and alcohol abuse, and various forms of hostile and aggressive actions.

To be optimally healthy, we must be able to cope with life's trials and tribulations while minimizing the detrimental effects of excess stress. Coping is any attempt to neutralize stress arousal. Coping systems include behaviors, physiological reactions, cognitions, perceptions, and motor acts. Coping can be healthy and growth producing (competent) or can be unhealthy (incompetent) and cause additional problems that persist long after stress arousal has diminished. Competent coping results in retaining optimal health and maintaining control while meeting life's demands. Incompetent coping results in the sacrifice of health and control and the inability to meet demands.

People characterized by incompetent coping are drawn to unhealthy physical or psychological means in order to cope. The psychological term for this is *recruitment*. There are numerous examples of recruitment. Bradshaw's (1990) examples of classic ego defenses people use when reality becomes intolerable include the following: conversion ("I eat, drink alcohol, or take drugs when I can't cope with reality"), denial ("It didn't happen," or "It's not really happening to me"), dissociation ("I can't remember what happened"), minimizing ("Oh, it wasn't really that bad"), projection ("It's your reaction, not mine"), repression ("It didn't happen"), and withdrawal from the world. These are all examples of incompetent coping.

We orient ourselves, what we know, what we feel, and what we value by banking it off the outside world. We learned the fear of rejection, the anger of being thwarted, and the guilt of unacceptable behavior, and we experience the anxiety of struggle between needs and what we have to do to fulfill them. Stress can change minds and mold bodies. It influences the length and quality of life. It determines the amount of peace we enjoy or struggle we endure. Interactions with other people are largely responsible for the amount of stress we experience. Until each person releases the tension between what they are and what they think they should be, anxiety and discomfort of stress will be their companions. Releasing this tension is the goal of stress management.

Stress Management

The stress that each person encounters throughout life may be seen as a battle among three elements: (1) beliefs and thoughts (the mental foundation of how we construct our world); (2) form and behavior (the physical manifestation of our thoughts and beliefs); and (3) spiritual awareness (how tuned in we are to our connection with spirit energy). The physical stress and pain we encounter and endure has its roots in old beliefs that are no longer beneficial to us, as seen through an emotional filter that affects our perception of "actual" events (more than previously thought possible, much of this emotional baggage is hardwired in our bodies). We respond with emotional behaviors that used to work but are no longer appropriate. We continue to try to resolve our stress problems because we know that peace and serenity, happiness and joy, love and compassion, healing and abundance are our birthright. When this knowledge becomes the core of our belief system and we live by the spiritual laws that will provide these dividends, stress diminishes and often disappears from our lives. Stress management methods such as meditation, visualization, and other introspective techniques are valuable aids in this process.

Intervention Points

At several points, intervention in the stressor-stress-disease cycle is possible. Remember that stress operates in many dimensions and is not always predictable. How stressfully we react to our environment is determined to a large extent by our attitudes, values, personality, and emotional development as well as by our ability to relax, our diet and physical activity patterns, and our ability to modify our lifestyles. Because stress reactions occur in various ways and on various levels, stress management should be holistic; that is, we should approach it from numerous and varied perspectives, incorporating mental, physical, spiritual, social, and environmental interactions.

Free Will and Mindfulness

In this first chapter we lay the foundation for learning to control the excess stress in our lives. All of the techniques, which are typically learned in a stress management course, fit under a large "umbrella" that can be conceptualized as free will. Free will is given to each soul; it is a spiritual birthright. It is the key element because it demands that we make conscious decisions about which thoughts to think, which feelings to nurture, which words to speak, and which behaviors to perform. We are constantly given the opportunity to shape experiences with the will. Little free will can be exercised when we depend on others to support us, so early survival depends on learning and doing what others want us to do. Adults become free when they discover that they have the ability to make free-will choices that affirm their real selves. The force of propensity or habit is stronger than the force of ideal action unless the will is awakened.

Figure 1.4 shows how the will affects decision making. On the left, decision making is a mindful, skillful response, and on the right the personality-based response proves to be less skillful, even stressful. The difference in the two responses lies in the motivation behind them. If motivated by wisdom and compassion, the decision becomes mindful. Through practice, one can develop stimulus-response types of skills, but mindfulness requires compassion and intention. Decision making in this context—that of exercising the will—we call *mindfulness*.

The goal in decision making, especially when it involves others around us, is harmonious coexistence in which there are no thoughts, feelings, and actions, that cause separation. Rather than using the personality to create separation, in mindfulness we use compassion to create union. Compassion is the key to mindfulness. The ultimate expression of compassion is forgiveness. To forgive is to no longer blame, and without blame, all that is left is the acceptance of responsibility. This means being responsible for your thoughts and feelings as well as your actions. It means shedding the psychological myth of conditioned responses, scripts, and roles that most of us

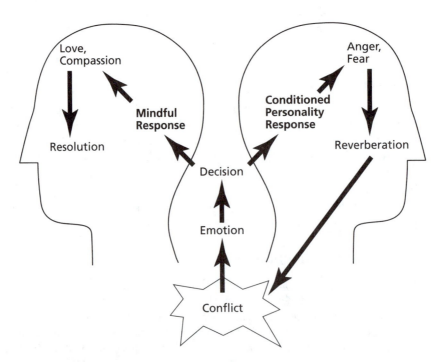

FIGURE 1.4   Mindful Choices

have been taught and have virtually constructed in our cells. It means taking responsibility for the trials and tribulations we cause ourselves and being gentle with the love and support of those who accompany us. It means choosing to act out of compassion and understanding. It means making mindful choices.

Mindfulness is demonstrated in subtle differences—not so much in technique but in motivation. Abraham Maslow (1968), generally accredited with founding the humanistic psychology movement, explains this fundamental difference as acting (1) from intellectual self-serving objectivism (usually fear based and competitive) or (2) from the intuitive belief in truths beyond ourselves, cooperation, and belief that humans can fulfill their highest potential.

Mindfulness is more a description than a prescription. It is less *what* to think and more how to think. The point on which this skill turns is the use of free will—being free enough from immediate gratification and debilitating emotions to make choices based on universal truths. This is not to say that one cannot consciously check decisions against the "yardstick" of options drawn from wisdom. One can understand the concepts involved and believe in both the possibilities and their own potential abilities and practice.

We are free to choose, and on our most basic physical level, we make the choices that seem to satisfy our most immediate physical needs. The hungry choose food and the cold choose warmth. At the next level, our choices are further influenced by other emotions. The lonely choose company or often self-nurturing with food, drugs, and alcohol. The fearful choose to withdraw or to hide in the emotional world of depression. Add to this physical-emotional mix a human's unique intellect, and the choices become even more complex. Knowledge can be translated into loving activities or spun into elaborate webs of revengeful deception.

Hidden from our immediate senses are myriad decisions about which thoughts to have, which feelings to nurture, and which words to say to elicit a desired reaction. Choices that are mindful do not follow the logic of the personality. Not seeking revenge when hurt or not insulting those who disagree with us are examples of mindfulness. Purposefully going against lifelong conditioning of personality by not choosing greed or prolonged grief are acts of mindfulness. The first step in moving toward a mindful response is controlling emotion. Separating emotion from the event produces detachment. Mindfulness is the freedom to be aware of the moment without reacting with old knee-jerk responses from the childhood, the unskillful past.

Choices

Like everything in life, stress management is about making choices. Consider first the most obvious arena—that of the world around you. The choice is between dancing to the beat of society's drum, getting swept up in the wave of humanity hustling to get ahead, mindlessly going along bombarded by the din of desire and perturbation, or choosing to quiet your external environment and learning to minimize the frequency of stress in your life.

Obviously, our environment is filled with stressors. The action or behavior of each individual or institution in the world becomes the input for other individuals. As we go about our daily activities, each individual with whom we interact presents some manner of stimulation. All of life's pursuits create potential stressors—from noise and pollution to competition for a seat on the bus, a place on the highway, or a position with a company. Generally speaking, more people means more complexity in social as well as in institutional organizations.

One of the easiest and most effective techniques of stress management is to identify stress-promoting activities and develop a lifestyle that modifies or avoids these stressors. These activities are designed to quiet the external environment in order to reduce the stressors in life. They should prompt a cognitive awareness of life events and then be utilized in restructuring your environment, thought patterns, and behavior.

Quieting the external environment to reduce stimulation of the individual produces the following effects:

- a cognitive awareness of life events and lifestyle
- a cognitive restructuring of the environment, one's thought patterns, and one's behavior

The next set of choices involves your internal world. The choice here is whether to learn techniques designed to allow you to better control your thoughts or to allow stressful, irrational thoughts and out-of-control emotions to dictate your behavior and to permit the chatter of your mind about worry, fear, "what ifs," and "should be's" to rob you of your ability to concentrate and to be quiet.

To a large degree, the amount of stress that society and the environment create depends on what information you take in and what you block; how you perceive, evaluate, and give meaning to that information; and what effect this whole process has on mental and physical activity. Attitude, which is the meaning and value you give to various events in life in combination with characteristic ways of behaving (behavioral patterns), has the awesome capacity to transform a normally neutral aspect of life into a psychosocial stressor. Few events are innately stressful, but we make them stressful by the way in which we perceive them. A person may alter stress-causing attitudes by learning how these attitudes are formed and then working to change that process. If this is effective, you will change the way in which you perceive a particular event to the point that there will be little or no physical arousal.

The stress response, which is physical arousal, can be elicited by conscious, voluntary action or by subconscious, involuntary (autonomic) activation, which keeps the body in a state of readiness. The constant state of readiness to respond with the fight-or-flight reaction when such a response is unwarranted is called "emotional reactivity." If the body remains in this state for long periods, organ systems become fatigued, and the result is often organ-system malfunction. Relaxation training can help reduce emotional reactivity. It promotes voluntary and autonomic control over some central-nervous-system activities associated with arousal and promotes a quiet sense of control that eventually influences attitudes, perception, and behavior. Relaxation training fosters interaction with your inner self, and you will learn by actual feeling (visceral learning) that what you are thinking influences your body processes and that your body processes in turn influence your thoughts. You will come to know your feelings and emotions as part of your thinking experience; your behavior will come more from what is within you rather than from how you feel you should respond to people and your environment. Primary therapeutic benefits of this phase of relaxation include learning to focus concentration on one thing at a time (especially on what is happening and what is being felt at the moment) and to quiet internal chatter that often comes from worrying about the future or feeling guilty about the past. When you have learned to stay in the present, to focus on what is happening right now and spend less time in needless worry and fantasy, you become more peaceful.

Quieting the internal environment in order to reduce sensory stimulation of the central nervous system has the following effects:

- decreased stimulation
- a calming or relaxation response
- a greater relaxation response

Yet another basic choice involves how your body handles stress once it occurs. You have the choice of sitting and stewing or getting rid of it by learning techniques to appropriately utilize the by-products of excessive stress arousal. The primary stress response is the fight-or-flight response, which has always helped ensure human survival and continues to do so today. In fact, no amount of relaxation training can diminish the intensity of this innate reflex. Stress is physical, intended to enable a physical response to a physical threat. However, any threat, either physical or symbolic, can evoke this response. Once the stimulation of the event penetrates the psychological defenses, the body prepares for action. Increased hormonal secretion, energy supply, and cardiovascular activity signify a state of stress, a state of extreme readiness to act as soon as the voluntary control centers decide what action to take. Usually the threat is not physical and holds only symbolic significance; our lives are not in danger—only our egos. Physical action is not warranted and must be subdued, but for the body organs it is too late: What took only minutes to start will take hours to undo. The stress products are flowing through the system and will activate various organs until these by-products are reabsorbed into storage or gradually used by the body. While this gradual process is taking place, the body organs suffer.

The simple solution is to use the physical stress arousal for its intended purpose—physical movement. The increased energy intended for fight or flight can be used for running, swimming, or bicycling. In this way one can accelerate the dissipation of the stress products, and, if the activity is vigorous enough, it can cause a rebound or overshoot after exercise into a state of deep relaxation.

Utilizing the stress by-products through physical exercise has the following effects:

- decreased arousal
- a sense of well-being and a feeling of imperturbability

Finally there is a choice that involves conditioning and learning to prevent future stress problems from developing. The choice is to be at the mercy of your environment or to build up your immunity to stress and decrease your susceptibility to future stressors by conditioning the mind to reduce stress-arousing thoughts and condition the body to be less reactive to stress. Stress arousal is a mind-and-body response to a social event. Throughout the day, each new stress situation leaves a residual amount of tension in the body, the accumulation of which cannot all be dissipated. The longer you practice relaxation exercises, the more you dissipate your residual tension and increase your general state of relaxation. Gradually, the relaxed state becomes a stable part of your personal choice and lifestyle. Representative techniques include many varieties of meditations. These activities are designed to train the mind to reduce arousing thoughts. They reduce stress-arousing memories and anticipations and instead direct thoughts to produce a peaceful and tranquil state. Meditation training yields the following effects:

- reduced mind chatter, fewer arousing memories and anticipations
- thoughts that produce peace and tranquillity
- increased philosophical awareness

SOURCES CITED

Bradshaw, J. (1990). *Homecoming*. New York: Bantam.
Cannon, W. B. (1939). *The wisdom of the body*. 2d edition. New York: W. W. Norton.
Deutsch, F. (1959). *On the mysterious leap from the mind to the body*. New York: International Universities Press.
Dubos, R. (1965). *Man adapting*. New Haven: Yale University Press.
Dunbar, H. (1935). *Emotions and bodily changes*. New York: Columbia University Press.
Maslow, A. (1968). *Toward a psychology of being*. New York: Van Nostrand Reinhold.
Pert, C. (1995). *Neuropeptides, AIDS, and the science of healing*. Alternative Therapies, 1, no. 3 (July). 70–76.
Pert, C. (1999). *Molecules of emotion*. New York: Simon and Schuster.
Selye, H. (1956). *The stress of life*. New York: McGraw-Hill.

CHAPTER

2

Systems That Control Stress Arousal

The Purpose of the Stress Response

The body responds to new stimuli by preparing to take physical action in order to protect life. The stimulus (the stressor) alerts the body (the stress response), and as a result the body performs at a higher level. Early science liked to think that the brain was in charge of the stress response, yet the newer paradigm discovered through research in neurophysiology, endocrinology, and immunology allows us to suspect that the whole body is aware of stress at once (Pert 1999) and that the response occurs on many levels. The higher brain centers, especially the frontal cortex, add perception and meaning to new information, and action may or may not be initiated. If there is perception that the new information is a threat to physical or psychological survival, the stress response is continued through additional outpouring of the informational substances. These substances in turn affect not only neurons but also cells throughout the body that have receptors for messenger molecules.

What are these receptors and molecules of communication? Virtually all cells contain many receptor sites whose function is to receive information from other cells of the body. They act somewhat like the scanners in a grocery store, except each scans for a specific molecule that has specific information for that cell. The information comes in the form of amino acid molecules (or *ligands*) that Pert (ibid.) breaks into three classifications. The smallest, simplest molecules are the *neurohormones*, such as norepinephrine and acetylcholine, that carry information across the synapse between nerve cells. The second category consists of steroids such as the sex hormones and the stress hormone cortisol. The third category, the peptides, is the largest, comprising perhaps 95 percent of all the ligands. They are involved in regulating practically all life processes.

Receptors are located on the surface membrane of a cell and have roots deep into the cell's interior. When a specific ligand communicates with the receptor, a message is sent to the interior of the cell that may either initiate or halt production of an enzyme, cause the cell to become more or less permeable, or any one of the myriad functions of that cell.

If the response to stress is physical action, the stress products within the body are utilized and dissipated. This is what nature intended. If the stress is not resolved and the products of the alarm reaction are not used for their intended purpose

15

(action), all the systems of the body continue to react and over time will show the adverse effects of the stress response. The purpose of this chapter is to promote an understanding of this alerting and arousal response. When one understands the mechanisms of stress, one can better accept and adopt measures to prevent it.

The Basic Systems of Control

Currently, scientific research supports the existence of three basic systems in the human body that are highly implicated in the control of the stress and disease process. These are as follows: (1) the central nervous system (CNS), particularly that portion that is called the autonomic nervous system (ANS), (2) the endocrine system, especially the pituitary and the adrenal glands, and (3) the immune system and its interaction with the rest of the body. The informational substances, or *neuropeptide system*, connect these three systems, indeed, all the systems of the body.

> *Neuropeptides:* short strings of amino acids produced by nerve cells. When neuropeptides lock into receptors attached to cells throughout the body, they cause physiological reactions. Neuropeptides and their receptors form an extensive network that the body uses to communicate with itself. This network is the biochemical substrate of emotions and provides a scientific explanation for mind-body healing.

Historically, the brain was the main focus of stress research. It could be scientifically demonstrated that stimulation of various brain structures brought about both immediate and delayed stress responses. Research found that the center of physical control was the hypothalamus, deep within the brain, which receives constant input from the limbic system. This concept of a limbic-hypothalamic center is sometimes extended to include the pituitary gland and referred to in the literature on mindbody disease and psychoneuroimmunology (PNI) as the limbic-hypothalamic-pituitary axis. Figure 2.1 illustrates the portions of the central nervous system that this section discusses. Our intention in this discussion is to elaborate on the two central nervous systems highly implicated in the stress response.

The Autonomic Nervous System (ANS)

Actions of the central nervous system—the brain, brainstem, and spinal cord—can be classified as either autonomic or voluntary. Autonomic functioning is automatic or reflexive: It regulates heart rate, body temperature, respiration, and other vital functions without our having to think about doing so. The voluntary system allows us to think before we act.

There are two main classifications within the autonomic nervous system: (1) the sympathetic nervous system, which sets off the alarm response that in turn energizes

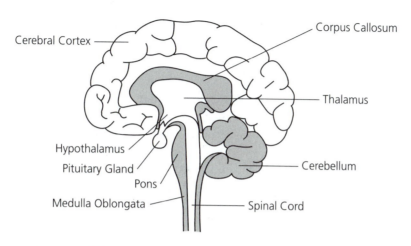

FIGURE 2.1   The Central Nervous System

the body to respond to stress, and (2) the parasympathetic nervous system, which reverts the energized systems to normal, more relaxed, function.

The sympathetic system is best known for its lifesaving fight-or-flight capacities. When this system is stimulated, all its parts react with a mass neural discharge to accomplish a common purpose—enabling the body to act above and beyond its normal, everyday function. For example, in a fight-or-flight situation, the body needs more blood, more oxygen, and more energy. Therefore, the heart beats faster and pumps more blood per beat. At the same time, the body makes more efficient use of the available blood supply by constricting blood vessels in organs, such as the gastrointestinal tract, that are not essential to the stress response. This decreases the function of the unneeded organs and allows an increased flow of blood to essential organs such as the heart and skeletal muscles. In the lungs, the bronchials (which carry air) expand, and breathing becomes deeper, faster, and generally more efficient. The pupils of the eyes enlarge, improving visual sensitivity, and salivary secretion increases. The adrenal glands, sitting atop the kidneys, secrete adrenaline, which reinforces and prolongs the sympathetic effect and stimulates the liver to release more glucose to fuel the action. Adrenaline also stimulates the adipose tissue to release fatty acids to fuel the muscles. See Table 2.1 for a summary of the effects on the body of the fight-or-flight response. In short, stimulation of the sympathetic system increases the activity of the organs needed for the fight-or-flight response and inhibits the organs that are not essential. Prolonged stimulation or inhibition of organs can cause malfunction and in turn promote stress-related illness.

The fight-or-flight response, mediated by epinephrine, norepinephrine, and dopamine (hormones of the sympathetic and adrenal systems), demands an integrated adjustment of many processes, as Table 2.1 shows. This response is facilitated

TABLE 2.1   Physiological Changes in the Fight-or-Fight Response

Organ	Change
Fat tissue	Increased breakdown of stored fat, more fatty acids, and glycerol in the bloodstream
Brain	Increased blood flow, increased metabolism of glucose
Cardiovascular system	Increased heart rate and force of contraction, vasoconstriction of peripheral blood vessels
Lungs	Increased respiratory rate, dilation of bronchi, increased oxygen supply
Muscles	Increased breakdown of glycogen to glucose for immediate energy supply, increased contraction, decreased uptake of glucose, increased uptake of fatty acids for energy
Liver	Increased glucose production via gluconeogenesis
Skin	Decreased blood flow
Gastrointestinal tract	Decreased protein synthesis
Genitourinary tract	Decreased protein synthesis
Lymph tissue	Increased breakdown of protein

Source: Adapted from Martin et al. (1990).

by other hormones of the endocrine system, the central nervous system, and by the various peptides.

The parasympathetic system, in contrast to the sympathetic system, does not exhibit a mass reaction to stimulation. It acts on specific organs, increasing the action of some while inhibiting that of others. Parasympathetic stimulation of the organ systems listed in Table 2.1 has the following effects: The heart slows down, most blood vessels expand, and the functions of the gastrointestinal system increase. The bronchials constrict, as do the pupils, and salivary secretion increases. After the arousal response, the parasympathetic system normalizes the function of all the organs involved.

Most organs in the body respond to both the sympathetic and parasympathetic systems. Some organs, however, are stimulated by only one. In this case, the controlling system determines whether the organ is activated or inhibited.

Structure and Function of the ANS.   The lower-brain structures of the autonomic nervous system respond to the physical world and are basically reflexive. These structures include the spinal cord, the cerebellum (the center of muscle coordination), the medulla oblongata (which controls heart rate, circulation of blood, respiration, coughing, and sneezing), the pons (a network that sends nerve impulses to various parts of the brain), the thalamus (the "switchboard" that sends incoming signals to proper brain areas), and the hypothalamus (see Figure 2.2). Throughout this area of the brain is a specialized system called the *reticular formation*, which we will discuss later.

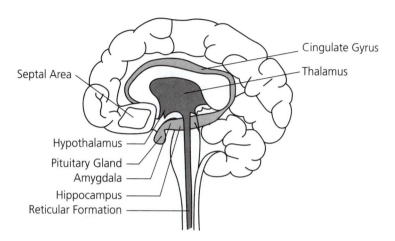

FIGURE 2.2   The Inner Brain

If humans have any resemblance to other animal species, it is in the basic programs stored within these lower centers., which govern actions or behaviors that are natural, direct, and open, without a great deal of learned inhibition. Activities centered in survival and reproduction (such as preparing a homesite, establishing and defending territory, hunting, homing, hoarding, mating, forming simple social groups, and doing routine daily activities) are instinctive and performed by lower animals as well as humans. But with their higher level of brain evolution, humans have shown the ability to override some of these basic responses for psychological and social survival.

The Hypothalamus.   Located at the base of the forebrain, the hypothalamus is not so much a distinct, identifiable organ as it is a combination of tissues with a somewhat vague boundary. These tissues are made up of a number of nuclei, or nerve centers, that control the basic autonomic functions.

The hypothalamus is at the very center of the limbic system and has profuse communication pathways with all levels of this system (Ganong 1995). It sends neural signals in two major directions: (1) down through the brainstem, mainly to the reticular formation within the pons, medulla, hypothalamus, and thalamus, and (2) up to many areas of the cortex. The hypothalamus affects the cortex indirectly, but dramatically, through its control of the brainstem portion of the reticular activating system.

The hypothalamus is the major integrator of the body's regulatory systems (such as hunger, thirst, temperature, blood pressure, heart rate, and sex drive). Stimulation of appropriate areas of the hypothalamus can activate the sympathetic system strongly enough to increase arterial blood pressure by more than 100 percent. Other areas control temperature by allowing more or less blood to flow to the surface of the skin. Still others increase or decrease salivation, control sexual responses, and regulate the digestive process and other responses to physical threat.

The hypothalamus is a major part of the "physical" brain: It receives physical messages and responds on a basic, physical level. When it receives messages that are either threatening or new and unique, it responds with a sympathetically controlled alarm reaction. When the threat abates or the new message is somehow integrated, calming messages are sent through the parasympathetic system to the excited organs so that their function is normalized.

Consider, for example, the response to noise. A noise is first perceived by the lower centers before it is registered in the cortex. Once the hypothalamus is stimulated, it prepares for possible action by increasing the discharge of hormones, increasing the availability of energy, preparing the cardiovascular (heart and circulatory) system by shifting blood flow to essential organs, and at the same time tensing the muscles. The conscious cortex may ultimately prevent the action, but the body is prepared for any eventuality and is technically in a state of stress. So, now you know why parents or roommates may respond so adversely to loud, obnoxious music.

The hypothalamus, with its intimate relationship to the pituitary gland, links the nervous system with the endocrine system. The hypothalamic-controlled ANS communicates through *neurotransmitters*, or *neurohormones*, with the parts of the body it affects. The sympathetic-system nerve endings secrete the neurotransmitter norepinephrine to activate receptors on the cells of the organs that the nerve endings modulate, and parasympathetic-system nerve endings secrete acetylcholine. These neurotransmitters bind with receptors in the cell walls of the target organs, changing the permeability of the organ's cell wall and causing targeted internal events to occur. In addition to changing cell permeability, neurohormones, peptides, polypeptides, and other messenger substances may activate receptors on the cell membrane of the target organ, thereby causing enzymatic events to initiate the autonomic response characteristic of that organ.

The Limbic System.   The limbic system offered its evolutionary predecessor, the physical brain, a measure of freedom from stereotyped behavior. Primarily, this newer system added the concept of feeling and emotion, which further ensured attendance to basic survival activities by making activities pleasurable or displeasurable. Feelings such as fear, anger, and love became attached to certain situations, guiding behavior toward that which protected and away from that which threatened. Understandably, two of our major neural pathways (those governing eating and reproduction) have intricate connections to the pleasure and unpleasure centers of the limbic system (Pert 1999). The concepts of reward or pleasure and punishment or displeasure are important to the concept of stress.

Because stress is an integrated response of the body, it must have an integrative conduit, and fifty years ago that area was demonstrated to be the limbic system (MacLean 1949). The limbic system is the hub of the central nervous system and the human stress response as well. This system (particularly the septal, hippocampal, and hypothalamic areas) integrates cognitive appraisals from the prefrontal cortex with the higher-order emotions arising in the cingulate and amygdaloid areas. The result of this input is neuromuscular articulation and stress-related symptoms and signs (Glaser and Kiecolt-Glaser 1994).

The Cerebral Cortex.   As biology has shown, the brain continued to develop with the addition of the cerebral cortex, also called the *neocortex*, or *forebrain* (Figure 2.3). The addition of a vast number of cortical cells allowed the development and storage of analytical skills, verbal communication, writing ability, fine motor control, additional emotion, memory, learning, and rational thought, as well as more sophisticated problem-solving and survival abilities. New dimensions were added to oral and sexual behaviors, and vision replaced smell as the primary sense. Voluntary control of movement made reactions more than mere reflex responses. For better or worse, an individual's reality could be determined by his or her own perceptions. Behavior could be weighed against possible outcomes. Symbolism, goals, motivation, and anticipation became part of the functioning human being.

Even though the brain developed in three stages, its three areas do not function independently. Although the lower centers deal mainly with survival and the higher centers permit the existence of complex society, we cannot view the lower centers as primitive entities requiring control by the higher centers. It helps to understand the function of each of these specific nervous-system structures in order to understand stress and how to overcome it. At the same time, it is important to think of stress as the response of an integrated whole brain.

The Reward System.   The reward system may help us to understand the drive to cope with our internal and external environments. Major reward areas are located at the limbic and hypothalamic levels and are involved with how easily we are aroused, our motivation, and our emotional memory.

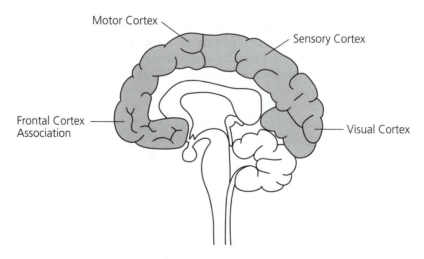

FIGURE 2.3   The Cerebral Cortex

Coping with adversity is an attempt to move our emotional, physical, mental, or spiritual being away from pain or toward pleasure and reward. CNS reward systems have developed over time, presumably to reinforce useful behaviors and extinguish harmful ones. In addition, these reward systems regulate the basic drives related to pleasure, pain, emotional comfort, sexual satisfaction, hunger, satiety, and thirst. If we learn to throw our reward systems off balance, we subsequently strive to bring them back into balance from a very deep subconscious level throughout the body up to an intentional conscious level in the brain.

The middle limbic area has a specialized area of intense reward, mediated by dopamine, the neurohormone that normally controls homeostasis. This area provides such intense reward that laboratory animals will stimulate themselves to death with intravenous psychomotor stimulants. Although scientific controversy exists as to whether there is one main reward pathway or many redundant pathways, it is accepted that the experiencing of pleasure most likely includes dopamine effects in the brain.

In recent years the costs of cocaine, heroin, and other drug addictions (and the crime that accompanies them) have spurred research on the natural reward systems. It has been found that the body produces its own opiatelike substances (*endorphins*) to help alleviate pain and produce pleasure. Since then, receptors for nicotine, cocaine, marijuana, and other drugs have also been discovered. The relationship between drugs and stress management is not subtle—human beings seek pleasure and avoid pain. This is a driving principle of human behavior.

The Reticular Formation.   The reticular formation is often referred to as the reticular activating system (RAS) or the ascending reticular activating system (ARAS). It is a network of nerve cells (or neurons) that extends from the spinal cord up through the thalamus. The RAS itself is categorized as neither sensory (connected to the sense organs) nor motor (connected to the muscles), but it links sensory and motor impulses. It is a two-way street, carrying impulses from brain to body and from body to brain.

The RAS was discovered by Moruzzi and Magoun (1949), who noted that its nerve connections projected to the limbic system, the hypothalamus, the thalamus, and throughout the cortex in order to stimulate or alert the brain. The RAS receives information from all of the body's incoming nerves, filters this input, and then forwards to the brain only new or persistent information (Bloom, Lazerson, and Hofstadter 1995; Robinson 1996). When RAS centers in the pons area of the brainstem signal new stimuli, the message immediately heightens awareness both in the cortex and also in the limbic-hypothalamic center, which integrates memory and houses reward or pleasure mechanisms. At the same time neuropeptides may be carrying the message throughout the body. In the brain, perception is added to the stimuli, and we may consciously choose to either ignore or attend to the stimuli.

A unique feature of the messages that pass through the RAS is that they are general as well as specific. In hearing, for example, once a sound is perceived by the auditory mechanism, it sends both specific and general impulses through the appropriate parts of the RAS. The specific arousal alerts the brain for increased attention to the sound, while the alerting, or general, impulses cause a general arousal of the cortex. Even before the cortex appraises the potential threat of the sound, this general arousal stimulates the limbic system and the hypothalamus, which in turn prepare the body for potential action. Muscle tension and hormonal and metabolic action increase before the cortex identifies the source of the stimulus. These increases are sensed by, and further alert and arouse, the RAS. If action occurs, the arousal was purposeful, and the products of arousal are utilized. If the sound is never consciously appraised or if no action is pursued, the RAS has become aroused (stressed) for no reason, and the products of arousal must circulate until they can be reabsorbed or otherwise used up. Figure 2.4 illustrates this process.

Of great importance in the study of stress and disease is the capacity of the RAS for reverberation (prolonged vibration) of an impulse, which will prolong a response. This means that the RAS can maintain a resting level of activity reflecting the general state of the other brain structures. A high level of resting activity increases and prolongs arousal, whereas a lower level of resting activity inhibits and shortens potential arousal. If you live a stressful life and find you are stressed many times during the day, the parts of your brain that become aroused to deal with that stress also affect the RAS, which adapts to frequent arousal by staying aroused. It is as though the RAS were saying, "Well, if you are going to be aroused so often, I might as well just stay aroused and save the time and energy of going up and down." The RAS also has the capacity to recruit impulses from other brain structures, and it will adapt to stimuli. Partly because of this ability to adapt, repeated situations cause less conscious stress than do novel experiences. For example, the noise of a city is less stressful for the permanent resident than it is for the visitor from a quieter environment.

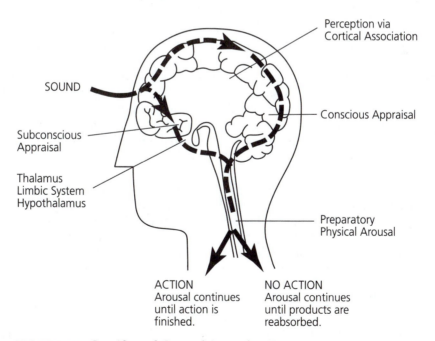

FIGURE 2.4 Specific and General Arousal in Response to Stress

The RAS is an essential part of the integrated limbic-hypothalamic-pituitary axis, which is responsible for an integrated physiological response to a life situation perceived as threatening. This response allows the organism to cope with the situation in a way that ensures its survival. However, when the response is chronically elicited, changes occur in the individual's normal physiological state. Under repeated stimulation (prolonged vibration) of the limbic-hypothalamic-pituitary axis, the transient elevations of activity become permanent. This phenomenon can be thought of as a hypersensitivity to stimulation, or a lowered threshold for activation of emotional arousal. Gellhorn (1970) called it "tuning." With chronic stimulation, the level of tuning increases in the part of the sympathetic nervous system that involves activity; the increased tuning is thus described as work. Gellhorn noted that this sympathetic tuning serves as a nervous predisposition to stress arousal, anxiety, and related stress disorders such as were mentioned in Chapter 1.

As we have seen, however, the activity of body organs is controlled by the relative level of activity of the sympathetic and parasympathetic nervous systems (as well as by endocrine activity). Tuning may be thought of as a balance between these two parts of the nervous system. According to Gellhorn, tuning dominated by sympathetic stimulation is *ergotropic tuning* (meaning work or action related). As ergotropic activity or tone increases, a reciprocal decrease in tone in the opposing trophotropic system occurs, and vice versa. Increasing ergotropic tone through constant stimulation (thus decreasing the tone in the opposing trophotropic system) augments dysfunction and pathology in the enervated organ systems. Increasing the activity in the trophotropic system through relaxation training reduces the tone in the opposing ergotropic system. Thus, any relaxation activity, especially those involving skeletal muscles, can charge the trophotropic system and discharge the ergotropic tuning, providing protection against chronic arousal and significantly reducing anxiety and other conditions related to arousal.

> *Ergotropic tuning:* stress-response tuning governed by the sympathetic (fight-or-flight) nervous system. The nervous systems of a chronically irritable person or a dog trained to attack are tuned ergotropically.
> *Trophotropic tuning:* relaxation-response tuning governed by the parasympathetic nervous system. A person becomes trophotropically tuned through relaxation training.

John Weil (1974), another pioneer in the study of the neurophysiology of stress, elaborated on Gellhorn's tuning model by broadening the concept of sympathetic versus parasympathetic tuning. He wrote that aspects of both systems work in concert with various hypothalamic-limbic structures on the basis not so much of anatomical structure as of physiological activity that results in either arousal or tranquillity. Weil suggested that the arousal system can be "charged" by high-intensity stimulation or by an increased rate of repeated low-intensity stimulation.

Once charged, the limbic-hypothalamic-reticular hub is capable of sustaining a high level of arousal through the discharge of impulses, providing general tonic activation. Gellhorn and Keily (1972), Benson (1992), and Weil (1974) suggest that decreases in proprioceptive input to the RAS and the limbic-hypothalamic-pituitary axis may be the underlying mechanism in relaxation training that charges or tunes the trophotropic system.

Pert (1999) also explains that when receptors are flooded with a particular ligand (neuropeptide), the cell membrane changes so that the probability of an electrical impulse crossing the membrane at the point is facilitated or inhibited, thus defining the bioelectric circuitry in that area. We become more easily stressed when we have this wiring.

Autonomic Control of the Stress Response

The autonomic nervous system ultimately controls how the body responds to new information. When the senses (sight, sound, touch, smell, and taste) and neuropeptides bring new information into the brain, the lower-brainstem areas orchestrate an immediate low-level physical arousal. The conductor of this orchestration is the hypothalamus, which immediately prepares the body with the arousal response. Background theme is added by the limbic system, which lends a feeling of pleasure or unpleasure. The intensity of response depends on the tone that has been set by the firing of RAS neurons. The cortex then assesses the physical arousal and tone and either enhances or inhibits them with conscious thought, tapping both conscious and subconscious memories. If the new information triggers a feeling of threat or a need for increased sensitivity, the stress response is heightened; if it triggers a feeling of safety, the stress response is allowed to diminish.

The fight-or-flight response is by no means the only contributor to the stress response. Actually, many emotional situations can alter the body's function, and different emotions evoke different physical states. When we feel anger, we become flushed, excited, and full of energy. Wolf and Wolff first reported in 1947 that in anger situations, the mucous membranes of the nose and stomach redden, swell, and become congested to the point of hemorrhage. Often gastritis can be traced to this cause. Fear has its own symptoms. When we are afraid, we tremble, our knees feel weak, and we often have difficulty speaking. Here, the mucous membranes of the nose and stomach become pale and shrunken.

It is difficult to generalize about how the nervous system affects stress-related disorders, for both stimulation and inhibition of the organ systems involved in the stress response can lead to body malfunction. Moreover, the nervous system both controls and is influenced by the another major system that controls the stress response of the body—the endocrine system. It is particularly harmful when these two systems get caught in a positive-feedback cycle, with each exciting the other and thereby increasing the stress response.

The Endocrine System

The endocrine system consists of glands that secrete substances called hormones into the bloodstream. These various hormones influence virtually all bodily activities. The glands we are most concerned with in this section are the pituitary gland and the adrenal glands, although all the glands are involved to some extent in the stress response.

The Pituitary: The Master Gland

The intimate relationship between the hypothalamus and the pituitary gland can be seen in Figure 2.1. As various areas of the hypothalamus are stimulated, it in turn stimulates corresponding areas in the pituitary. Thus, thoughts, anticipations, and nervous-system responses can and do become hormonal actions. Some portions of the hypothalamus stimulate the parasympathetic nervous system and inhibit the stress response. Other areas of the hypothalamus activate the sympathetic nervous system and increase the stress response.

Hormone-releasing factors are produced in the hypothalamus and released into a local bloodstream to the anterior pituitary, which releases pituitary hormones into the bloodstream and on to their target organs. This is an example of hormonal stimulation of the pituitary gland. The hypothalamus also executes nerve control over the pituitary through neurological connections between select nuclei in the hypothalamus and the posterior portion of the pituitary gland. The hypothalamic cells that produce hormone-releasing factors and the ones that stimulate neurological release of pituitary hormones are neurologically linked with the limbic system and the cortex. These links constitute a basic connection between our thoughts and emotions and psychosomatic disease (Rossi 1993).

The Adrenal Glands

Although all the endocrine glands may eventually become involved in the stress response, the adrenal glands are responsible for most of the physical manifestations of stress arousal, such as increased heart and respiration rates. There are two adrenal glands, one sitting over each kidney. The adrenal consists of two parts: an inner section called the medulla and an outer layer called the cortex (Figure 2.5).

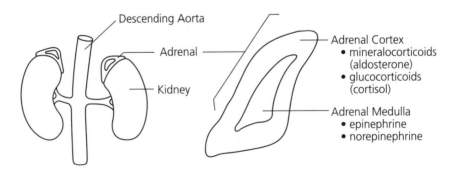

FIGURE 2.5   Adrenal Glands and Hormones

The medulla responds to the hypothalamic messages that travel along sympathetic nerves extending into the medulla. When the hypothalamus is alerted, an impulse is sent to the adrenal medulla, and this area immediately releases the hormone epinephrine (commonly called adrenaline), which primarily affects the cardiovascular system. With the effects of this hormone, along with its close kin, norepinephrine (noradrenaline), and a third hormone, dopamine, the stress response is fully manifested throughout the body. As long as the control centers of the brain perceive the need for arousal, stimulation of the adrenal medulla continues. Prolonged stress can eventually fatigue the medulla.

The hypothalamus acts on the adrenal cortex not through nerve impulses but by means of a hormone secreted by the pituitary gland in response to a hypothalamic hormone-releasing factor. This hormone, ACTH (adrenocorticotropic hormone), circulates through the bloodstream to the adrenal cortex. Once the adrenal cortex is stimulated, it in turn secretes hormones into the blood that manifest the stress response in a number of ways. The two primary secretions of the adrenal cortex are *glucocorticoids* (primarily cortisol) and *mineralocorticoids* (primarily aldosterone). Cortisol affects metabolism (that is, the total body processes) by increasing the availability of energy (in the form of glucose, fatty acids, and amino acids), either for the stress response or for recovery from an extreme period of overactivity. It increases, as much as tenfold, a metabolic process of the liver called *gluconeogenesis*, through which the body forms glucose out of available glycogen and amino acids. This assures the body, especially the central nervous system, of an adequate supply of the most efficient energy source (blood glucose) for use during this period of heightened need. Furthermore, during gluconeogenesis, cortisol decreases the use of glucose by muscles and fatty tissue, probably by making the system insulin resistant, thus producing a mild diabetic effect.

During the stress response, cortisol mobilizes both fatty acids and proteins in the blood. The mobilization of protein reduces the stores of protein in all body cells (except in the liver and the gastrointestinal tract, which is where the mobilization takes place). Hence, if the stress response is maintained for a long period, the supply of protein available for the formation of mature white blood cells and antibodies diminishes to the point of disease susceptibility. In this way, prolonged stress can promote muscular wasting and impair the immune system.

When fatty acids are mobilized from adipose stores, they circulate through the bloodstream in order to be available as an energy source for muscle tissue. When fatty acids are actually used for physical resolution of the stress response, they present little health threat. However, high levels of fatty tissue in the blood appear to promote *atherosclerosis* (fatty plaquing of the arteries), especially when they are present over time. In this day of "pseudostressors" such as caffeine, nicotine, sedentary lifestyles, and nonassertive response to stress, the fatty acids called out during the stress response may circulate in the bloodstream for hours until they are taken up by the tissues and stored away for future use. There is some evidence that the body prefers to store fat near the liver, which processes it, and fat cells near the abdomen appears to be particularly sensitive to glococorticoids. Thus people under chronic stress may tend to deposit more fat around their abdomen even when they are not particularly overweight. As we have mentioned many times, the body is an extremely efficient organism and will change its form and function to realize efficiency. In this case it is to keep fat near where it is needed, and in general, it is to maintain arousal if that appears needed to solve ongoing threats, whether real or imagined.

Aldosterone is the other major adrenal cortex hormone secreted in increased amounts during the stress response. The body reacts to aldosterone by preparing itself for increased muscular activity and better dissipation of heat and waste products. It does this by retaining extra sodium (salt), which results in increased water retention. This leads to increases in blood volume, blood pressure, and the amount of blood the heart pumps out with each beat. As with other body systems, prolonged manifestation of the stress response can endanger the cardiovascular system.

SOURCES CITED

Benson, H. (1992). *The relaxation response.* New York: Avon.

Bloom, F., Lazerson, A., and Hofstadter, L. (1995). *Brain, mind, and behavior.* New York: W. H. Freeman.

Ganong, W. (1995). *Review of medical physiology,* 14th ed. Los Altos, CA: Lange.

Gellhorn, E. (1970). *The emotions and the ergotropic and trophotropic systems.* Psychologische Forschung, 34, 48–94.

Gellhorn, E., and Keily, W. F. (1972). *Mystical states of consciousness: Neurophysiological and clinical aspects.* Journal of Nervous and Mental Diseases, 154, 399–405.

Glaser, R., and Kiecolt-Glaser, J. K., eds. (1994). *Handbook of human stress and immunity.* New York: Academic Press.

MacLean, P. D. (1949). *Psychosomatic disease and the "visceral brain": Recent developments bearing on the Papez theory of emotion.* Psychosomatic Medicine, 11, 338–53.

Moruzzi, I., and Magoun, H. (1949). *Brain stem reticular formation.* Electroencephalography and Clinical Neurophysiology, 1, 455–73.

Pert, C. (1999). Molecules of emotion: Why you feel the way you feel. New York: Simon and Schuster.

Robinson, D. L. (1996). *Brain, mind, and behavior: A new perspective on human nature.* Westport, CT: Praeger.

Rossi, E. L. (1993). *The psychobiology of mind-body healing.* New York: Norton.

Weil, J. L. (1974). *A neurophysiological model of emotional and intentional behavior.* Springfield, IL: Charles C. Thomas.

Wolf, S., and Wolff, H. G. (1947). *Human gastric function,* 2d ed. New York: Oxford University Press.

CHAPTER

3

The Body's Response to Stress

The Stress-Response Pathway

Stress follows a predictable route. A leads to B, and B leads to C. If A is stress, B is system dysfunction, and C is disease and premature death. This was known to the Greek philosopher Epictetus, who wrote that death was a "common consequence of chronic perturbation" and that anxiety was a disorder of the "will to get." He believed that it was better to die of hunger exempt from grief and fear than to live in affluence with perturbation. The exact path and mechanisms of this relationship between stress and premature death have been identified. This chapter discusses how the body's major systems respond to stress.

Although the central mechanisms for short-term arousal, as outlined in Chapter 2, are basically the same for everyone, each person reacts to prolonged stress arousal in different ways. Why some individuals respond to their stressors by developing ulcers, others by becoming hypertensive, and others by exhibiting behavioral effects such as depression, withdrawal, abuse of alcohol, drugs, or other people has been questioned since the inception of the study of stress. How a person "assigns" the stress response to a particular organ is called organ specificity. Franz Alexander (1965), one of the early pioneers in mind-body medicine, proposed that just as pathological microorganisms have a specific affinity for certain organs, so also do certain emotional conflicts afflict certain internal organs and behaviors. Bernie Siegel (1994) more recently concluded that individuals suffering from stress-related disease sensitize specific organs of the body. Ernest Rossi and Milton Erickson (Rossi 1993) propose that the person who experiences stress reacts in an appropriate way to alleviate that original stressful situation. However, the individual then becomes conditioned to that mind-body response, so that even when the original stress is over, the body tends to continue to react in this newly learned way. Eventually the organ or system that is responding to prolonged stress arousal breaks down due to exhaustion, or, as we explain in Chapter 4, emotional patterns become conditioned, and individuals tend to continue to react inappropriately long after the initial arousal.

29

Regardless of whose theory of organ specificity is "right," the points that are important to the discussion of stress-related disease include the following:

- Stressful events, situations, or experiences elicit the generalized stress arousal discussed in Chapter 2 and summarized in Table 2.1.
- The stressor is appraised immediately at the hypothalamic level, and the arousal response begins.
- Simultaneously, the hypothalamus alerts the limbic system and the higher cortical levels.
- Feeling tone is added by the limbic system and fed back to the lower centers of the brain, and in this manner the stress response may be prolonged. The cortex adds perception and conscious thought, further stimulating arousal.
- Depending on the emotional value (positive or negative) along with the conscious appraisal of the stressor, the appropriate systems of the body are asked to help solve the stressful problem.
- Upon solution of the problem or disappearance of the stressor, the trophotropic system attempts to return the system(s) to normal.
- RAS arousal may continue, increasing the reactivity tone of the central nervous system.
- If a person is often confronted with stressors causing central-nervous-system arousal, the system develops a higher resting nervous reactivity.
- Upon responding to the initial stressor, the body learns a response that, although appropriate at the time, may continue to be elicited by prolonged arousal.

Prolonged duration of the stress response is the factor that causes the most harm. It is not so much the one-shot, generalized alarm reaction that brings about illness; it is the prolonged state of arousal in response to which we somehow "choose" one or more systems to defend the body against stress. These systems become susceptible to all kinds of stressors and keep fighting until exhaustion. The resulting diseases and conditions might be called diseases of prolonged arousal. Figure 3.1 illustrates the flow of stress arousal from the brain to the stress response.

Harold G. Wolff, an early proponent of stress management, considered stress to be an internal or resisting force that is usually stirred to action by external situations or pressures that appear as threats—especially symbolic threats (i.e., threats involving values and goals). However, mobilizing our physical defenses (which were originally designed for battling physical threats) in response to symbolic (social or psychological) sources of threat produces an inappropriate response. To determine whether a response is appropriate, we must consider the outcome. Physical arousal to physical threat is appropriate: It is usually short lived and is usually dissipated with action. Physical arousal to symbolic threat is problematic in at least two ways: (1) in our modern society we can seldom resolve psychological threats to the ego with physical activity in order to resolve stress, and (2) symbolic threat tends to last longer because of

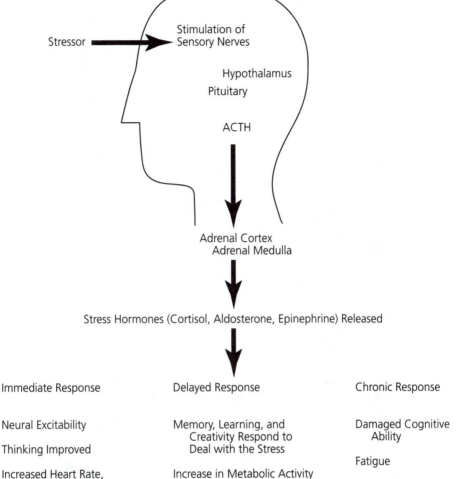

FIGURE 3.1   The Stress-Response Pathway

emotional input and internal dialogue and therefore is not as easily dissipated. When physical action is not warranted, it is not performed, and the reaction becomes detrimental to the body.

Hans Selye, perhaps the most noted stress researcher of the twentieth century, contributed a concept that is fundamental to the understanding of stress-related disease. In 1926, as a second-year medical student, he first noted that patients suffering from a number of diverse diseases displayed a common set of symptoms. At the time, he called this the "syndrome of just being sick" (Selye 1974).

Selye took his interest in the "sick syndrome" into the laboratory, where he injected impure and toxic gland preparations into laboratory animals. Regardless of the gland tissue and hormones injected, the animals developed a stereotyped syndrome (a set of symptoms that occur at the same time). These symptoms included increased activity and enlargement of the adrenal cortex, atrophy of the thymus gland and lymph nodes, and development of ulcers in the gastrointestinal system. Selye soon found that this same syndrome occurred in response to other kinds of stress: heat, cold, trauma, infection, and many others. This syndrome identified by Selye became known as the biological stress syndrome or the general adaptation syndrome (GAS). The three stages of the GAS, seen in Figure 3.2, are alarm, resistance, and exhaustion (Selye 1956).

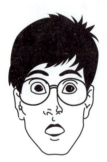

1 Alarm Phase

Complex physiological response initiated by presence of stressors triggers release of adrenalin, muscle tension and increased heart rate and blood pressure.

2 Resistance Phase

Body mobilizes to combat stressor.

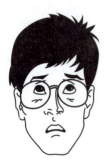

3 Exhaustion Phase

Resources become depleted; resistance breaks down; disease or death may result.

FIGURE 3.2   General Adaptation Syndrome

Alarm is the initial response to a stressor. In the alarm stage the body shows generalized stress arousal. This stage is characterized by widespread sympathetic discharge, increased ACTH secretion by the pituitary, and stimulation of the adrenal glands. Adrenal stimulation in turn assists in the full-blown fight-or-flight response. The body shows generalized stress arousal, but no one specific organ system is affected, although most, and in some cases, all of the body systems show measurable changes.

The resistance stage is marked by the channeling of the arousal into one or several organ systems. This is the body's unique intelligence of directing the stress response into the specific organ system most capable of coping with the stressor. Dealing with the stressor is a complex phenomenon encompassing physical, mental, emotional, behavioral, and philosophical coping mechanisms. In addition to mustering the forces to deal with the stressor, the body begins to adapt to the stress arousal. This process may be thought of as bending a little so as not to remain rigid and break. However, this adaptation process contributes to stress-related illness. The specific organ system becomes aroused, and with prolonged arousal and chronic resistance it may fatigue and begin to malfunction. As the system deteriorates, problems specific to the system begin. For example, stress arousal in some parts of the nervous or cardiovascular systems can produce life-threatening debilitation in a short time.

The resistance stage becomes particularly troublesome when resistance goes beyond responding to the initial stressor. It is as though the body has learned a new mode of defensive adaptation and continues it until it becomes a disease or condition in itself.

Exhaustion occurs after prolonged stress because the organs and systems of resistance have been depleted of their energy to perform. During this final stage, the organ system or process involved in the repeated stress response breaks down. ACTH secretion increases, and the response takes on the generalized character of the alarm stage.

In the exhaustion stage, disease or malfunction of the organ system or even death may occur. Sometimes exhaustion of one weakened system will shift the resistance to a stronger system, forcing that system into the adaptation process. To illustrate the damage that can be caused by adaptation, let's consider hypertension as a response to stress. The body must react to the stressor, so it needs to pump more blood to the muscles. This is accomplished by increased blood pressure. The increased blood pressure sets off another set of alarms so the body can eventually normalize the pressure. If the stress is prolonged and increased blood pressure is part of the response, the body will adapt and shut off the alarm, thus decreasing its internal struggle of lowering the pressure. It learns to live with the elevated pressure—it adapts. The body can adapt to high blood pressure without constantly eliciting an alarm reaction, but the increased pressure promotes kidney and heart damage, which can eventually kill the individual if the situation is allowed to continue. Adaptation may be a lifesaving process, but it must also be recognized as a type of disease process. In fact, Selye often referred to stress-related symptoms as "diseases of adaptation."

What has intrigued researchers for years is that the stress symptoms can provide information about the nature of the stress. There are noticeable differences between anger and fear responses, for example. As outlined by Selye, there are two arousal paths that lead to physical symptoms. One pathway is that of abnormal physiological processes provoked by the failure of general coping abilities. The other is triggered by appraisals of specific threats, which may be channeled to specific organ systems for resolution. If resolution does not occur, and the threat continues, a symptom of continued arousal of the specific organ will eventually become noticeable. A specific symptom is merely the specific locality in the body that has taken up the stress response. The brain is responsible for thinking and for emotional storage and retrieval, but it cannot move or act. Action belongs to the organs, especially the muscles. In a stressful situation, all emotional and thought processes occur in a directed attempt to resolve conflict. Organ systems are activated in an attempt to resolve stress arousal; however, coping strategies can misfire. Even when behavior or action is inhibited, the physiological aspect is expressed as getting ready (background action). Inhibited behavior can still leave a person excited. The physiological aspects of a blocked action can be continued or repeated because no appropriate cutoff signal is received. Throughout the day, each new stressful situation leaves a residual amount of tension in the body, the accumulation of which results in an inability to dissipate all the residual tension.

Individuals can remain in a phase of active coping or resistance almost indefinitely. Patients with stress-related symptoms show many signs of being in an active coping phase too long. In the muscle system there is excessive muscular contraction as the individual prepares for a specific intentional response. Emotions, defined as "directed energy," are often the cause of prolonged muscle contraction. Emotional energy is intentional, meaning it is directed at resolution of the problem. Sometimes general arousal is used for resolution, and other times very specific mechanisms are targeted for coping with the emotional problem. For example, anger can result in generalized muscle contractions needed for a total body response to run away from danger, or the anger may result in contraction of the hand muscles to make a fist to strike back.

As one might expect, understanding of stress symptoms vary with an individual's experience and beliefs. Some individuals make an instant connection between a particular symptom and their lifestyle and stressors. They intuitively understand the symptom and are ready do something about it. They understand that they are responsible for their health, just as they are responsible for their economic well-being, their relationships, and their happiness. They are willing to be responsible for the positive and the negative behaviors and events in their lives.

The body is so hardy and programmed for survival that it takes months or years of stress arousal, incompetent coping and unhealthy lifestyles to break down organ systems. If we choose to listen to these symptoms—the messages from the body—we may be able to prevent more serious conditions from developing. If we listen to the symptoms and make changes in our lifestyle, we can create good health. These conditions present an important learning component and they appear to be closely related to the stress, struggles, and coping endeavors of everyday life.

To Selye, stress was more than a response; it was a process that enabled the body to resist the stressor in the best possible way by enhancing the functioning of the organ system best able to respond to the stressor (Rosch 1997). Understanding the body's response can be the first step in mapping out a competent coping strategy.

The following sections describe how the body's major systems respond to stress.

The Muscles' Response

The muscles are our only means of expression. We cannot move toward pleasure or away from danger without muscle movements. Speech, facial expression, eye movements, indeed every mode of expression, feeling, and resolution of an emotion is achieved through muscle movement. Yet the muscles are under the command of the will, awaiting orders and obligingly obeying them. Oddly enough, many of the orders are given subconsciously, are counterproductive, and contribute significantly to stress and tension. This is because chronically tense muscles complete a feedback loop and further stimulate the mind, resulting in increased stress, which appears as irritability and hostility. Chronically tense muscles also result in numerous stress-related disorders, including headache, backache, spasms of the esophagus and colon (the latter resulting in either diarrhea or constipation), posture problems, asthma, tightness in the throat and chest cavity, some eye problems, lockjaw, muscle tears and pulls, and perhaps rheumatoid arthritis.

It is important here to reemphasize the word *chronic*. Stress disorders are caused by chronic, long-term overactivity. Acute, even violent, muscle contractions are not as harmful to the body as are slight or moderate contractions sustained over a long period.

Muscles have only two states, contraction and relaxation—although varying degrees of contraction, called tension, occur. Relaxation occurs when there is an absence of muscle contraction or tension. In this sense, activities that we commonly call *relaxation* (as in the sentence "I am going to the movies to relax") are better termed *recreation*. Movies may be recreational, but seldom do they produce muscle relaxation.

A muscle is a mass of millions of cells that can shorten when stimulated by nerve impulses. This shortening moves bones, traction occurs, tension develops, but no work is done. This situation is referred to as muscle tension and is linked with the stress-related disorders previously mentioned. Pain develops when a partially contracted muscle closes a blood vessel, causing an inadequate amount of blood to be delivered to the tissues. Pain can also develop when a chronically shortened muscle exerts an abnormal pulling pressure on a joint; when a chronically shortened muscle is overexerted and its fibers thereby torn; or when the proper function of an organ is disrupted, which is the case in smooth-muscle disorders such as diarrhea, constipation, and esophageal spasms.

Even though muscles maintain their own resting level of contraction, purposeful movement is under the control of the central voluntary parts of the brain, primarily the cerebellum and motor cortex. The most specific and exacting control comes from the motor cortex, which contains specific areas corresponding to particular areas of the body, such as the finger area, leg area, and neck area. Stimulation of any of these areas of the brain results in the movement of muscles in the corresponding body area. When the brain finally decides on an action, impulses are directed from the motor cortex, and the muscle contracts.

Remember that muscle cells receive only two commands—contract or relax; this is the limit of their capabilities. A finely coordinated action involves an unbelievable number of contract and relax commands, the sequence of which must be learned, practiced, and stored in the memory. Even then a coordinated movement is impossible without constant feedback about the result of the contraction. This feedback allows a person to instantly approve and refine the muscle action until the brain can accomplish the act without conscious control. A person has only to think, "Pick up the pencil," not figure out how to accomplish the act.

Let's now consider this in relation to stressful muscle tension. Imagine a potentially threatening situation in which you are contemplating some defensive action. You think defensively, you prepare to move, and you automatically assume a defensive posture. Whether you are correct in interpreting the situation as a threat is not important. What is important is that you have *engrams* (learned patterns) for this type of reaction, and they can be assumed without your consciously thinking about it. The muscle action for bracing, defensive posturing, or preparing for action can be completed even though your mind is not consciously considering such action. Thus you can see how hidden fears or anger can result in chronic stressful muscle tension.

Although anticipation is necessary for preparation, it has been found that muscle tension develops and remains until a task is completed or until the mind is diverted to a new thought process. Interestingly enough, successful completion of a task results in more rapid resolution of muscle tension than does failure to complete the task. Also, if you imagine a muscle movement or an action (for example, a defensive posture), you will experience the same preparatory muscle tension that occurs when you are actually engaging in the activity. This may explain why highly anxious people who are often in a high state of expectation often prove to have a great amount of muscle tension.

The muscle tension and movements described in the last few paragraphs are controlled by the motor cortex of the brain. Impulses from the motor cortex are normally carried to the muscles by the spinal cord and a cable of neurons called the *pyramidal tract*. In addition, a pathway called the *extrapyramidal motor system* sends signals from the hypothalamus and upper limbic area to the muscles. Stimulation through this pathway causes a variety of unconscious postures and rhythmic movements. Like the reticular formation, discussed in Chapter 2, this system seems to be both specific and nonspecific. Nonspecific activation may result in *nonspecific tonus*, or increased general tension throughout the system. This hidden state of tension may last over time and can augment a "voluntary" bracing action or cause a muscular overreaction. Either stimulation results in chronic muscle tension, which can lead to illness. Of course, relaxation can replace tension if the inherent rhythm is dominated by a low-arousal, tranquil rhythm. Such is the purpose of the relaxation exercises and techniques given in later chapters.

The Gastrointestinal Response

When Hans Selye conducted his classic experiments on stressed laboratory animals, he found ulcerations of the stomach lining to be one of the responses. But why would the gastrointestinal (GI) system be involved? It serves no function in the fight-or-flight response and logically should not be controlled by the parts of the brain that anticipate or interpret possible threats. Nevertheless, GI disorders are responsible for filling more hospital beds in the country than any other disorders, and science has clearly established that many GI disorders have stress-response roots.

The gastrointestinal system (Figure 3.3) is responsible for accepting food; mechanically breaking it down by churning it in the stomach; moving it through the intestines; and supplying enzymes that will finally convert small food particles into the blood sugar, simple fatty acids, or amino acids the body uses for energy or for building tissue. The GI system has an inherent rhythm and is governed by numerous automatic reflexes that control its movements, its emptying, and its secretion of enzymes. The GI system is also associated with the motivation system, in that hunger must lead to food-gathering behavior. The centers that control hunger and appetite are located in the hypothalamus and are closely related to pleasure and displeasure (see the discussion of the limbic system in Chapter 2). Hunger and satiety are definitely emotional states and, as such, affect the functioning of the GI system.

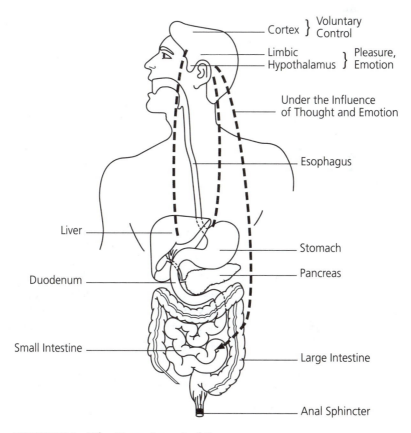

FIGURE 3.3   The Gastrointestinal System

The GI system responds to emotional situations in a more complex manner than the typical sympathetic versus parasympathetic process described in the preceding chapter. Also, an understanding of the GI system dispels the stereotype that the sympathetic system arouses and the parasympathetic relaxes, for overstimulation of either of those two divisions of the autonomic nervous system can result in disease.

Response to stress arousal can be measured in every structure along the alimentary canal, starting with the mouth. Since Pavlov's classic studies, it has been clearly demonstrated that emotional states influence the flow of saliva. You may have had the experience of getting up before an audience to deliver a speech and finding your mouth dry. This occurrence has long been used as a measure of fear: In ancient China suspected criminals were made to chew rice, and the lack of a mucous wad was taken as an indication of guilt. On the other hand, seeing the dentist preparing to drill a tooth often turns on saliva to the point that the dentist must continuously vacuum it away.

The emotions can also induce spastic contraction of the muscles in the esophagus, which leads to the stomach. These contractions disrupt peristalsis (the rhythmic movement that carries food through the digestive system) and make swallowing difficult and in some situations impossible. The stomach, too, has been recognized as part of the emotional response system. Most anxiety tests take into consideration the state of the stomach. Statements such as "I have no appetite," "I have a gnawing feeling in the pit of my stomach," and "I feel nauseated" are the most often described physical symptoms of anxiety and emotional arousal.

Doctors have been able to observe the activity in the stomach lining. They have noted that in situations producing anger, resentment, or aggression, the lining increases its secretions of hydrochloric acid and various enzymes and becomes engorged with blood. The membrane eventually becomes so frail that eruptions occur spontaneously and ulcerations develop. Situations producing fright, depression, listlessness, and withdrawal produce the opposite reaction—the stomach lining functions below its normal level. But even that situation is not without problems: Decreasing the blood flow to the secreting glands reduces the natural protection of the area against certain harsh substances such as hydrochloric acid, which helps break down food in the stomach.

In the intestines, similar patterns have been observed. Stress arousal has been shown to alter peristaltic rhythm. This alteration in normal peristalsis in both the small and large intestines is responsible for two of the most classic stress responses: diarrhea, if movements are too fast and normal drying through water absorption does not take place; and constipation, if movement through the intestines is very slow and excessive drying occurs. Chronic constipation can lead to more severe intestinal blockage. Blockage of the bile and pancreatic ducts as well as inflammation of the pancreas (pancreatitis) have been linked with stress arousal, although little research has been conducted in this area.

Pert's study of neuropeptides indicates that from top to bottom, the gut has receptors that respond to the various molecules of emotion (1999).

The Brain's Response

Although we discussed the brain as part of the control system (see Chapter 2), we can also view it as a response system because its electrical activity can be analyzed. First, we should understand how its nerve cells function. These neurons constantly exchange ions (atoms that carry tiny electrical charges) across their cell membranes. This activity forms wave patterns, which can be followed through the use of an electroencephalograph (EEG). This instrument measures the frequency or rate of the wave pattern in cycles per second, or hertz (Hz). Unlike the muscles, which remain electrically inactive until they are stimulated into action, the cells of the brain emit a constant electrical rhythm.

The dominant, quiet rhythm of the brain has been designated the *alpha wave pattern*. It is characterized by a wave pattern that fluctuates at the rate of 8 to 13 cycles per second, and it emits energy that typically varies from 25 to 100 microvolts. An increase in the brain's activity changes this basic alpha rhythm, producing a wave pattern that is higher in frequency (13 to 50 cycles per second) but emits less energy. This faster wave pattern of lower voltage has been designated *beta*. Another common wave pattern, called *theta*, fluctuates at the rate of 4 to 7 cycles per second, and an even slower wave pattern, *delta*, fluctuates at fewer than 4 cycles per second and usually occurs only during sleep.

Analysis of complex brain-wave patterns has been used to diagnose abnormal brain states. More recently, the practice of referring to wave patterns to describe various activation states has become popular. The alpha wave has been associated with the absence of meaningful cause-and-effect thinking; this is a quiet state of mind in which stress arousal is at a minimum. The beta pattern is characterized by a focusing of attention, problem solving, and relating the self to the external world. Although this is not necessarily a stressful state, stress arousal is more possible in the beta state. Less is known about the mental state associated with the theta pattern, although researchers report that the thought patterns are directed internally and are less related to specific external events. Daydreams, fantasies, and what some researchers call "creative images" are more likely to occur during the theta state. More information on the brain wave and its associated mental states is presented in the chapters on relaxation and meditation.

Apart from the more measurable physical responses of the brain to stress, psychological or mood responses occur as well. Besides the "hardwiring" of the brain (such as we see in axons, dendrites, and the synaptic activities between them) is the constant chemical exchange in the brain cells, especially in the nerve complexes, or nuclei. Receptors for endogenous mood changers (from endorphins and myriad other neuropeptides) are found in abundance in the pleasure-pain pathway from the hindbrain to the forebrain, in areas where the five senses bring their information to be shared, throughout the forebrain where ethical decisions must be made, even the supportive glial cells. Emotional states and moods are produced by the various neuropeptide ligands (Pert 1999).

During rest and relaxation, the brain is said to be in *homeostasis*, which means that the subjective moods of the individual are in harmony, promoting a healthful relationship between mind and body. During stress, the psychological mechanisms of the mind are thrown into turmoil. A "mood disturbance" is one common characteristic of the stress reaction. Stress commonly elicits confusion, fear, extreme emotional sensitivity, and feeling of ego threat.

The Cardiovascular Response

Not all diseases are stress related. However, in the case of cardiovascular disease, stress is highly implicated. The question is exactly how much of a contributor stress is in relation to the other risk factors. The indirect nature of stress and the long-term development of this chronic disease obscure the answer.

Diseases of the cardiovascular system (Figure 3.4) include problems related to the heart itself (its basic structure and rhythm), to systemic blood flow and blood pressure, to the structure of the blood vessels, and to the constituency of the blood. It is obvious that each aspect cannot be considered separately from the others; they are all intricately related, and malfunction of one affects the others.

The heart's job is to pump blood to the body's cells. The blood contains oxygen and energy-producing substances that are the basic necessities for the life of the cell. To pump blood, the heart, a cavity surrounded by muscle, must contract. As the muscle contracts, the cavity becomes smaller. This increases the pressure of the blood within the chamber. When the pressure in the cavity is greater than that outside it, the blood is ejected into the miles of blood vessels, arteries, and veins that travel to every part of the body. Each blood vessel contracts in a similar manner, thus helping to maintain the pressure and aid the movement of the blood traveling through the system. Once ejected, the blood is pushed along under pressure, which in the average adult male is about 120 millimeters of mercury (slightly less for females). When the heart completes its contraction phase, it relaxes, and the pressure in the system drops to about 80 mmHg in the average male (again, slightly less for females). These pressure indications (120/80) are used to express blood pressure, which is easily measured by a cufflike instrument called a *sphygmomanometer*.

It should be obvious that the fewer times a heart must contract or beat to accomplish the necessary supply functions, the more rest it will get. The heart has an inherent rhythm that is determined by the membrane potential of a special area in the right atrium called the *pacemaker*. Even when the heart is denied nervous stimulation, it is capable of independent action; however, the heart is constantly receiving impulses from the brain, and its inherent rhythm is continually influenced by the central nervous system. The heart receives impulses from both the sympathetic and parasympathetic nervous systems (see Chapter 2). Thus, it is under moment-to-moment control by various centers of the brain that are in touch with the body's metabolic and physiological demands. In addition to neural regulation, the heart can also be influenced by the hormone epinephrine, which can increase the contractibility of the heart muscle (the *myocardium*), increasing the speed and strength of the contraction.

Research evidence suggests that chronic stress is implicated in enhanced cardiovascular reactivity, elevations in stress-related hormones, and depressed immune function.

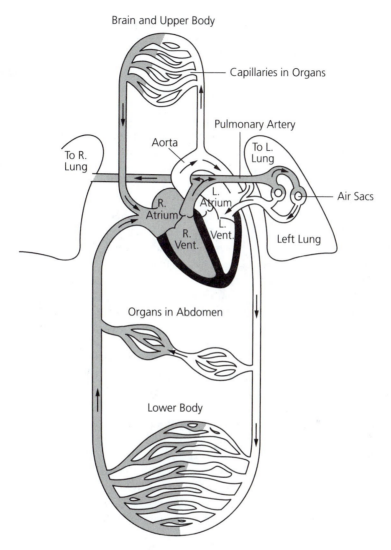

FIGURE 3.4   The Cardiovascular System

Uchino and colleagues (1992) studied older subjects who were long-term caregivers for Alzheimer's disease patients and found that the chronic stress of care giving increased cardiovascular reactivity. (See also Baum, Cohen, and Hall 1993). Caregivers had a substantially greater incidence of depressive disorders than matched control subjects, and the caregivers were also found to have poorer immune function than controls. Chronic stressors seemed to produce longer-term autonomic, immune, and endocrine alterations.

A significant survival mechanism of the cardiovascular system is that the heart is capable of anticipating physiological and metabolic demands by increasing its action before it actually has to. As we have seen, however, the anticipation of such demands very often increases the activity of the system, but then the final action is thwarted by the conscious cortex. In this case, the cardiovascular response is to no avail. Similarly, many psychological states increase cardiovascular activity when no action is actually required. A new or unusual experience frequently elevates the heart rate, as do fear, anger, anxiety, and most situations that threaten the ego. You will recall Harold Wolff's definition of stress as a physical response to a psychological or symbolic threat that is inappropriate in kind and intensity in our complex society; stressors are usually symbolic, requiring no physical action. The response, nevertheless, is physical. Thus, a chronically stressed person often has a chronically overworked heart.

Another cardiovascular problem related to stress is chronically elevated blood pressure, or *hypertension*. It has been estimated that perhaps 15 to 20 percent of the adult population suffers from hypertension, usually considered to be a pressure above 160/95. Approximately 90 percent of the cases are called *essential hypertension*, meaning the origin is unknown. Because the primary work of the heart is to overcome the pressure in the arteries through which the blood must flow, high blood pressure greatly increases the work of the heart and contributes to cardiovascular problems.

Like the heart, the blood vessels have an inherent tone that can be altered moment to moment by both parts of the autonomic nervous system and by hormones (epinephrine and norepinephrine) to reflect the physiological demands placed on the system. Anticipation and psychological states such as fear, anger, and anxiety will alter the diameter of blood vessels, producing a physical response to symbolic or imagined threats.

A third problem concerning the cardiovascular system is *atherosclerosis*, the destruction of the vessels by the infusion of fatty plaques, which contain cholesterol, triglycerides, and other fatty elements. The relationship between stress and vascular problems appears to be that during stress arousal, the hormones epinephrine and cortisol mobilize fats and cholesterol for use by the muscles, and the fats and cholesterol circulate in the bloodstream until they are used or reabsorbed. (The process was described in Chapter 2.) Although there are many factors in the development of atherosclerosis, constantly saturating the system with unneeded fats through the stress mechanism can only exacerbate the problem. An artery infused with such plaques will eventually lose elasticity and harden, producing *arteriosclerosis* (an advanced form of atherosclerosis). This disease is directly responsible for over half a million deaths annually in the United States.

When an artery in an advanced state of disease loses its elasticity, it elevates the blood pressure, thus contributing to hypertension and disease of the heart itself. In addition, atherosclerotic plaques, by narrowing the diameter of the blood vessels, diminish oxygen delivery and may bring on a *myocardial infarction*, or heart attack, if the coronary arteries are affected. Many factors contribute to the development of atherosclerosis and hypertension, including a diet high in cholesterol and saturated fats, which add to the amount of potential fatty deposits in the blood vessels; lack of exercise; smoking, which mimics sympathetic nervous system stimulation, narrowing the blood vessels and increasing the heartbeat; obesity; sex (males are more at risk); age; heredity; and, of course, stress, which underlies many of the others.

Another vascular problem associated with stress is the vascular headache, also known as the migraine headache. Migraines are thought to be caused by an exaggerated constriction of blood vessels in and around the brain. This constriction is followed by a reflex dilation or enlarging of those vessels, which causes the release of toxic chemicals that irritate local nerve endings and add to the pain. The root of this type of attack is complex and appears to involve, in a headache-prone individual, a psychogenic trigger of the sympathetic nervous system, which then causes the initial constriction of the blood vessels. This phase, known as the prodromal phase, is characterized by nausea, increased irritability, and an unusual sensitivity to noise and light. Physiologically, this phase seems to deplete the level of the hormone serotonin in the system. It may be the loss of this hormone that causes the reflex dilation of the vessels and the accompanying intense pain. Little is known of the underlying cause of migraine. The migraine-prone individual may have abnormal metabolism of serotonin or may be deficient in an enzyme that oxidizes this hormone. Recent clinical investigations have shown that certain types of migraine headaches can be alleviated by controlling the central nervous system through elaborate relaxation training. This points not to the alleviation of any chemical imbalance but to control over the initial psychogenic trigger.

The Skin's Response

It is sometimes difficult to think of the skin as a separate system capable of responding to stress arousal, but its complex function and intricate nervous control make it a sensitive response system, and its accessibility makes it a convenient window into the body. When you observe the stress response of any body system, you are looking through that system into the mental activity responsible for the response.

The skin has two basic response patterns that show the world what is going on in the body and in the mind. One is often referred to as electrical language because it seems to speak if you have the proper listening device. Each of the millions of cells that constitute the skin system contains chemicals that have an electrical nature. As the body expresses itself, the chemical activity of the skin cells changes, producing different patterns of electrical activity. This electrical activity can be measured on the skin surface. The constant but ever-changing activity of the skin appears as "chatter," and although complex and sometimes difficult to interpret, it is used by police authorities in most lie-detector systems and by health professionals to help understand an individual's emotions, motivations, and problem-solving techniques.

The second basic response system of the skin is its temperature. Under the skin are small blood vessels that change in response to emotion. During tense, anxious periods they shut down and allow less blood to pass, causing the skin to appear pale and the skin temperature to decrease. At other times, the blood vessels open and allow the skin to flush with blood, thus increasing the skin temperature. Determiners of blood flow in the skin include the neuropeptides.

With this type of response pattern, it is not hard to visualize how prolonged emotional responses could change the activity of the skin long enough to result in malfunction and disease. Certain skin conditions or illnesses have been found to have roots in our psychological response patterns. For example, eczema, a skin lesion characterized by redness, swelling, itching, and fluid discharge, has been associated with emotional stimulation. The reddening and itching are indicative of abnormal blood flow to the area, while the fluid discharge is indicative of an increased rate of fluid production by the skin cells. Laboratory studies have established that in eczema-prone individuals, emotional arousal increases the amount of fluid exuded by the skin cells, whereas relaxation diminishes it. Eczema patients have been classified as being restless, impatient, and unduly irritable, but the relationship of these characteristics to the skin condition has not been clearly established. Similar preliminary work has been done with patients suffering from urticaria (hives), psoriasis, and acne, but these investigations are still in their infancy.

The Immune System's Response

Structure and Function of the Immune System

The immune system (see Figure 3.5) provides natural and acquired defense against foreign elements that enter the body through the air we breathe, the food we eat, or in other ways. The immunity we are born with, *innate immunity*, is provided by the skin, the acidic secretions of the stomach, mobile white blood cells, and other natural body structures and biochemicals that defend against all invaders in a nonspecific manner. Also, we develop what is called *acquired immunity*. This is a process whereby

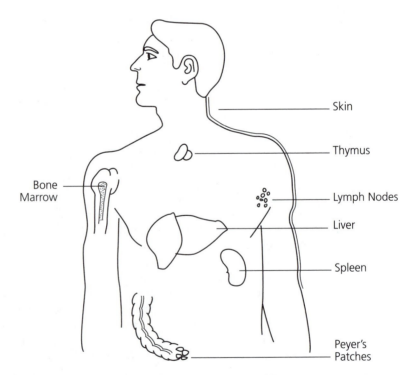

FIGURE 3.5   Major Centers of Immune System Tissue

the body recognizes foreign agents called *antigens* (bacteria, toxins, and viruses) and responds to each by producing antibodies specific to it. Two lines of acquired immunity defense, *humoral* and *cellular,* are very important to our discussion of stress and psychosomatic disease. Both originate in the bone marrow, where undifferentiated stem cells are produced.

In humoral immunity, the stem cells migrate from the bone marrow to the various lymphatic tissues throughout the body, where they mature into white blood cells called *beta-cell lymphocytes* (B-cells). When an antigen enters the body and is taken up by the bloodstream, it is detected by the B-cells as the blood is filtered through the lymph nodes, spleen, and so on. The antigen stimulates the B-cells to evolve into plasma cells that then synthesize specific antibodies that attack the invading antigen. Figure 3.6 depicts this process.

The development of cellular immunity is similar to that of humoral immunity, except that the stem cells of the bone marrow travel to the thymus gland, where they mature into *T-cell lymphocytes* (T-cells) that attack invading antigens directly. Some of these T-cells travel to the skin to make the entire surface of the body part of the

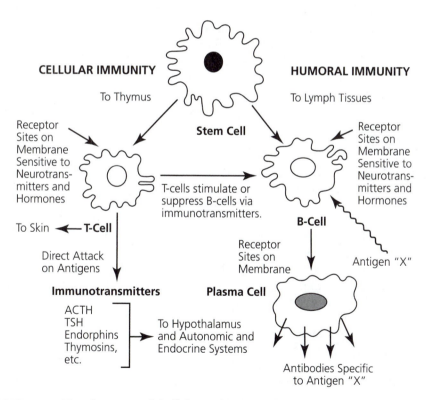

FIGURE 3.6   Development of Cellular and Humoral Immunity and Production of Immunotransmitters

immune system (Glaser and Kiecolt-Glaser 1994). It is important to the discussion of stress and disease to note that T-cells and B-cells have receptor sites that respond to neurotransmitter substances of the autonomic nervous system, to hormones of the endocrine system, and other informational substances that keep the whole body's communication network up to speed. This means that the immune system can influence and be influenced by the control systems discussed in Chapter 2.

In the 1960s immunology came of age as a science, and it is now one of the most exciting branches of research into illness and disease, especially with the AIDS threat. For years immunologists were so busy discovering the complexity of the immune system itself that they paid little attention to its communication with the other systems of the body. More recently, however, research in psychoneuroimmunology (PNI), has begun uncovering the physiological mechanisms that control the intimate communication among the nervous, endocrine, and immune systems. It is this research that gives us the missing link between how our thoughts and emotions influence our health and disease states.

Immunological research has found that neurotransmitters (such as epinephrine and norepinephrine) can attach to immune cells and change their ability to multiply and destroy invading agents. Furthermore, research has identified the "hard-wiring" system of nerve fibers that transmit messages between the brain and lymphocytes that fight infection and cancer in the body (Pert 1999).

In addition to immune-cell response to neurotransmitters and hormones of the endocrine system, the immune system apparently talks to the other control systems through immunotransmitters such as ACTH, thyroid-stimulating hormones, and other polypeptides such as the endorphins and thymosins. T-cells also have the ability to stimulate or suppress B-cells.

Stress and the Immune System

Our current knowledge of the coherent mechanisms of communication among the nervous, immune, and endocrine systems is altering the old medical belief that thoughts and emotions had nothing to do with disease. The medical findings of world-renowned physicians and researchers such as O. Carl Simonton, Stephanie Matthews-Simonton, Bernie S. Siegel, Joan Borysenko, and Norman Shealy, to name a few, have led to widespread recognition that thoughts, emotions, attitudes, and beliefs have a great bearing on health, disease, and the ability to rebound from illness. Candace Pert might be called the "mother of emotional research" with her groundbreaking study of the neuropeptides published in her book, *The Molecules of Emotion* (Pert 1999).

The immune system may become dysfunctional and lead to stress-related illnesses in basically three ways: (1) underactivity, (2) hyperactivity, and (3) misguided activity (Rossi and Cheek 1994). Characteristic diseases caused by these three types of dysfunction are, respectively, cancer, asthma, and rheumatoid arthritis. Underactivity or depression of the immune system occurs in response to stress-induced release of adrenal cortex hormones. Various researchers (Cohen et al. 1995; Zakowski et al. 1992) have found that even slight depression of the immune system greatly increases susceptibility to pathogens. The hyperactive immune response seen in asthma involves a highly irritable mucosal lining of the lungs. When the lining is irritated, the resulting hyperimmune response can cause symptoms ranging from mild discomfort to respiratory failure. Autoimmune diseases are examples of a misguided immune system that attacks its own tissues as well as those of invading antigens. Autoimmune disorders are often associated with immune-deficiency syndromes, injuries, aging, and malignancies (Rossi 1993). Breakdown in communication within the nervous, endocrine, and immune systems through neurotransmitters, endocrine hormones, and immunotransmitters is basic to all immune dysfunctions (Kiecolt-Glaser and Glaser 1995).

Studies in which volunteers were exposed to pathogens such as cold viruses provide direct evidence that stress modulates the speed and potency of immunological defenses. For example, to study the effects of academic stress on immune response, Glaser and colleagues (1992) gave a series of hepatitis B inoculations to forty-eight second-year medical students on the last day of a three-day exam series. Students who were less stressed, less anxious, and who reported greater social support demonstrated a stronger immune response.

If stress arousal is prolonged, any or all of the biochemicals, organs, and systems involved will be affected until fatigue occurs. At that point, infections, common colds, and slight skin conditions appear. As the fatigue continues, the conditions worsen and more serious illnesses develop. When the immune response to disease elements is diminished by 50 to 60 percent, the body may respond with persistent and repeated infections requiring antibiotics, with summer colds, with serious skin-disease inflammation, and with chronic respiratory conditions such as bronchitis, asthma, or tuberculosis. Immune-system fatigue diminishes the body's ability to resist all invading viruses, bacteria, and toxins.

The Prevention and Treatment of Diseases of Arousal

The *allopathic* or traditional medical system continues to be perplexed by mind-body diseases of adaptation. Selye (1974) suggested that medication could be given to counteract stress hormones that ravage the system or that the adrenal glands could be removed surgically. He also noted that if a nonspecific shock could cause these conditions (which he characterized as "getting stuck in a groove"), perhaps various forms of nonspecific shock therapy could counteract the conditions. Because such clear evidence exists of a mind-body connection in the genesis of disease, there is growing acceptance in the medical community of the addition of more holistic practices in the fight against mind-body disease.

One of the most highly researched mind-body diseases is cancer, which will serve here as an example of how holistic modalities based on mind-body theory may facilitate healing. A major line of evidence of the mind-body connection in cancer centers in studies of life-change stress (Dohrenwend and Dohrenwend 1974; Meador 1992). It appears that any form of trauma involving a significant life change can activate the cortical-hypothalamic-pituitary-adrenal response, producing the adrenal cortical hormones that suppress the immune cells that continually search out and destroy cancer cells in the system. In addition, a negative self-concept, depression, and anxiety are all associated with immune-system suppression or underactivity. Coping ability is also a significant factor in whether stress will have an immunodepressant effect (Poikolainen, Kinerva, and Lonnquist 1995).

A recent research study to show the influence of behavioral intervention on cancer development or progression involved health education, enhancement of problem-solving skills regarding diagnosis, stress-management techniques, and psychological support for stage I or II malignant melanoma patients (Fawzy et al. 1993). Intervention patients who were seen in groups of seven to ten for ninety minutes every week for six weeks exhibited reduced psychological distress and more significant immunological changes than the control group. The intervention group showed significant increases in the percentage of natural killer cells, as well as increased natural killer cell activity. A six-year follow-up of these patients showed a trend toward greater recurrence and a statistically significant higher mortality rate in control patients than in the intervention group patients.

Data suggest that psychological and behavioral outcomes for women with gynecologic, breast, and colorectal cancers and men with digestive tumors, prostate, and bladder cancers can be improved with psychological interventions, and it is likely that even greater gains could be achieved if more health behavior components were added (Anderson 1994). To address the stress component of this disease directly, prevention of prolonged stress arousal is the first line of defense. Prevention can take the form of learning to avoid stressful situations, restructuring or reframing events previously thought of as stressful (through assertiveness training, realistic setting and attaining of interpersonal and professional goals, and so on), and learning to reduce the arousal tone of the central nervous system through meditation or other quieting activities.

If disease has become apparent, these preventive measures are also used in treatment (Siegel 1994). In addition, active intervention in the form of imagery has been found helpful in some cases of cancer. The reasoning behind the use of imagery in fighting disease is that mind modulation of body processes is considered to be a psychoneurophysiological fact; if the mind can contribute to the sickness, it can also contribute to getting well. Matthews-Simonton and colleagues (1992) and Simonton (1994) have successfully used imagery and the technique of cognitive reframing to treat cancer and found that their methods seem to enhance cellular immunity. While such therapists and researchers as Matthews-Simonton, Simonton, and Creighton have found the use of active imagery to be successful, others such as Seigel (1994) and Benson (1999) have approached prevention and treatment through quieting the mind. Herbert Benson's "relaxation response" was designed to bring about an inner stillness of central origin. The combination of imagery and some form of meditation is used by most current practitioners of psychosomatic medicine (Rossi and Cheek 1994).

SOURCES CITED

Alexander, Franz (1965). *Psychosomatic medicine.* New York: Norton.

Anderson, B. L. (1994). *Surviving cancer.* Cancer, 74, 1484–96.

Baum, A., Cohen, L., and Hall, M. (1993). *Control and intrusive memories as possible determinants of chronic stress.* Psychosomatic Medicine, 57, 274–86.

Benson, H. (1992). *The relaxation response.* New York: Avon.

Benson, H. (1999). *Timeless healing: The power and biology of belief.* Audiocassette. New York: Simon and Schuster.

Borysenko, J. (1999). *Fire in the soul: A new psychology of spiritual optimism.* Elizabeth, NJ: Replica Books.

Borysenko, J., Borysenko, M., and Kramer, J. eds. (1994). *The power of the mind to heal.* Los Angeles: Hay House.

Cohen, S., Doyle, W. J., and Skoner, D. P., (1995). *State and trait negative affect as predictors of objective symptoms of respiratory viral infections.* Journal of Personal and Social Psychology, 68, 159–69.

Dohrenwend, B., and Dohrenwend, B. eds. (1974). *Stressful life events: Their nature and effects.* New York: Wiley.

Fawzy, F. I., Fawzy, N., Hyur, C., Elashoff, R., Guthrie, D., Ashey, J., and Morton, D. (1993). *Malignant melanoma: Effects of an early structured psychiatric intervention, coping and affective state on recurrence and survival 6 years later.* Archives of General Psychiatry, 50, 681–89.

Glaser, R., and Kiecolt-Glaser, J. K., eds. (1994). *Handbook of human stress and immunity.* New York: Academic Press.

Glaser, R., Kiecolt-Glaser, J. K., and Esterling, B. A. (1992). *Stress-induced modulation of the immune response to recombinant hepatitis B vaccine.* Psychosomatic Medicine, 54, 22–29.

Kiecolt-Glaser, J. K., and Glaser, R. (1995). *Psychoneuroimmunology and health consequences: Data and shared mechanisms.* Psychosomatic Medicine, 57, 269–74.

Matthews-Simonton, S., Simonton, C. O., and Creighton, J. L. (1992). *Getting well again.* New York: Bantam Books.

Meador, C. K. (1992). *The person with the disease.* Journal of the American Medical Association, 268, 1, 35.

Myss, C., and Norman Shealy, C. (1998). *The creation of health.* New York: Three Rivers Press.

Pert, C. (1999). *Molecules of emotion.* New York: Simon and Schuster.

Poikolainen, K., Kanerva, R., and Lonnquist, J. (1995). *Life events and other risk factors for somatic symptoms in adolescence.* Journal of Psychosomatic Research, 39, 1, 53–62.

Rosch, P. J. (1997). *Reminiscences of Hans Selye, and the birth of "stress."* Health and Stress: The Newsletter of the American Institute of Stress, no.9.

Rossi, E. (1993). *The psychobiology of mind-body healing.* New York: Norton.

Rossi, E. L., and Cheek, D. B. (1994). *Mind-body therapy: Methods of ideodynamic healing in hypnosis.* New York: Norton.

Selye, H. (1956). *The stress of life.* New York: McGraw-Hill.

Selye, H. (1974). *Stress without distress.* New York: Signet.

Siegel, B. S. (1994). *Love, medicine and miracles: Lessons learned about self-healing from a surgeon's experience with exceptional patients.* New York: Harper and Row.

Simonton, O. C. (1994). *Healing journey: The Simonton Center program for achieving physical, mental, and spiritual health.* New York: Bantam.

Uchino, B. N., Kiecolt-Glaser, J. K., and Cacioppo, J. T. (1992). *Age and social support: Effects on cardiovascular functioning in caregivers of relatives with Alzheimer's disease.* Journal of Personal and Social Psychology, 63, 839–46.

Wolff, H. G. (1968). *Stress and disease.* Springfield, IL: Charles C. Thomas.

Zakowski, S. G., McAllister, C. G., and Deal, M., (1992). *Stress, reactivity, and immune function in healthy men.* Health Psychology, 11, 223–32.

CHAPTER

4 Stressful Emotions, Thoughts, and Beliefs

Negative emotion is the tinder that feeds the fire of stress. Emotion is expressed in the contraction of fear and the explosion of anger; it is the slow cooker of revenge, the cancer of depression, the stealth of guilt, the blanch of terror. Everyone experiences negative emotion, and some cultivate it until it kills them. At some point in life, most people decide that negative emotions are luxuries that they cannot afford and begin to give them up.

What is emotion? In its broadest definition, emotion includes the commonly used terms such as anger, fear, joy, guilt, jealousy, love, courage, and sadness; the drive states such as hunger and thirst; and basic sensations of pleasure and pain. Early scientific arguments between Walter Cannon and William James questioned whether emotions originated in the brain and then messages were sent out to the body so that it would respond appropriately, or whether emotions originated in the body on a feeling level and then were worked on by the brain. As in all great arguments, each side probably offers something to ponder. From Pert's research (1999) on what she terms the "molecules of emotion," we find what Oriental healers and philosophers have proclaimed for centuries: The body and mind are one. Although various parts of the body have their own specificity of action (the heart pumps blood, the lungs aerate the blood, etc.), an interconnecting network of neuropeptides allows all cells of the body to have their own mobile phone, so to speak, to talk with everyone else—the human internet.

We do learn (become accustomed to using specific neural and chemical pathways) to expect emotions to feel a certain way and lead to certain outcomes, yet it is a total mind-body learning rather than memories laid down in certain parts of the brain. Once an emotional response is formed and stored away in the limbic part of the brain, it colors later actions and decisions. We know the amygdala (a walnut-shaped structure deep in the limbic system) has emotional "hot spots" or nuclei. When something scares or otherwise upsets us, the amygdala is at the center of the brain's circuits for stamping that moment in memory. Thereafter, when something seems to resemble that original moment of distress, the amygdala recognizes that similarity and dictates our response in a few hundredths of a second, even before the forebrain has had time to fully mull over what is going on—or what the consequences of our reaction will be (Goleman 1997, 1998).

Emotion is an energy complex involving nerves, muscles, gut, bone marrow, glandular activity, and other diverse cells of the body. Over time it may be learned as a physical pattern that readies the body for confrontation, retreat, expression, or no expression. Emotions are instantaneous forms of experience and reaction. When people are being emotional, they express immediate physical reality, and this expression takes place before they can even be consciously aware of it. Emotions are forms of immediate experience. When individuals experience emotion, they are in direct contact with physical reality.

Emotional responses learned in early life are reactions to basic needs and external stimuli, and as people grow older they also learn to create emotional patterns from their thoughts. Even before emotional patterns are learned by any kind of cognitive conditioning, however, there is an innate feedback system that is designed to keep the mind-body in balance. We call this the "wisdom of the body," or perhaps *homeostasis*. In early life babies practice emotional patterns until they are fairly habitual reactions. Because children are taught directly or indirectly to not show their emotions, especially unpleasant ones, they develop negative self-talk (an inner dialogue with one's self) that also becomes part of their emotional patterns. If children do not like the way an emotion feels or are not allowed to have it, they may "block" it out of their consciousness altogether. Emotional reactions become part of the basic personality.

The Development of Human Emotion

MacLean explains that, anthropologically, the brain developed as three distinct parts (see Figure 4.1): (1) a brain that relates to the physical world, (2) a brain that relates to the inner world, and (3) a brain that relates to abstraction and creativity (1990). We might think of these parts as physical, emotional, and mental. The evolution of the brain began as brain 1, the physical brain. It helped us survive for hundreds of millions of years by registering and responding to physical input. It was merely instinctual and reflexive. Following the adage "ontogeny recapitulates phylogeny" (meaning that, as an organism develops, it passes through, or repeats, each phase of the evolution of its species), the physical brain was complemented with brain 2, the emotional brain. The emotional brain wrapped around the physical brain, and these two areas developed an intimate communication network. Now, explains MacLean, in addition to responding to physical stimuli, humans began to place an emotional value on their relationship to the physical world and to each other. The emotional brain handles not only emotions but all internal images. It receives concrete, physical images from the lower brain and abstract images from the cortex, and its job is to make some kind of cohesive relationship out of those images. Pearce (1994) calls the midbrain the "heart" of the central nervous system, for it handles love, hate, fear, attraction, aversion, bonding, and all other relationships. Finally, with further evolution, the third brain (the thinking brain, or cortex) enveloped the other two parts. It enabled us to work with abstract imagery, think on an intellectual plane, and create thoughts and forms not necessarily based on physical input. The thinking brain, or cortex, makes it possible for us to analyze, synthesize, create, compute, and otherwise play with the information furnished by the two lower brains. Especially important to our study of stress is

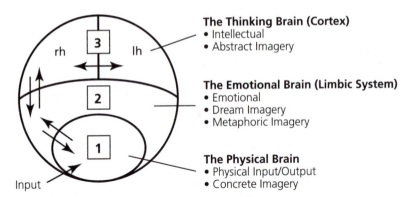

The Thinking Brain (Cortex)
• Intellectual
• Abstract Imagery

The Emotional Brain (Limbic System)
• Emotional
• Dream Imagery
• Metaphoric Imagery

The Physical Brain
• Physical Input/Output
• Concrete Imagery

FIGURE 4.1   The Triune Brain and Its Intercommunication Links (adapted from Pearce 1985)

the development and functions of the forebrain or frontal cortex. This area of the brain is responsible for our being able to be consciously responsible. It gives us the ability to plan for the future, to delay gratification, to formulate intent and make changes toward intent, and make conscious decisions. Pert (1999) explains that this part of the brain does not fully develop until the early twenties in humans, which might explain unsocial behaviors of youth.

The two hemispheres of the cortex are not connected at birth and therefore undergo concurrent development. At about age one, the corpus callosum begins to provide a communication link between the two hemispheres, and specialization begins to occur in each (see Figure 4.2). Before the development of the corpus callosum is completed (somewhere around age four), the two hemispheres communicate only with their respective parts of the lower brains. Once the corpus callosum is developed, the hemispheres can communicate freely without any input from the physical and emotional brain functions, making it possible for us to think and plan without emotional and physical interference. This ability has created the double-edged sword of being able to think and create on a very high plane but without compassion for the physical body or for human relationships and ethics.

A very important aspect of emotional health rides on the lines of communication among the three parts of the brain. The physical and emotional brains communicate in both directions, showing the constant synchrony of these two areas. There is also strong bidirectional communication, although not as complete a synchrony, between the emotional brain and the *right* hemisphere of the cortex. However, that same bidirectionality is *not seen* between the emotional brain and the left hemisphere of the cortex; in fact, it appears that the two are only casually connected. Therefore, the lower-brain nerve signals that reach the left hemisphere must travel through the right hemisphere and across the corpus callosum (Pearce 1985).

In other words, the emotional brain is in close neural communication with the functions of the right hemisphere but not with the functions of the left hemisphere. In a culture that rewards left brain functions very highly, it is likely that neural mes-

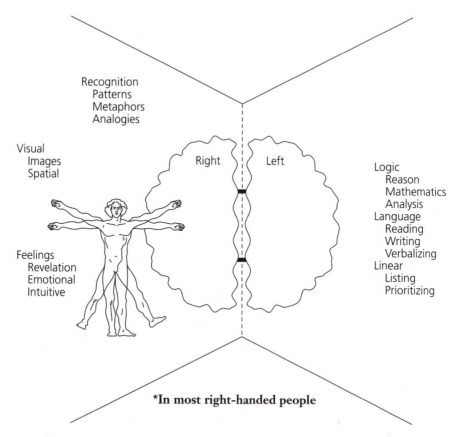

Recognition
Patterns
Metaphors
Analogies

Visual
Images
Spatial

Right

Left

Logic
Reason
Mathematics
Analysis
Language
Reading
Writing
Verbalizing
Linear
Listing
Prioritizing

Feelings
Revelation
Emotional
Intuitive

*In most right-handed people

FIGURE 4.2   **Right and Left Brain Functions***

sages are neither received, recognized, nor communicated by the rational, left hemisphere. The right hemisphere of the brain cannot write or speak, so it must send emotional messages via the body (i.e., physical signs and symptoms).

By understanding the original nature and development of these three parts of the brain, which in current terminology are the *thalamus, hypothalamus,* and *brain stem* (the physical brain), the *limbic system* (the emotional brain), and the *cortex* (the thinking brain), we are afforded insight into the neural connections of mind-body disease. Beyond the neural connections, the neuropeptide system is also at work. These peptides are important keys to the understanding of emotion in that their receptors are found in extremely high concentration not only in the hippocampus, amgydala, and hypothalamus but also throughout the autonomic nervous system, in nerve ganglia on either side of the spine, in internal organs, on the surface of the skin, in the dorsal horn of the spinal cord (which is the first synapse where all somatic-sensory information is processed), and other locations (Pert 1999). With this information, it no longer holds that the emotional brain is housed only in the limbic system and hypothalamus.

According to Pearce, during the first year of life, babies develop and use primarily the physical brain to sense and respond to their world. At about age two the emotional brain centers begin to develop. The physical brain still receives all the outside messages, but the emotional linkage now begins coloring the information with "like" and "dislike" immediately upon receipt of the information from the physical brain. With the development of emotional learning, the child becomes not only a physical self but also an emotional self, relating outside events with feelings of joy and laughter, fear and crying, love and happiness. These actions take on a stimulus-response form as memory patterns develop. For example, a child may form a negative emotional memory pattern from being left with a sitter when the parents go out. After the first traumatic time, the child may begin to cry whenever either parent merely prepares to leave. In fact, the child's reaction to early separations from the parents becomes the basis for his/her reaction to all separations and losses later on in life.

As growth and development continue, the functions of the neocortex are added to the functions of the midbrain and old brain. This makes it possible for the child to just think about the parents leaving him/her alone, which elicits the emotional habit form of fear, anger, and even rage. In this instance nothing external or physical has actually happened, such as the parents preparing to leave, calling a sitter, or telling the child that they plan to go out. Because the child can now think in "what if" terms, any emotional pattern with an experiential base can be voluntarily brought back. Accompanying this pattern may be subconscious beliefs such as "They must not love me, or they wouldn't go away without me," and an even more basic belief, "I must be an unlovable person," or "I must be a bad person." Unless these beliefs and thought forms are changed, they are carried into adulthood and used as a belief in other negative emotional experiences. It is not difficult to imagine how traumatic real abandonment or abuse can be and what long-term risk factors can develop. Individuals tend to block emotional memories of childhood traumatic experiences, and when emotional energy is blocked, the mind loses its full capacity to analyze, evaluate, and synthesize situations and experiences (Viscott 1997). When negative emotions are blocked, the mind cannot integrate the experience, and what is more, the blocked emotional energy continues to build with new experiences that resemble the original traumatic experience. This further diminishes the mind's ability to function clearly, and behavior in response to the new stimulus becomes less logical because it is based on an old experience that probably happened when the child was not old enough, powerful enough, or skilled enough to do anything about the situation.

Because emotional patterns learned in response to actual, physical stimuli are stored in the mind and body, they can later be stimulated by merely thinking about them or by having a certain part of the body (where we hold the stress) stimulated. Through the ability to relive stressful situations, people learn how to scare themselves to death, worry themselves into an anxiety attack, and catastrophize even the most harmless situation. By the same token, however, people can retrieve pleasure, joy, love, and happiness by thinking about times when they felt those emotions.

SELF-ASSESSMENT EXERCISE 1

Place your answer to each of the following questions in the space provided before each number.

_____ **1.** I know when something is emotionally upsetting me.
   a. almost always   c. seldom
   b. often   d. almost never

_____ **2.** My choices are strongly colored by my emotions.
   a. almost always   c. seldom
   b. often   d. almost never

_____ **3.** When anger or depression strikes, it overwhelms me.
   a. almost always   c. seldom
   b. often   d. almost never

_____ **4.** When I'm angry, everyone around me pays for it.
   a. almost always   c. seldom
   b. often   d. almost never

_____ **5.** I have the ability to wait long periods of time to get what I want.
   a. almost always   c. seldom
   b. often   d. almost never

_____ **6.** I experience test anxiety.
   a. almost always   c. seldom
   b. often   d. almost never

_____ **7.** Set-backs don't keep me down for long or keep me from doing my job.
   a. almost always   c. seldom
   b. often   d. almost never

_____ **8.** I can tell just by watching when someone around me is upset.
   a. almost always   c. seldom
   b. often   d. almost never

_____ **9.** I find it impossible to handle emotional conflict within relationships.
   a. almost always   c. seldom
   b. often   d. almost never

_____ **10.** I can put the emotional tension around me into words and help release the tension.
   a. almost always   c. seldom
   b. often   d. almost never

_____   Total Score

Scoring: For Numbers 1, 5, 7, 8, and 10: a = 1, b = 2, c = 3, d = 4
            For Numbers 2, 3, 4, 6, and 9: a = 4, b = 3, c = 2, d = 1

Results: 32 or ABOVE: Time to improve your emotional responses.
            20–31: Average level of emotional response.
            19 or UNDER: You probably experience good emotional health.

Yale psychologist, Peter Salovey proposed the concept of "emotional quotient" in the early 1990s, and Dan Goleman (1997, 1998) subsequently popularized the topic in an effort to help people understand the role that emotion plays in successful interactions with others. He pointed out that an individual may have a high intelligence quotient, yet be emotionally inept. The emotionally inept suffer poor interpersonal relationships, whether they be at home, work, or school.

Goleman found five basics that are involved in emotional intelligence: (1) self awareness: being aware of what you feel and using inner knowing to make skillful decisions; (2) self-management: being able to control anxiety and impulses and to use anger appropriately; (3) self-motivation: using inner zeal and optimism when setbacks occur; (4) empathy: being able to recognize unspoken emotional states in others and being able to respond in a compassionate way; and (5) interpersonal skills: skillfully interacting with and handling emotional reactions of others.

Pain and Pleasure

Broken down to basic physiology, initial emotions arouse only two feelings: pain and pleasure. Psychiatrist David Viscott (1997) reduces the emotional complexity of young and old alike to a single process that is repeated time and time again in everyone's life. The process begins in the present where only pain or pleasure are felt. It ends up with feelings such as guilt, anger, and depression, which are centered in the past. The following is a progression that you may be familiar with:

Pain in the present is experienced as hurt. If released here, it goes no further.
If held, the pain of the past is remembered as anger.
Pain created by thoughts of the future is perceived as anxiety.
Unexpressed anger redirected against one's self and held inside is called guilt.
Anger directed inwardly toward one's self creates depression.

The main insight from Viscott's work is that much of our stress and distress comes from stored hurt, which disguises itself as anger, anxiety, guilt, and depression and manifests itself as behavioral patterns. Look under depression and you will find anger. Look under guilt and you will find anger. Look under anger and you will find hurt and sadness. Look under hurt and sadness and you will find fear, what you have been hiding all along.

Emotional Energy

Deepak Chopra (1998) explains emotional energy with the most dynamic of new sciences—quantum physics—and also through ancient Indian spiritual philosophy. Chopra makes a convincing case that we all exist in a common field of intelligence in which solid material structure, time, and space are merely concepts. Further, the body is a field of intelligence, or mind, that has produced a physical body through thought. When a thought occurs, the message is known to all parts of the body—

every cell—simultaneously. All parts of the body then produce the hormone(s) responsive to the particular thought. When an individual thinks of an experience as exhilarating, all cells respond with the physical (neuropeptide) correlate of exhilaration. When the thought response to a situation is depression, the entire body hormonally expresses depression. Thoughts produce emotion; emotion produces thoughts.

Emotional energy carries messages that each individual names fear, anger, and so forth on the basis of experience. Lazarus (1998) and Morse (1995) observe that regardless of whether there is a label or a universally correct word for an emotion, all of us have had the following emotional experiences:

1. anger
2. anxiety
3. sadness
4. guilt
5. shame
6. envy
7. jealousy
8. disgust
9. hope
10. pride
11. gratitude
12. happiness
13. love
14. compassion

These experiences are stored in the mind-body in the form of memory patterns, and when the body is triggered, it responds with a pattern. To illustrate, take a moment to gasp as though surprised or frightened. The body instantaneously braces itself. Muscles contract, the lungs and heart modify their action, and if taken to great extent, this "as if" situation can cause all the systems involved in this emotion to alter their functions. Through nerve stimulation, the muscles tense, the heart beats faster and/or harder, respiration quickens and/or deepens, the pupils dilate, and glands are stimulated to either reduce or increase their secretions, depending on the function of the gland. The adrenals are stimulated and begin dumping out hormones to help answer the emergency signals that have been given at the brain level. The emergency signal is the perception of a situation that demands attention. It may be a situation wherein joy or humor is perceived, or the signal may be perceived as danger. Also, it may have its roots in the external world or within a thought pattern that has little external base. The response to the emergency signal is the emotional reaction pattern, or—as we first identified it in this book—the stress response.

Emotions such as anger, happiness, and jealousy are expressed more actively than fear, guilt, and contentment; yet all of them have a total-body response pattern. Pert (1999) explains that all emotions have a neurological-hormonal profile and that we can categorize emotional response patterns as either healthy or unhealthy by their impact on the immune system. Furthermore, each person's learning experience and cognitive control may help to place all of his or her emotions in the healthy category through recognition, restructuring the meaning of the emotion, and letting go of an "unhealthy" emotion once the associated emotional experience is over.

If the emotion you experience is positive, tension builds and then is released as a shout or laughter, perhaps. Pleasure is felt with the release of emotional tension. When the emotion is negative, tension builds up and tends to be stored. Usually, during this time, negative self-talk increases the tension. Pain is caused by extreme and unrelieved tension.

Emotional messages do not dissipate until they are delivered, and delivery means that the message is recognized and allowed to play itself out. When blocked-up emotional energy is released, certain body aches and pains may also go away.

Stressful Emotional Patterns

At a very early age little girls and boys learn that very few emotions are acceptable. At first, laughter and giggling are usually highly prized by adults, but as children grow into adolescence, they quickly learn that loud laughter and silly giggling are not acceptable in public. Children are rewarded for not crying, reprimanded harshly for displaying anger, and chided for being fearful. They are asked to not show that they have been emotionally hurt, to be selective about whom they should love, and to contain their exuberance. Thus, it is no wonder that most adults engage in negative mind-talk when they get angry, are hurt or fearful, or even want to shriek in happiness and joy.

Because of the years of negative mind-talk that accompany emotions, everyone denies negative emotions to some degree or another. When a person gets angry and says, "This is really silly to get mad," the emotion is not honored. But it happens anyway. And it is stored in a favorite place (or places) in the body, with all the other anger that has been denied and not released. Release of an emotion is necessary before the body can go back to a relaxed state, or back into balance. Most people know the effectiveness of a good laugh or cry as a release to make them feel better.

Bradshaw (1992) points out that dysfunctional families deny their children the right to feel or to talk about feelings. This keeps the children from being in touch with what they are feeling because, first of all, they are shamed out of expressing any feelings and, second, they aren't allowed to talk about their feelings. In some families, children are allowed to express only certain emotions, such as guilt. This early learning forms the child's emotional quotient.

By studying your own behavior you may be able to identify which emotions are your primary stress responses. Fear and anger are the two emotions that when chronically used, most negatively impact your health. Fear is a lifesaving response, and anger can also be an appropriate response. However, when either of these emotions becomes a chronic response to life, it becomes inappropriate. Fear is a "flight" stress mechanism; it is a constriction, a contraction, a pulling inward away from confrontation. All negative emotions may be based on fear. Anger is a "fight" stress mechanism that explodes outward. In order to target these emotions for resolution, complete the Emotion Recall exercise that follows. Count how many times fear or anger is mentioned. If one response predominates, there is a message there for you. Techniques that will help you get a handle on fear and anger follow later in this chapter.

Emotion Recall Exercise

1. Think of a situation that has occurred in your life recently that stirred up negative emotions in you (these are usually stressful situations). Now close your eyes and take yourself back into that situation. See in your mind's eye where this occurred and who was there; get a very clear picture of the situation; listen to what everyone was saying, including what you were saying to yourself; allow yourself to experience the feelings you felt then and immediately afterward. Also remember what you were saying to yourself after the experience.

2. Now identify all of your feelings involved during and after the situation by putting a check *in front of* any/all of the following emotions that apply.
"The situation that I am remembering made me feel. . . . ."

_____ Anxious _____	_____ Lonely _____
_____ Submissive_____	_____ Confused _____
_____ Inadequate_____	_____ Irritated _____
_____ Miserable_____	_____ Critical _____
_____ Discouraged _____	_____ Foolish _____
_____ Depressed _____	_____ Rage _____
_____ Helpless_____	_____ Guilty _____
_____ Furious _____	_____ Hostile _____
_____ Bewildered_____	_____ Embarrassed _____
_____ Insecure_____	_____ Bored _____
_____ Jealous _____	_____ Ashamed _____
_____ Hateful_____	_____ Insignificant _____
_____ Rejected_____	_____ Stupid _____
_____ Inferior _____	_____ Weak _____
_____ Frustrated _____	

3. The two major negative emotions are <u>Anger</u> and <u>Fear.</u> On the line after each feeling you have checked, write in the basic emotion that best fits your feelings at the time.

Example: __✓__ Rejected <u>Anger</u>

__✓__ Insecure <u>Fear</u>

4. Count the incidence of your responses, and identify which of the two basic emotions (Anger and Fear) you identify with most often in the list of feelings.

5. Write down some of the phrases you were saying to yourself *during* your situation:

6. Write down some of the phrases you were saying to yourself *after* your situation:

Breaking Unhealthy Emotional Cycles

Because most negative emotional responses are old, habitual responses to perceived dangers, people can learn to break those patterns in various ways. One is by relaxing. Movement of energy occurs in the body as it carries out an emotion. The instantaneous constriction of muscles becomes such a part of the emotional response that the physical reaction to stress cannot occur if the muscles will not respond. Therefore, one way to break the emotional stress response is to RELAX. A time-honored, efficient, and effective way to relax in any situation is to do deep, diaphragmatic breathing. Chapter 12 describes the use of breathing exercises as a method of general relaxation.

Another way to break old negative emotional-response patterns is to act on them as soon as you notice that you are thinking negative thoughts or saying negative things to yourself. At that time, tell yourself, "Stop it!" Then, after noting your negative thinking pattern, replace it with relaxation and/or positive thoughts, or just focus on and enjoy what you are doing and experiencing at the present time.

As you are learning how to break negative emotional-response patterns, those patterns will still occur. However, it is healthy to experience the patterns, honor them, and learn to release the tension that could otherwise lead to poor health. If the emotional energy is not released, disease or behavioral symptoms will occur. The following exercise gives explicit directions for turning unhealthy emotional responses into healthy ones:

1. Allow yourself to focus on the emotion; really focus on how it feels.
2. Ride out the unpleasant feeling, allowing it to vibrate throughout the body, even if it appears as physical symptoms.
3. Assist the process by finding the thought form that is blocking you. Test thoughts and phrases that come to you to determine whether they are the cause. Sample phrases might be: "I am scared," "I am lonely," "Quit picking on me!" "I give up," "No, No, No!" Scan your body for the feelings that come up with each one of the statements.
4. When you discover the restricting thought, change it into a new, productive one, such as "I can work through this," "I am happy to spend some time with myself," "There is nothing to fear."

5. Continue to work on using the old thought form less and less as the new thought form is patterned by use. Imagine making a new path through the grass and letting the old one you used to take grow over. If you do not change the causal situation (the old, negative thought form), any symptom relief is temporary.
6. Write your experience as a journal entry.

Thoughts and Beliefs

Once we have recognized an emotional pattern, we can learn from it something about our basic attitudes and opinions in life. An emotional response to a situation is always produced by a belief, attitude, or opinion. Most of the time we are not aware of the thought pattern because the reaction is a habit, not a well-thought-out response.

Thoughts

Our state of health, physical development, coping behaviors, moods, feelings, emotional response, and level of stress are all expressions of our thoughts. They are also subject to alteration by a change in thoughts (Damasio 1994, 1999). Our thinking or belief system can be the ultimate control system in our lives. The conscious mind attempts to control our stress by controlling our actions and behaviors. Control is the way we function to get our needs met. When the mind focuses on some goal, our thoughts can control and manipulate our world (including our unconscious mind) until the goal is achieved.

If we do not wish to display our emotions, we can suppress them with the mind. The left hemisphere of the brain has the ability to bypass feeling input, and we learn to do that well when there are negative consequences of emotional feelings. If the body cannot be controlled by covering up symptoms (such as wearing deodorants or by taking drugs), the conscious mind can choose to ignore the symptoms up to a point of endangering health. On the positive side, the thought system can change stressful situations into controlled ones. When people are depressed or unhappy, they can choose to do activities they did when they felt good, and this activity is likely to make them feel better (Glasser 1994, 1999).

Thoughts allow us to anticipate a situation, assume a defensive posture, and increase background arousal if necessary. In a situation of prolonged stress arousal, thinking efficiency may be decreased due to overload. What you believe dictates how you will react to a stressor and what you will experience from the situation. Control is maintained by taking small steps that do not exceed your ability to cope.

Small steps may mean engaging in new behaviors that you can manage. Large steps, in the form of behaviors that challenge deep beliefs, usually force individuals beyond their normal ability to cope. At this point recruitment occurs. Recruitment is the use of negative maladaptive behaviors—for example, ego defense, rationalization, withdrawal, and illness—as helpers in the attempt to cope. Attempts at controlling stress in these times of overload usually result in what is known as incompetent coping. When one feels out of control, it is usually the result of too much input demanding too many responses.

Thus far we have noted that the physical body is aroused by emotions. Emotions may be thought of as the "middle man" between the body cells and the mind. In the final analysis, most causes of stress stem from the thought process, how we perceive our world. Patent (1998) points out that we have 50,000 or more thoughts a day (most of them being the same ones we had the day before) and that the majority of our thoughts are in the form of beliefs, which are necessary to interpret the world around us.

Beliefs

Beliefs are enduring patterns of thought. Most beliefs are learned early in life from parents, relatives, peers, and authority figures. The beliefs that are accepted from others and formed on our own become the programs that determine behavior on emotional, mental, physical, and spiritual levels. A true belief is a nonconflicted, solid idea that governs our day-to-day thoughts and actions. The beliefs that people hold about themselves and about life in general are the foundations upon which they base all their behavior. Beliefs provide a framework through which experience is measured, analyzed, and evaluated, and that determines the response to experience. As such, they provide a sense of security even when an experience is negative.

If information about reality is not consciously rejected by the mind or if it does not directly conflict with existing beliefs, then an individual accepts it as true. Once incorporated as a belief it is generally forgotten even though it continues to operate. This does not mean that beliefs are lost to conscious awareness, only that the mind no longer pays attention to them. It is something like having money in the bank. Even though you may not be using it right now, it influences how you live and affects many of your decisions. In the case of beliefs, they become such a familiar way of interpreting the world that they are completely taken for granted.

The self-image is an example of a belief, a base, or a foundation upon which an individual's entire personality and behavior (and eventually their reaction to stressors) are built. For example, if self-image is strong and positive, day-to-day experiences will seem to verify, and thereby strengthen, self-image. If the self-image is weak or negative, day-to-day experiences will seem to verify that and thereby weaken the self-image.

Beliefs act as guidance systems for the flow of life. Where there is conflict, the flow is distorted, and this distortion may lead to acute or chronic tension, often expressed on the muscular, organ, or cellular level. Such tension can lead to pain and illness, and this is the basis for the mind-body philosophy. Some experts in the field believe that the source of all illness is in conflicting personal beliefs, ideas, and actions.

Milton Erickson, the famous hypnotherapist and behavior-change artist, believed that every person has his or her own unique map of the world, an inner belief system that is unconscious and constitutes a kind of hypnotic trance. It is as though we go through life with a posthypnotic suggestion that we act in a certain way to certain stimuli. It is the "inner child" who forms this core belief system. Core material, according to Kurtz (1997), is the way our internal experience is organized. It is composed of our earliest feelings, beliefs, and memories that are made in response to the stresses of our childhood environment. This *core material* is nonlogical and primitive; it was the only way a child knew how to survive. Once these core beliefs, feelings, and memories are formed, they become the basis of future responses.

Deepak Chopra explains this concept in another way, using the term *premature cognitive commitment* rather than core material. He notes that the brain and body form an early response to an object/situation and that response is embedded there. It becomes an actual neurophysiological pattern. All future experiences in any specific area are based on this premature cognitive commitment.

Two examples given by Chopra in his book, *Ageless Body, Timeless Mind* (1998) are the following:

1. When newly hatched fish are placed in an aquarium that has been separated down the middle by a Plexiglas divider, the fish learn to stay on their own side of the divider. When the divider is removed, the fish still stay on their side of the aquarium.

2. One litter of newborn kittens was reared in a "vertical" environment—all the objects and lines in their space were vertical. Another litter was reared in a "horizontal" world—all the objects and lines in their space were horizontal. When the kittens were grown and placed in the opposite environment, they actually could not see physical barriers that were different from those where they were reared. That is to say, kittens from the "horizontal" world ran into the vertical legs of chairs and tables. Even though there was nothing wrong with their sight, these animals had given premature cognitive commitment to their early environment.

What motivates the child in early infancy are the first rungs on Maslow's motivational hierarchy: getting physical needs (such as hunger) met and feeling safe and secure. In order to do that, the baby is at the mercy of the older people in its environment. It must meet the demands and adapt to the reality of significant others. In computer language, this becomes the hardwiring of the individual (Maslow 1968).

At the core of our being is the basic belief structure that has guided our thoughts and actions throughout our lives. Positive changes must be made at this level so that they reflect a change in our perceptions and, in turn, the way our bodies react to the mental and emotional input. In order to use beliefs and thoughts to change an emotional reaction, we must perform four basic operations:

1. Recognize and honor the emotion rather than deny, repress, rationalize, or otherwise not honor it.
2. Identify the negative thought complex that is behind the negative emotion. Every stressful situation in life has an old, outdated, negative belief behind it. That belief was formed when it was useful. In adulthood it is no longer so.
3. Break the habitual loop that the emotion triggers.

4. Replace the negative thought complex with a new, positive thought complex.

5. Respond to situations from the new belief complex.

Exercises to Decrease Emotional Stress

Anger and fear are the two negative emotions that we most frequently encounter. It is as though they are ends of a behavioral continuum: We either strike out in anger, or we pull back in fear. As noted earlier in this chapter, anger is an emotion we use when we do not resolve feelings of being hurt. Hurt is generated from fear. When first encountering a new situation, do you move toward it, or do you shrink back in fear? Everyone uses anger and fear when more appropriate behaviors could reduce the stress of potentially hurtful situations. Here we offer a few alternatives to add to a stress management program.

Learn Anger Management

1. Keep an anger diary for one week. On a three-by-five index card, for each incident jot down what precipitated the anger; how you reacted; how you felt before, during, and after the incident; what you expected from others in the situation; why you think others acted the way they did; your self-talk before, during, and after the incident; and how long the self-talk lasted.

2. Write a list of coping self-talk statements. Under the headings "Before the incident," "When physiologically aroused," "During the encounter," and "After the encounter," write four or five statements you can use to help you stay calm during that time. For example:

> Before: I don't need to get angry in this situation.
> Physiological Arousal: Relax now and stay centered. Breathe . . .
> During: What is my outcome here? Honey catches more flies than vinegar.
> After: I did the best I could. That could have been worse. I did a great job.

3. Choose the incident that provoked the least anger, and review it in your mind.

4. Use a relaxation technique that works for you (deep breathing, neuromuscular relaxation, and so forth), and while relaxed, mentally review the incident you have chosen. As you play through it, insert an appropriate positive coping-statement at the four points outlined in #2.

5. When you can relive this incident with no feelings of anger, choose the next least stressful situation from your diary, and repeat the procedure using your positive coping self-statements.

6. When old incidents can be relived without anger, transfer the technique to future potential anger situations in your life.

Examine Beliefs Regarding Anger

An underlying cause of anger is not getting what we expect. Therefore reducing the incidence of anger involves examining beliefs about expectations. Typical anger-inducing expectations are based on beliefs such as the following:

- I know how to do it best and quickest.
- If it's not done my way, it's done wrong.
- If you can't do it quickly and excellently, get out of the way.
- If I do everything "by the book," I'll be appropriately rewarded and live happily ever after.
- If I hurry faster, I'll get everything done.

After an anger situation, review your thoughts and behavior. What must you believe in order to think and behave that way? On identifying an irrational or negative belief behind the anger, change it to a positive one such as "People have their own ways of doing things that are right for them."

Explore Your Fear History

To learn more about responding in an anxious manner to stressful situations, write your history of fear. When frightened as a child, how did you react? How did your parents react when they were fearful? Was there any one incident from which you seemed to learn the fear reaction? According to David Viscott (1997) the basic questions that reflect the predominant fears of most people are as follows:

- Am I good/Am I bad?
- Am I lovable/Am I unlovable?
- Am I strong/Am I weak?
- Am I smart/Am I stupid?
- Am I right/Am I wrong?
- Am I worthy/Am I unworthy?

Whenever fear or anxiety experiences arise, even in adulthood we go back to these basic questions.

Choose an anxious situation from your childhood and identify the basis of that anxiety. It may have been a realistic reaction for you as a child, but is it still a realistic response now that you are an adult and have more knowledge and experience?

Take Action

Fear constricts. The opposite of constriction is expansion or movement. When anxiety strikes, make an immediate plan of action so that you change the old, patterned response to fear. An example of this is the person lying in bed who hears a noise outside the window. An anxious reactor may become terrified and paralyzed in his or her bed. Making this situation nonstressful calls for getting up immediately, turning on the lights, and looking for the source of the noise. If the source is found to not be harmful, laughter and a pleasant goodnight to the source can end the incident. If the source is not found, an affirmation of "there is nothing here to be afraid of" can end the incident. If the source is found to be harmful, taking action to correct the situation is the only path to follow.

Give Away Fear

1. Write a lengthy, scary letter to yourself about your fear. Make it as fearful as possible. Catastrophize. Put it away for a day.
2. Come back the next day and make the letter even worse than it was. Follow the fearful feelings as deeply as you can. Again put it away for a day.
3. Come back the third day with a red pen or pencil and identify the parts of your letter that have no rational basis.
4. After identifying which of your fears may be rational and which parts are not, release all the unrealistic, unfounded fear that you have put into the letter by burning it in a ceremonious manner.
5. Take action regarding the fear that is real.

Examine Beliefs Regarding Fear

What are your beliefs about what others can do to you? About your own strength and ability to maintain your security? What is the basis of such beliefs? Change the beliefs to positive statements, and begin to affirm that you are always safe and secure. Nothing can harm you.

SOURCES CITED

Bradshaw, J. (1992). *Homecoming*. New York: Bantam.
Bradshaw, J. (1999). *Men and women are from earth after all: Effective ways to deal with ten problems inherent in all relationships*. Audio cassette. Houston: Bradshaw Cassettes.
Chopra, D. (1998). *Ageless body, timeless mind: The quantum alternative to growing old*. New York: Three Rivers Press.
Damasio, A. R. (1994). *Descartes' error: Emotion, reason and the human brain*. New York: Putnam's Sons.
Damasio, A. R. (1999). *The feeling of what happens: Body and emotion in the making of consciousness*. New York: Harcourt Brace.
Dusek, D., and Girdano, D. (1995). *Emotional risk factors*. Winter Park, CO: Paradox.
Glasser, W. (1994). *Control theory manager*. New York: Harper and Row.
Glasser, W. (1999). *Choice theory: A new psychology of personal freedom*. San Francisco: HarperCollins.
Goleman, D. (1997). *Emotional intelligence*. New York: Bantam.
Goleman, D. (1998). *Working with emotional intelligence*. New York: Bantam.
Jackins, H. (1993). *Reclaiming the power*. Seattle: Rational Island Publishers.
Jackins, H. (1997). *Body-centered psychotherapy*. Mendocino, CA: LifeRhythms.

Kurtz, R. (1997). *Body-centered psychotherapy: The Haikomi method.* Mendocino, CA: LifeRhythms.

Lazarus, R. (1998). *Fifty years of the research and history of R. S. Lazarus.* Hillsdale, NJ: Lawrence Erlbaum.

MacLean, P. D. (1990). *The triune brain in evolution: Role in paleocerebral functions.* New York: Plenum Publishing.

Maslow, A. (1968). *Toward a psychology of being.* New York: Van Nostrand Reinhold.

Morse, D. R. (1995). *Love and hate: Their many guises and stressful effects.* Stress Medicine 11:177–97.

Patent, A. (1995). *You can have it all.* Piermont, NY: Money Mastery Publishing.

Patent, A. (1998). *Bridges to reality.* New York: Celebration Publishers.

Pearce, J. B. (1985). The magical child matures. New York: Bantam.

Pearce, J. B. (1994). Magical child, magical adult. New York: Sound Horizons.

Pert, C. (1995). *Neuropeptides, AIDS, and the science of mind-body healing.* Alternative Therapies, 1, no. 3, 70–76.

Pert, C. (1999). *Molecules of emotion: Why you feel the way you feel.* New York: Simon and Schuster.

Viscott, D. (1992). *Emotionally free.* Chicago: Contemporary Books.

Viscott, D. (1997). *Emotional resilience: Simple truths for dealing with the unfinished business of your past.* New York: Crown Publishing.

CHAPTER

5

The Human Spirit

A decade ago it may have been strange to see a chapter devoted to the human spirit in a book about stress and stress management. Within that time frame, though, acceptance of matters regarding the human spirit have become more commonplace, even highly sought by men and women of all ages and religions. Spirituality is one of the four basic areas of health (physical, emotional, mental, and spiritual), and it can be described in either secular or religious terms. The common thread to all religions is the desire to help people live a more spiritual life and to learn about spiritual leaders and their living examples of a spiritual life. The Buddha preceded Jesus by about 500 years, and both professed a philosophy not unlike the ancient Taoists or the Native Americans: Live simply with loving kindness and equality toward all. As the people of the world parted into various religions and their particular dogmas, separation of one sect from another became the norm, and we often still see religious rivalry, persecution, and death as a consequence. As we have seen throughout history, strict or fanatical adherence to religious dogma tends to separate, whereas our true spiritual nature is to connect, to join, and to love unconditionally without judgment.

Spirituality is our relationship with some higher power or source of energy and also our relationship with others and the environment. Spirituality develops over time, and that development goes through a number of stages, beginning with an egocentric and unprincipled life. This is characterized by young children and self-serving adults. The next stage is characterized by strong belief in religion and church-going. The individuals here are strongly tied to their religious dogma and are not tolerant of spiritual practices that differ from theirs. The next stage is the questioning stage, when the individual begins to examine set religious practices and keeps only those that seem right and truthful to him or her. The last stage is one of universal loving and acceptance, and it can occur within one's religion or outside of a set religion. People at this stage accept all others, regardless of their religion, race, age, economic class, sexual preference, status, or any other divisive classification. In this stage people see the spirit that connects all living things.

Deepak Chopra, in discussion with noted physicists, persists in asking whether there is not a universal intelligence that governs all of life. Either there is a plan or there is no plan. Even molecules in seeming chaos, when gently nudged, fall into order.

Living the Spiritual Life

Simple words of wisdom that contain the essence of the spiritual life come from the ancients. Their descriptions of the serene and happy life appear more as philosophical reminders of how one should live than as a specific dogma of what one must think and do in order to receive the rewards of a possible later life. Somehow we know that spirituality has something to do with truth, caring, trust, and loving kindness.

Consider the spiritual direction given by Lao Tsu on Taoism and by a Cheyenne medicine man regarding the medicine wheel:

The Tao.   Famous quotes from the *Tao Te Ching* by Lao Tsu include, "The Tao that can be told is not the eternal Tao," and "The nameless is the beginning of heaven and earth." Such is the difficulty of defining spirituality. The *Tao Te Ching* is thought to have been written in the sixth century B.C. and has been translated more than any work other than the Bible. It is the epitome of a spiritual treatise, a philosophy of how to live a life of health and happiness. The philosophy of Lao Tsu was simple: Accept what is in front of you without wanting the situation to be other than it is. Study the natural order of things, and work with it rather than against it because to try to change what is only sets up resistance. Nature provides for all without discrimination—therefore let us present the same face to everyone and treat all as equals, however they behave. If we watch carefully, we will see that work proceeds more quickly and easily if we stop trying, if we stop putting in so much extra effort, and if we stop looking for results. In the clarity of a still and open mind, truth will be reflected.

The Medicine Wheel.   The Native American philosophy of life, with its own colorful images and symbols, brings the nature of spirit closer to our times and place. Hyemeyohsts Storm, in his book *Seven Arrows*, offers insight into the spiritual life of the Plains Indians. The Medicine Wheel is a sacred symbol of the Plains Indians that shows how each person must make a conscious journey for spiritual fulfillment.

As the very Way of Life of the People, the Medicine Wheel gives an understanding of the universe. It is the Great Shield of Truth, the Heart, and the Mind. The Medicine Wheel Way begins with the touching of the brothers and sisters, then of touching the world around (all living things), and finally of teaching to Sing the Song of the World in order to become Whole (Storm 1972).

The Medicine Wheel is to be thought of as a mirror in which everything is reflected: nature, ideas, and other people. Figure 5.1 depicts a simple Medicine Wheel. Usually constructed of small stones, each stone of the Wheel represents one of the many things in the universe and differs from person to person, depending on who is constructing it. Stones might represent family members, animals, religions, philosophies, or even nations. All things within the Medicine Wheel are equal, as it is in the universe. In order to become whole, everyone must learn harmony with all the spirits

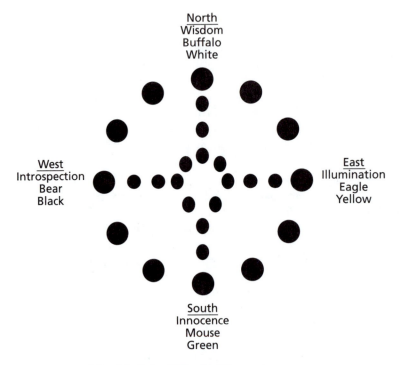

FIGURE 5.1   The Medicine Wheel of Seven Arrows

of the Universe. To do this, they must learn to seek to find their place or purpose. They must learn to Give-Away (give the gift of themselves as the buffalo or deer gave of itself so that people might eat).

The basic starting place for the journey is the direction of birth on the Medicine Wheel. Each of the four directions, or the Four Great Powers, has a symbolic color, animal totem, and philosophic meaning. As described by Storm, the top of the Medicine Wheel is North. Its color is white, the buffalo is its medicine animal, and its meaning is Wisdom. The South is represented by the color green, the mouse is its medicine animal, and it is the place of Innocence and Trust and for being close to what has heart and meaning. The West is the place of Looks-Within or introspection. Its color is black and the bear is its sign. The East is the Place of Illumination, where we see clear and far. Its color is yellow and the symbol of place is the Eagle. We are each born to a starting place that gives a way of seeing and experiencing the world. Our starting place will be the easiest way for us to relate all our lives, but in order to be whole, we must visit all four directions and learn how to live each. The Four Great Powers, when lived, give wisdom, heart or passion, illumination, and the ability to look within. Those powers integrated described their spirituality.

Stress in Seeking Spirit

This brings us then to the connection between stress management and spirituality. Perhaps the deepest roots of human stress—buried, invisible, and unconscious to many—are the four basic spiritual questions of humankind:

1. What is the basic energy that moves the universe?
2. What is life, where did it come from, and where is it going?
3. What is the human role on this earth, and where are we going as a species?
4. Who am I? What is my purpose, my function, and my destiny?

Spiritual philosophy (as in, "We are spirits that happen to be living inside human bodies") teaches us that the answers to these questions are inherent in every human being. Spirit and individual souls are indivisible partners in the power that moves the universe, and all material things are produced by that power. This knowledge is buried in the "mind" of everyone, and this knowledge is real and true for all time. It urges us toward fulfilling our spiritual goal. It is almost as though we just have to know the part of us that is forever unchanging. Aldous Huxley called it the "Perennial Philosophy," that there is something beyond the world of change, and philosophers from every age seek to know what that is.

The previous chapters regarding physiology, emotions, thoughts, and beliefs underscore the necessity that we concentrate most of our lives on survival of the psyche and the physical body, and so the spiritual questions often go unanswered. As egocentric beings, we spend most of our time on question 4: "Who am I?" and as a subset, "Why are all these other people making it so difficult for me?"

In birth as we move from soul energy to human energy, we are set apart from others, we are divided against one another by our selfishness and competition, yet we yearn for harmony and togetherness. We have a need to love and be loved, yet few among us obtain the harmonious loving state of unified separateness until we have paid our dues. Individualization, self-discovery, feelings, risk taking, and confiding are part of the process of relating to others who act as mirrors for us so that we can learn to do it better next time. Our emotional relationships become a win/loss column, a see-saw process that ebbs and flows between sublime comfort and intense stress.

After birth, the human infant is in servitude for months upon months, learning how to get its needs met. It learns that behaving in certain ways can be bartered for being fed, held, loved, and cared for. In order to survive in this world of other people, many of whom hold the reins of acceptance or denial, we learn to judge and compete. We orient ourselves, what we know, what we feel, and what we value by banking it off the outside world. From the earliest of times and the very depths of our knowing come comparison and judgment (also called reflection, relativity, or relationship).

To become human means to be separate from all other material things. Our goal is to use the other material things as teachers to remind us how to get back to a perfect soul state. It is trial-and-error learning, and it takes as long as it takes. Until the

process is a gift and a friend, anxiety and stress fill the mind. Mindfulness, or consciousness, becomes the path to peace.

In our search for love, we want to grasp, to hold, to cling, and to possess. We
know that we are part of something larger and want to belong. But does peace come
from the conditional type of loving that we see in most human relationships? More
likely such relationships are fraught with unmet expectations and unspoken barter and
become the breeding ground of stress.

Most of us think of relationship as in "significant other," family, and friends. Yet,
relationship occurs between us and all other aspects of our lives, such as money, time,
religion, and, yes, even ourselves. Some believe that love relationships are primarily
and simply to ensure the propagation of the species. In fact, we must seek relationships in order to learn to think and behave skillfully. Doing so brings the rewards we
require on a soul level.

Seriously searching for "who we really are" slowly turns our head toward the
more philosophical questions. When we begin to consider the meaning of life, the
power that moves the universe, and the collective human role, our human relationships come into perspective, and we become more skilled in our behavior.

Managing stressful behavior begins at a survival level. We do what we have to do
to save our skin! We become more skillful as we learn about human psychology and
apply it to ourselves and others. The continuum of skillful behavior continues as we
move toward worldly understandings and on to universal philosophical understandings.

We learn the fear of rejection, the anger of being thwarted, and the guilt of
unacceptable behavior, and we experience the anxiety of struggle between needs and
what we have to do to get our needs met. Until each person releases the tension
between what they are and what they think they should be, anxiety and the discomfort of stress will be their companions.

Stress will change their minds and mold their bodies. It will influence the length
and quality of life. It will determine the amount of peace they enjoy or struggle they
endure. Interactions with other people will be largely responsible for the amount of
stress they experience. Purposefully seeking the answers to life's basic questions and
constructing a conscious philosophy to live by will concomitantly enhance the quality
of human relationships.

Two Insights from Science

For those of a scientific bent, two scientific paradigms offer insight into the mystery,
definition, and interpretation of spirit and spirituality. The earlier of the two is that of
quantum physics. Einstein presented to the world an equation that allowed the inter-
changeability of mass and energy ($E = MC^2$). At the quantum level, where energy can
become mass and mass can become energy, all material things begin. The human body
is energy that has been materialized. The macro human body and all its cells are surrounded by and infused with energy that is not as visible as the material self. Each
level of manifestation is characterized by its own degree of consciousness, which is one

octave removed from the other. This is discussed at greater length later in the chapter under the topic of personality and individuality.

The second paradigm is that of psychoneuroimmunology or mind-body medicine. Although this laboratory research has identified the amino-acid structure of many ligands or neuropeptide messengers that influence cells all over the body via receptors on cell membranes, it brings up questions that pique the minds of spiritual philosophers. If all cells of the body are "in on" everything that happens (or has ever happened) to it, is the physical body, in fact, the mind? We know that the body remembers traumas and that those traumas can be released during bodywork of various kinds. Then the big question: What is the intelligence or wisdom that directs the physical body toward balance, health, or homeostasis? When Walter B. Cannon coined the term "homeostasis," was he talking merely about the physical feedback mechanisms that keep the body in balance, or was he philosopher, asking the question, "Do we have consciousness, or does consciousness have us?" Is there invisible life energy that originally programs the body toward health and happiness?

Personality and Individuality

To use quantum physics to describe our world, we would note that the molecular masses that vibrate the most slowly are those that we can see and touch, that is, that we can use our physical senses to explore. There is little doubt that there are human energy fields that we cannot so easily explore with the physical senses. Emotions and thoughts are energy fields, and although we may interpret them through overt behavior, their very essence is extrasensory. The most elusive of the human energy fields is the spirit.

Ouspensky, Gurdjieff, James, Jung, and countless other philosophers/psychologists since their time speak of two coexisting entities within humans: One is *personality*, consisting of the physical body, its emotional makeup, and its mental makeup (see Figure 5.2). The physical or material layer of our existence is the most basic. It includes not only simple mass but also the vegetative state wherein the mass searches for food, takes it in, and digests it. The physical body is often our focus because we can see it, touch it, and understand its physiology down to the microscopic functioning of RNA and DNA. For most people it is difficult, if not impossible, to comprehend the idea of the other "invisible" supportive energy layers around the physical body. The early Greek philosophers Socrates, Plato, and Aristotle (as with modern physicists) sought to define what was "real" by being able to physically measure it. Only through deductive reasoning could they examine spirit (Wolf, 1999).

The next layer of energy out from the physical is the emotional (sometimes called the "animal") layer that adds emotion, drives, antipathy, and desires to the physical. Next, the mental layer adds intellect and consciousness. In some teachings these three layers are simply called "man," characterized by his intellect. Others, including the great psychiatrist Carl Jung, called it the personality.

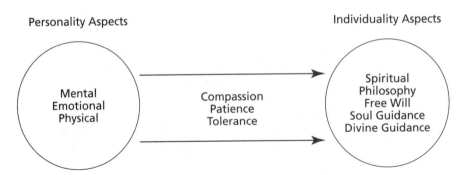

Personality Aspects   Individuality Aspects

Mental
Emotional
Physical

Compassion
Patience
Tolerance

Spiritual
Philosophy
Free Will
Soul Guidance
Divine Guidance

FIGURE 5.2   Personality and Individuality

The second of the two coexisting entities is *individuality*, which consists of free will, the soul, and divine energy (see Figure 5.2). Jung felt that the purpose of life was far greater than just learning how to cope with maladjustment in one's psychosexual makeup: There was also a challenge to cooperate with a profound impetus from deep within one's own being, an impetus toward wholeness. He proposed that there was a level of mind that contained "archetypal" or universal themes, a collective unconscious to which we all have access. One of those archetypes is the "Self," that part of humans that seeks to find its spiritual purpose and connection.

The behaviors that issue from the personality and the individuality are quite different. The response from personality is more of a childhood-learned behavior, whereas an individuality response stems from wisdom, compassion, and a higher consciousness. It is a higher order of being, of eternal dimension, richer in meaning and relationships. It is the awakening of the human will, connecting us with a higher order of behavior. Individuality is ever present and available to guide the personality. It is one's individuality that more closely defines the real self, who we really are. Its nature is to be innovative, creative. Free will is a spiritual birthright. It is a key to advancement because it demands that conscious decisions be made; conscious decisions about which thoughts to have, which feelings to nurture, and which behaviors to perform. It is not just knowing what your mission is but also how to live it. Will allows us to give attention to specific ideas beyond mere physical survival. We are constantly given the opportunity to shape experiences with the will.

Connecting the personality and one's individuality is a *compassionate/intuition* energy, which is also called the genius level, characterized by intuition. Compassion, or listening to our inner voice, puts us in touch with our higher spiritual nature, which is ever present and available to guide the personality layers. If the personality does not allow feelings and thoughts that nurture spiritual search, the process may be delayed for a lifetime. Living one's life at a higher level requires that one get past the knee-jerk reactions of the personality and learn more skillful responses to painful experiences. Compassion guides this process, especially compassion for oneself.

The human spirit is the very essence of being. It motivates us, guides us, and coaxes us toward consciousness. Stress-producing behaviors we engage in and observe in others are all the proof we need that we spend much of our time in the unconscious state. To become conscious (or mindful) is a choice we must make, and then we must practice it as a skill to eventually become a living art. In Chapter 1 we spoke of mindfulness or conscious choice as a means of gaining peace. Much of this book gives direction for solving stress issues in accepted cognitive-behavioral ways, yet the human spirit draws us to the ultimate stress management techniques—compassion, love, kindness, faith, honesty, and trust.

The Forces

Within us are several basic forces or voices. First is the voice of our social environment—family, friends, church, and other institutions. As we become enculturated or socialized by these people, we adopt their belief system or pay the consequences. We are taught what we must do in order to survive in this social environment. This is the "tribal power" Caroline Myss describes (1998) that is instilled early in life and seeks to control the group's behavior. The mind of the tribe changes slowly, over decades or even centuries.

A second voice, the individual voice that recognizes that all is not well, begins to speak within us when we accumulate the knowledge, experience, and self-esteem to question the tribe's power and decisions. Many times it is awakened by a stressful situation. This is the individual voice of the human spirit, and it begins to speak to us when we are no longer content to be controlled by money, acceptance, or other external rewards. The individual mind can change much more quickly than the tribal mind. Reading a book, taking a seminar, or talking with a mentor may change one's outlook. An epiphany may come overnight.

The third voice is a voice of divine guidance. We are so thoroughly trained to obey the laws of the people and then urged by inner desires to take command of own lives that it is difficult to switch to a release of the self to the divine. From the third voice we learn that we are not the ocean, we are a droplet of water in and of the ocean and that there are universal laws that bring happiness and peace.

Lama Surya Das (1999) calls these the outer, inner, and innate powers or voices.

Steps toward Enlightenment

How many experts does it take to change a light bulb? Many or few, depending on whether it wants to change. How do we get to conscious behavior? We do not just trip over it and then pick it up when we turn twenty-one or forty or some magical age. The motivation to become conscious comes first. Consider the man who could not dance:

> There once was a man who couldn't dance, yet he imagined he could. He invited a woman to go dancing with him, and although they enjoyed each other's company as they dined and chatted, the dance floor experience was a disaster. He stepped on her toes, bumped into other dancers, twirled her into walls, and the beat of the music completely evaded his feet. On the dance floor he realized he had made a terrible mistake: He had chosen a woman who could not dance! It took him dozens of women before he realized that it was he who could not dance. He went to a dance studio and learned all the steps and became quite a dancer and lived happily ever after.

How long does it take to recognize that what we are doing is not working? How long do we curse and blame others when things continue to turn out poorly? It takes the willingness to look at our life and admit that something is not working here. Perhaps it is a habitual anger response or jealousy or how we shrink back in fear. Whatever stresses a person gives them a clue that change is due. If the stressor can be perceived as a gift and a piece of information, it propels a person forward.

As physical beings, we all inevitably experience pain. How long we suffer from it depends on our perception. Much of suffering is caused by trying to avoid situations that we expect will be painful. Suffering is like an untreated disease that festers and gets worse, yet it is the suffering that finally gets our attention. The cataclysmic events in life act as lightning rods that draw insight to those who are willing to understand the message that comes with the event.

What causes suffering? A two-and-a-half-century-old response given by Eastern spiritual masters would be ignorance, craving, and hatred—the three poisons of the mind. Ignorance was defined as not having the perception of the true nature of the self or soul; craving (or greed) defined as an insatiable overwanting; and hatred encompassed fear, anger, jealousy, and envy. All of these poisons stem from attachment—attachment to material things, relationships, and mental states to which the person has become accustomed. Change becomes the enemy, yet change is so constant that if befriended, it becomes the expected rather than the rending surprise.

Ignorance may be the first hurdle—ignorance of the true nature of the self. The true nature of the human spirit cannot be explained in personality terms. The spirit does not necessarily follow the physical laws that humans have established trying to ensure "civilized" societies. The spirit follows divine law that truly makes all people equal, sharing universal intelligence and benevolence. Divine law puts us all in the same pool; no one soul is better or worse than another because the true self is a part of this divine pool. Each person has ideas and beliefs about this pool. Many call it God/Goddess, the Great Spirit, Allah, or universal benevolence or goodness.

The first step toward enlightenment is the step from outer control to self-control. At some time each person makes the decision to listen to an inner voice rather than to external voices. The tribe has a great deal of power, and the individual must go beyond that power. Each person must make his or her own decisions, even though these decisions may cause trouble. The "mistakes," however, are the individual's own mistakes, and they are lessons to be learned.

It is as though the individual knows we all have the birthright of happiness, yet the person keeps putting up roadblocks with fear, anger, greed, procrastinations, and prevarications. The individual does this because his or her personality (our conditioned physical, emotional, and mental aspects) has learned to protect and to ensure the survival of the psyche and physical body. Human spiritual nature pushes us toward refining our thoughts and actions to uncover the soul. It does this by helping us find ways to unlearn old, no-longer-useful personality behaviors that separate us from others and from our very own souls and to begin to become mindful of every choice we make.

This step may take the person out of his or her job, marriage, or family. Depression may occur. The fear of aloneness is often strong during this time, yet it is a time when learning to live happily with oneself is a high priority. It does not mean a life of celibacy or living alone in a cave; it is a time of getting to know and enjoy the self. Remember that this is the step from outer to inner guidance.

When self-concept is strong enough and the choice is made to continue toward finding spirit, the next step evolves. This is the step of losing the self and entering the symbolic, looking at things from a transcendent, universal, or spiritual view rather than a material view. Rather than depending upon the received, or heard, wisdom learned from others; or the intellectual wisdom that occurs after one has learned from others and then examines its rationality, benefit, and practicality for oneself; the individual finally depends upon personal experiences and has his or her own realization of truth. This is the step from inner voice to innate voice. It is governed by one's individuality, the spirit nature that has always been there even though it had been buried by material worries. This is where the true self resides. The last stage of this last step is living a life of appreciation or gratitude.

On a personal level, being off your spiritual course feels negative, and you may experience remorse for your actions, thoughts, or words. Remorse, like all negative feelings are signals that you have strayed off course. Joy, on the other hand, is a signal that you are keeping to the course you have charted. "Right action" is choosing the action that results in joy rather than in remorse, yet feeling remorse can motivate you to seek a different way to do it in the future. Remorse is often not apparent on a conscious level. However, it must be brought up to a conscious level in order to stimulate behavior change. When you are off your spiritual course, you create situations that become opportunities to bring remorse to your consciousness. Although remorse can be beneficial, lasting guilt is useless and paralyzing because it keeps one focused on the past. Even though glancing back may be useful, you cannot steer ahead while looking backward.

We all ultimately search for one thing: happiness. The key elements that contribute to happiness are health, wealth, and friendship, yet the master key is perception—how we think about what we have. True happiness is of the heart.

Exercises

Honor Code

What is your honor code with the universe? First, write in your journal or notebook the items that make up your personal honor code. Likely items would be truth, acceptance, loving kindness, and so on. List as many things that you can think of that govern your behavior.

Second, take each item and write about a recent scenario in your life in which you used that item. An example might be the item of "truth." You were asked why you did not like someone's response, and you told them the truth in a kind, assertive manner.

Third, after you have completed the first parts of the exercise, think about what you have written. Was it difficult to come up with examples that prove your honor code? Did it seem easier to come up with examples that disproved your honor code? Is your professed honor code different from the code you actually live by? Remember that you are as you act.

Lies I Have Told

In this exercise, keep a notebook handy for a full week to write down all the lies you tell during that time. Big lies, little lies, mean lies, and white lies. Leave some room between your lies. The second part of the exercise is to write an explanation of why you told the lie. Were you tired, scared, or ignorant? Also write down how you felt after you did the deed.

Then think again of your Honor Code (as in the first exercise). Was truth part of your code? What is happening in your life that keeps you from telling others the truth? Is there one particular aspect of your life where truthfulness is especially lacking? Is it easier to tell some people the truth than others? Who? Why?

The Four Major Questions

This exercise asks you to answer the questions outlined earlier in the chapter:

1. What is the basic energy that moves the universe?
2. What is life, where did it come from, and where is it going?
3. What is the human role on this earth? Where are we going as a species?
4. Who am I? What is my purpose, my function, and my destiny?

Write your answers and/or discuss them with someone else.

1. If you believe that a spiritual power esists, describe it. Is it an entity, an energy, nature, and so on? What are the characteristics of this power? Is it benevolent, all goodness? Describe the goodness. Is it a mixture of goodness and something else? Describe that. How does this energy affect you?
2. How did life originate? What is it? Was there a beginning? What came before the beginning? Is there such a thing as death? Life ever-lasting? Where do you go when you die? What do you think of reincarnation? Karma?
3. How did humans come to take on material life? Why do we have to come and take on the miseries of being human? Just what is it that we are supposed to do here as a human race?
4. What is your purpose in life? Do you know what it is? Is it merely a way to make a living, or is there a bigger reason why you are here? Did you choose your parents, or did they choose you? Do you choose your opportunities, friends, where you live, and other experiences in life, or do they choose you?
5. Did your philosophy of life change as you went through this introspection? How?

Mysteries and Miracles

Keep an ongoing journal of the mysteries and miracles in your life. Write about how your spiritual questions are answered, how unexpected good things happen to you, the "spooky" things that have happened to you and others you know well, when you feel out of spiritual alignment, and what you plan to do to realign yourself.

SOURCES CITED AND RECOMMENDED READINGS

Chodron, P. (1997). *When things fall apart: Heart advice for difficult times*. Boston: Shambhala Publications.

Cousineau, P. (1998). *The art of pilgrimage: The seeker's guide to making travel sacred*. Emoryville, CA: Conari Press.

Dalai Lama. (1999). *The art of happiness*. New York: Riverhead.

Dalai Lama Bstan-Dzin-Rgya-Mtsho. (1998). *The good heart: A Buddhist perspective on the teachings of Jesus*. Edited by R. Kiely. Boston: Wisdom Publications.

Epstein, M. (1998). *Going to pieces without falling apart*. New York: Broadway Books.

Jung, C. G. (1933). *Modern man in search of a soul*. New York: Harcourt Brace Jovanovich.

Keating, Father T., (1998). *Centering prayer in daily life and ministry*. Edited by G. Reininger. New York: Continuum Publishing Group.

Lama Surya Das. (1999). *Awakening to the sacred*. New York: Broadway Books.

Levine, S. (1998). *A year to live: How to live this year as if it were your last*. New York: Three Rivers Press.

Myss, C. (1998). *Why people don't heal and how they can*. New York: Three Rivers Press.

Pert, C. (1999). *Molecules of emotion*. New York: Simon and Schuster.

Speeth, K. (1976). *The Gurdjieff work*. New York: Harper and Row.

Storm, H. (1985). *Seven arrows*. New York: Ballantine

Welch, J. (1982) *Spiritual pilgrims*. New York: Paulist Press.

Wilber, K. (1998). *The eye of the spirit: An integral vision for a world gone slightly mad*. Boston: Shambhala Publications.

Wolf, F. A. (1999). *The spiritual universe*. Portsmouth, NH: Moment Point Press.

CHAPTER

6

Patterns of Behavior

"**A** man's fate is his character," said the famous philosopher Heraclitus. The study of character styles, that is, the study of personal behavior choices, offers some order and congruence to all the different kinds of stressful behavior in which the individual engages (Engler 1999).

One's response to stress is clearly affected by one's behavioral habits. The famous physician Sir William Osler once suggested that where malignant disease is concerned, it may be more important to understand what kind of patient has the disease rather than what kind of disease the patient has.

In this chapter we examine how selected features of personal behavior, habits, skills, and choices interact with stress. We examine self-perception and its role in health and disease initially. Next we consider one of the most often studied stress behaviors, the type A behavior pattern. We then examine anxiety as a response to stressors. Last, we examine the role of control in human stress. Each section is preceded by a self-assessment exercise; complete each one before reading about the topic relating to it, and learn about yourself as you learn about stress in general. Each section concludes with some effective stress management tools that have been reported in the literature.

Self-Perception

For many years psychologists have been pointing to self-concept, or the way we perceive ourselves, as perhaps the single most influential factor in behavior. It would follow that self-perception plays an important role in stress and stress management, also. Simply put, the stronger the self-concept, the more resources a person can bring to bear to avoid stressful situations and respond to stress arousal.

Your self-perception, or self-concept, is simply the image you hold of yourself. You form this image by evaluating your power and self-worth, based on input from your family, friends, and other people who hold significant places in your life. At a very early age (perhaps even before you begin to speak), you begin to accumulate information about yourself from these sources, and slowly but surely you form your self-concept. This formation may stop as early as the age of five or six or may continue until death.

SELF-ASSESSMENT EXERCISE 2

Choose the alternative that best summarizes how you generally behave, and place your answer in the space provided.

_____ **1.** When I face a difficult task, I try my best and usually succeed.
     a. almost always   c. seldom
     b. often   d. almost never

_____ **2.** I am at ease around members of the opposite sex.
     a. almost always   c. seldom
     b. often   d. almost never

_____ **3.** I feel that I have a lot going for me.
     a. almost always   c. seldom
     b. often   d. almost never

_____ **4.** I have a very high degree of confidence in my own abilities.
     a. almost always   c. seldom
     b. often   d. almost never

_____ **5.** I prefer to be in control of my own life as opposed to having someone else make decisions for me.
     a. almost always   c. seldom
     b. often   d. almost never

_____ **6.** I am comfortable and at ease around my superiors.
     a. almost always   c. seldom
     b. often   d. almost never

_____ **7.** I am often overly self-conscious or shy when among strangers.
     a. almost always   c. seldom
     b. often   d. almost never

_____ **8.** Whenever something goes wrong, I tend to blame myself.
     a. almost always   c. seldom
     b. often   d. almost never

_____ **9.** When I don't succeed, I tend to let it depress me more than it should.
     a. almost always   c. seldom
     b. often   d. almost never

_____ **10.** I often feel that I am beyond help.
     a. almost always   c. seldom
     b. often   d. almost never

_____   Total Score

Scoring: Items 1 to 6: (a) = 1 point, (b) = 2 points, (c) = 3 points, (d) = 4 points
            Items 7 to 10: (a) = 4 points, (b) = 3 points, (c) = 2 points, (d) = 1 point

            Place your total score in the space provided, and read the section "Self-Perception."

What is your image of yourself? Self-Assessment Exercise 2 was designed to provide some insight into your self-concept. If you scored from 10 to 19 points, you have a high self-concept. A score of 20 to 24 indicates an average self-concept. If you scored between 25 and 40, your self-concept appears to be in need of bolstering.

Components of Self-Concept

High self-concept is basic to all personal interactions. A healthy concept of self ensures confidence, worth, security, spontaneity, and other positive descriptors of the actualized person. Some use the terms *self-concept* and *self-esteem* interchangeably, but it would seem that total self-concept consists of many different components (including self-esteem), each necessary to complete the ideal self (Dusek and Girdano 1995). Six major components of self-concept, self-awareness, self-worth, self-love, self-esteem, self-confidence, and self-respect are discussed here.

Self-Awareness.   Being self-aware is realizing that you have an impact in this world and that your presence and actions can and do influence others and vice versa. This does not mean that you are responsible for the reactions of others; they may choose to feel enhanced or hurt by your presence, and this is their choice. Regardless of whether the smiles and intimacy, anger and criticism of others is intentional, every person has an impact on others.

What is the purpose of being self-aware? To see the interrelationship of all people and the part that you play in your own growth and development, and also in that of others.

Self-Worth.   Some parts of the self-concept are inborn, and self-worth is one of them. A basic tenet of the founders of the United States (and other democratic nations as well) was that all citizens are created equal: No one person is worth more or less than any other human on this earth, and all have the basic rights to life, liberty, and the pursuit of happiness. This is an instance in which the written laws of the land paralleled the spiritual doctrine of the founding fathers. It assumed that all people come into this world and travel through it with a worth that is equal to that of all others. Nothing can be added to make one person worth more than another. Conversely, no horrible deed can reduce the basic human worth of a person. The only thing that reduces worth is when the individual assumes from life experiences that he or she has less than the 100-percent worth inherited at birth. The gravest mistake one can make with self-worth is trying to earn it. No one can get more than 100 percent, and everyone already has that. It can be unearthed or realized by an individual, but it cannot be earned from someone else.

Self-Love.   Just as with self-worth, we all have an inborn capacity for self-love; it is not something one earns from others over a lifetime of struggle. Many believe that they have to earn self-love through sacrifice and punishment of self and through pleasing others. Those lacking in self-love must relearn compassion for themselves in all situations, through all emotions, and in all actions. This is done by letting go of judgments from outside: the self-judgments learned from parents, friends, teachers, and society.

Part of relearning self-love is learning self-forgiveness, which revolves around the basic belief that we all do the best we can with the skills we have at the time. This is not to say that we cannot learn more effective ways to behave; rather it means accepting that "this is who I am, and this is the way I behaved in that situation. I'm learning to do it differently, but no matter how I do it and how it turns out, I love myself."

Self-Esteem.   This is probably the most familiar component of self-concept, and many people use the two terms interchangeably. However, self-esteem is a compassion for self that is earned through one's actions (unlike self-worth and self-love, which are inherent). Because self-esteem is earned, it comes from success. Many earn self-esteem through their interpersonal relationships, academic accomplishments, sports, or successful job performance. Self-esteem that is rewarded internally is lasting, and it enhances the other self-concept components. However, self-esteem earned from the outside can be taken away at any time, which can be devastating. If an individual has earned esteem from the outside, the need for rewards and attention from others can become insatiable, and if that reward is removed or reversed (which happens from time to time within all relationships), feelings of powerlessness and anger from being powerless result. It follows that internal resources are truer and more helpful for enhancement of self-concept than are pats on the back from others.

Self-esteem is itself built on some basic components: honesty, especially with oneself; responsibility for one's perception of what is real; trust; listening to intuitions and acting on them; and positive intent toward others.

Self-Confidence.   Self-confidence is the earned or learned ability to cope with perceptions of the world (an individual's reality). Each person sets up his or her perception of the world and then handles those perceptions in a confident or not-so-confident manner. Success in this component comes from seeing planned outcomes develop into real outcomes by using past resources, trust, hope, and courage.

Self-Respect.   Self-respect is the ability to honor, or appreciate, one's emotional nature: to express fear, happiness, anger, love, and joy appropriately when they are felt. This does not mean "dumping" these emotions on someone else but expressing them when the need is felt. Holding back from expressing an emotion not only blocks its energy but also shows lack of self-respect. When a person respects who he or she is, expression of emotions is natural and appropriate.

Effects on Behavior

Researchers and clinicians have known for years that if, in a given situation, individuals devalue themselves and perceive themselves as helpless and certain of failure, this perception will virtually ensure failure in that situation. This concept has been referred to as the *self-fulfilling prophecy:* the likelihood of failure at some task will be greatly increased if you imagine yourself failing even before the task in question has begun. The converse of this relationship is true as well: If you imagine yourself succeeding at your task, your probability of success will be greatly enhanced. In his text *Self-Fulfilling Prophecies,* Russell Jones (1977) exhaustively reviews self-expectations (for example, the self-fulfilling prophecy) in terms of social, psychological, and even physiological outcomes. He concludes that interpersonal social success, psychological states such as depression and anxiety, and even physiological arousal (for example, stress) can all be dramatically affected by self-expectancies. In accordance with Jones, Seligman (1992) does not think that special intensive training will significantly raise a child's IQ or help the child talk three months early, but he is convinced that the social environment can produce a child who believes he or she is helpless and cannot succeed. When that happens, the child will perform stupidly, regardless of his or her IQ. However, if a child believes that he or she has control and mastery, that youngster may outperform more talented peers who lack such a belief.

Self-perception also has its effect on hostility. People with low self-esteem are more vulnerable to interpersonal insult than those with high self-esteem, and those with low self-esteem become angrier than those with high self-esteem when they are unsuccessful in getting an apology (Goleman 1998; Ingram 1998).

Effects on Disease

Not only are self-esteem and self-perception important both in the outcome of behavioral performance and in the severity of the stress experienced, but self-perception (especially the devalued, helpless, and hopeless image of self) may play a significant role in the eventual onset of disease.

The bulk of research done with patients concludes that there may indeed be such a thing as "proneness." This tendency is characterized by gross self-devaluation, helplessness, and feelings of hopelessness. In effect, this personal style sees itself in a totally passive and dependent role within its environment. These individuals tend to see themselves as stupid, clumsy, weak, and inept even though their achievements are often enviable (Siegel 1990, 1999). This is as good a description of low self-concept as one is likely to find.

In summary, it should be emphasized, first, that perceptions of helplessness and self-devaluation can lead to increased stress. Second, a poor self-concept may also play a significant role in the onset of various diseases. It may be that a poor self-concept generally increases one's susceptibility to many disease forms. Third, by improving your perception of control and self-worth, you may begin to reduce and eliminate stress. You may find that as an added benefit you begin to see your "luck" in all endeavors change as well. Finally, it is important to note that Self-Assessment Exercise 2 was not designed to give predictive insight into any particular illness; it merely gives you some feedback concerning your self-perception.

Enhancing Self-Concept

Everyone can work toward a more positive self-concept. Low self-concept is a result of negative beliefs about oneself, negative self-talk that fuels the old negative beliefs and the way life experiences are perceived. Until the negative spiral is broken, enhancement of self-concept is not possible. The following techniques present a number of levels of possible change.

List Your Resources

Write down all the resources that you have in your life. You are alive and have attained a certain number of years. What do you have going for you that has helped you get where you are now? In listing resources, remember to include physical and material resources such as income, clothing, housing, money; social support resources such as family, friends, teachers, and counselors; internal resources such as empathy, tenacity, sense of humor, honesty, being a good friend to others, and so on.

Once you have listed as many items in each category as possible, write each resource on a three-by-five card, placing a new card on the top of the deck each day. On reading the daily resource, repeat several times to yourself or out loud that you possess this quality or resource. Merely reading the words on the card is not enough to enjoy how you feel about yourself and thus enhance your self-concept—you must internalize the resource and accompany it with a positive feeling.

Enlist Subpersonalities

Having listed internal resources, name them and then use them to help you in stressful situations. This concept was developed in the psychosynthesis movement of the 1960s and 1970s (Vargiu 1977). For example, a list of internal resources might be the following:

caring for others	intelligence	sense of humor
tenacity	reliability	risk taking

Give each of the characteristics an alliterative name, such as Connie Caring, Tony Tenacity, Ina Intelligence, Roy Reliable, and so on. Each of these "people" is part of your personal behavior style and has been hard at work to help you throughout the years.

When a stressful situation comes up, internally scan your cast of characters and call upon one or more to help you through the situation. Talk to the subpersonality (or write a script between you and the character), and let that part of you donate its expertise to the solution of the situation. At first this technique may seem a little silly, yet given time and serious thought, your subpersonalities can become very helpful.

Affirmations

Affirmations are statements that you write and repeat affirming that you already have what you envision having. They are written in the first person, present tense. They are positive statements accompanied with positive feeling. Follow these steps:

1. Clearly get in mind what you want.
2. See yourself clearly in the situation where you have gained what you want (refer to Step 1). If you cannot see yourself having completely attained your goal, drop back to a point that you can see having accomplished. Work forward from there.
3. Experience the good feeling of having accomplished what you want.
4. Make a meaningful statement regarding the accomplishment of getting what you want.

"It's easy for me to . . ."
"I enjoy having . . ."
"I am becoming more and more . . ."

These statements should focus on the characteristic or quality you want ("I enjoy being self-confident"), not the ability to get there ("I can become self-confident"). They should be as specific as possible. An affirmation of "I am losing weight easily and quickly" is more specifically stated, "I am easily and quickly reaching my goal of 120 pounds." Putting words such as "easily" and "quickly" into action creates movement from the present situation to the affirmed situation. Words that trigger feelings (for example, *joyously*, *excitedly*, *lovingly*) are also helpful.

5. Write affirmations for all aspects of your life—social, emotional, spiritual, occupational, intellectual, and so on—so that you have a well-rounded life.
6. Say your affirmations at least once a day but optimally two, three, or more times throughout the day. On rising and before going to sleep are common times committed to affirmations. Other likely times are when waiting for appointments, while driving, or at scheduled times when at work, home, or school.

Compliments

1. Practice giving compliments to others, and make a study of how they accept them. Do they just say "Thank you," or do they add on a statement of humility? Make your compliments "real" by commenting on something that you really like. Begin with your friends, then expand to others in your work or study space, sales clerks, service people, and so on.
2. Begin to accept compliments by giving a smile and a "Thank you." Period. Make no follow-up statement unless it is a positive confirmation of the compliment, for example, "Thank you. I really like it, too."

Assertiveness

Verbal assertiveness is saying what you like or dislike about someone or something without using degradation; it is getting what you want but not at the expense of someone else's self-esteem. Assertiveness is "feel good" communication. Some people confuse assertiveness with aggression. Aggression is demanding in a bossy and demeaning way that someone obey your wishes. It is an act of verbal pushing and shoving with no consideration for the other person's self-esteem. When the other person does not comply or agree, the aggressor insists that he or she is "dumb," "stupid," or "crazy" for not agreeing. When people respond to a situation aggressively, they often receive counteraggression, alienation, and defensiveness from the other person. Communication is virtually blocked, and all who are involved come away from the situation feeling anxious, angry, and misunderstood.

At the opposite end of the scale from aggression is nonassertive or passive behavior (see Figure 6.1). Many have learned in childhood to be passive placaters who do not have the skill to ask for what they want. Their mode of operation is to manip-

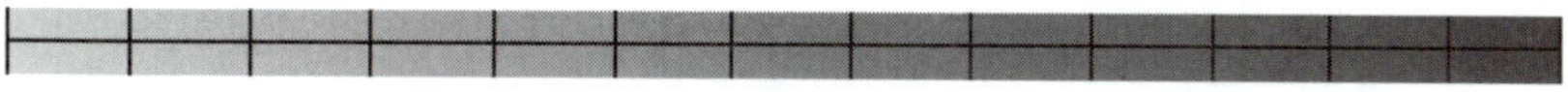

Passive	Assertive	Aggressive
This person is	*This person is*	*This person is*
• Shy	• Usually more extroverted	• Somewhat hostile
• Withdrawing	• Aware of rights and privileges and uses them constructively	• A vehement defender of own rights yet often violates or usurps the rights of others
• Reluctant to assert rights and privileges	• Socially productive	• Unmindful of where own rights end and the violation of others' begins
• Socially inhibited		• Socially destructive

FIGURE 6.1   Assertiveness Scale

ulate. They sit back wishing that someone would notice their needs and fulfill them, or they set up subtle and roundabout ways of getting what they want. Manipulators use guilt to get others to do what they want. They control others with *shoulds, oughts,* and *ifs.* Nonassertiveness is highly related to low self-concept. In becoming more assertive, it is important to know that you have certain inalienable assertive rights (Alberti and Emmons 1995), which include the rights to do the following:

- say no without feeling guilty
- change your mind
- take your time in planning your answer or action
- ask for instructions or directions
- demand respect
- do less than you possibly can
- ask for what you want
- experience and express your feelings
- feel good about yourself, no matter what

Assertiveness training in mainstream American culture involves operationalizing these rights.

The Assertiveness Ladder

The Assertiveness Ladder (Figure 6.2) is a hierarchy of assertiveness exercises that you might attempt in your daily contacts with other people. The exercises are listed in order from least to most difficult. Start slowly at the bottom and progress up through the list. You might spend a week or two practicing each one before moving up to the next. If you begin to experience anxiety, drop back to the previous exercise for another week, and then try to move up again through the list.

"Assertiveness"

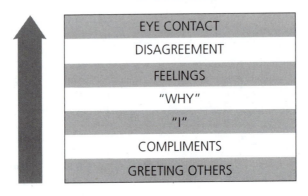

EYE CONTACT
DISAGREEMENT
FEELINGS
"WHY"
"I"
COMPLIMENTS
GREETING OTHERS

"Unassertiveness"

FIGURE 6.2   **Assertiveness Ladder**

Exercise 1: Greeting Others. Many unassertive people are too shy to greet others or initiate conversations. This exercise consists of initiating at least two exchanges or conversations per day with individuals whom you would not consider close friends. It may be difficult or seem "plastic" at first, but continue trying. You may meet some very interesting people.

Exercise 2: Complimentary Statements. This exercise involves giving others compliments. This is a social behavior that may lead to greater social horizons. Many unassertive people neglect to give compliments by rationalizing "Oh, that's dumb" or "Why would they care what I think?" Giving compliments is polite, and people probably do care what you think, so give it a try.

Exercise 3: The Use of "I" Statements. Many unassertive people are hesitant or afraid to use the word "I." The reason is that the use of "I" shows ownership, and disagreement with an "I" statement by someone else is often seen by the unassertive person as a personal rejection. This is not usually the case, however. Do not be afraid to take a position. Let your preferences be known; if you do not, they will never be realized.

Exercise 4: "Why?" This exercise involves asking "why?" Many unassertive people feel that to ask why represents a challenge—it does not. "Why?" simply asks for additional information. In this exercise, you should ask "why" at least two times a day from people you consider to be "above" you in status, position, or respect—your boss or a teacher, for example. If you think the word "why" may be too threatening to that person, substitute "What makes you think that?" or "How is that so?" or finally, "Could you help me to understand that better?"

Exercise 5: Spontaneous Expression of Feelings. Unassertive people often repress feelings. This exercise consists of having you spontaneously react on a feeling level to someone else's statement or behavior. Repressed feelings are hazardous to your health and well-being; therefore, express them a little at a time. Try to express your emotional reaction at least two times a day. You will find it gets easier the more you practice. Remember, sometimes it is better to take the risk of hurting someone else's feelings than to keep your feelings bottled up. If that person is your friend, he or she will understand.

Exercise 6: Disagreement. This exercise involves disagreeing with someone when you feel that person is wrong. Many people take such disagreement personally, but that is a problem they must work out for themselves. If the other person is secure, he or she will know that disagreement can be a healthy and positive force for new ideas. Give it a try, but be sure not to be arbitrary—if you disagree with someone, make sure you really believe in what you are saying.

Exercise 7: Eye Contact. Maintaining eye contact is often one of the most difficult things for the unassertive person to do. You may find it awkward at first, but continue trying. The best way to attempt maintaining eye contact is to start with short intervals two to three seconds in length. Eventually extend it to four to five seconds, then nine to ten seconds. It is important that you not stare at people; this is too often interpreted as a challenge. Therefore, use this time interval technique. When you break eye contact, it is important not to look down; maintain your basic eye level. Do not look down!

When you can successfully climb up this Assertiveness Ladder, you will be well on your way to becoming an assertive individual and will have done much to improve your self-concept. Remember that not all assertive behaviors will result in rewards; other people may simply be defensive or aggressive. But do not allow their problems to hinder you. Feel good about yourself and your new assertive personality.

Interpersonal Effectiveness Training

One of the most useful tools you can find for enhancing self-perception may be referred to as Interpersonal Effectiveness Training. Psychologists have used techniques for decades to help their patients improve their self-esteem and overcome dysfunctional passivity and the depression that may result.

Interpersonal Effectiveness Training is best understood within the context of helping people become more interpersonally effective and avoid the problems of passivity and of aggressive behavior (look again at Figure 6.1). As such, Interpersonal Effectiveness Training may also be thought of as a form of assertiveness training but far broader in scope. It should be used in any interpersonal situation in which you feel yourself pulled toward passive or aggressive behavior. It is critical to understand that the goal of such an exercise is not merely to "get your way." Rather, the primary goal is to avoid passivity or aggression toward others, both of which lead ultimately to interpersonal dysfunction. However, by avoiding passivity and aggression, you will find that your chances of obtaining what you seek will be enhanced and you will feel better about your own interpersonal effectiveness.

Any interpersonal situation in which you feel yourself pulled toward interpersonal passivity or interpersonal aggression is an appropriate situation in which to use interpersonal effectiveness training techniques (refer again to Figure 6.1).

Recognition

1. Experience the presence of an emotional cue, for example, guilt, anger, loss of self-esteem, or even confusion.

Analysis

2. Analyze the situation:
   a. Has the other person done anything to violate your interpersonal rights? Try to see the situation from that person's eyes. If your rights have not been violated, do not continue this exercise. Similarly, do not continue if you decide it is really not worth discussion or if you feel it to be unwise from the "interpersonal politics" perspective. Otherwise, if your interpersonal rights have been violated and you feel the issue is worthy of discussion, then continue.

Action

3. Describe to the other person what they have done or what has happened that has violated your rights. Simply describe the facts.
4. Continue by telling the other person how the incident has made you feel, for example: "I felt . . . cheated, betrayed, stupid, foolish, angry, worthless, sad," and so forth.
5. Now inform the other person what you would like to see done to correct the situation, that is, to change it so that your rights are no longer violated. Use the principle of "minimal corrective action." This involves requesting that the situation be corrected but without making anyone else feel or look bad (for example, without punishing anyone). Be careful not to become aggressive here.
6. A final, optional step that you may employ if your wishes are not met and you feel your rights have still been violated is escalation. Escalation simply means that you inform, not threaten, the other individual of more action-oriented steps you will pursue if satisfactory action is not taken: For example, you may call someone of higher authority, and so on.

Remember, practice makes perfect, so start slowly at first. Also remember that no matter how interpersonally persuasive you may be, you cannot make anyone do anything that he or she does not really want to do. So, if after Step 6 you still have not gotten satisfaction, be proud of yourself; you have done all you could without resorting to passivity or aggression.

Common situations in which this exercise may be useful are the following:

1. Disputes with clerks while shopping
2. Disputes with repair persons
3. Times when friends or family have hurt your feelings or violated your rights in some way (it is okay to ask for an apology for Step 5)
4. Encounters with "pushy" salespeople, and so forth

Avoid Negative Self-Talk

Negative self-talk perpetuates negative feelings about the self and also continues to affirm negative self-beliefs. This exercise consists of the following steps:

1. Monitor yourself for one day, and write down all the words and phrases you say to yourself that are negative. You might also enlist the help of others around you—have them identify statements they hear you say about yourself.
2. For each negative phrase you have identified over the period of a day, write a positive follow-up. For example, a negative phrase might be: "You big dummy." Follow it with, ". . . and I like you anyway."
3. After this exercise, each time you hear yourself saying something negative about yourself, add something positive.

After mastering Step 3, each time you begin to say something negative about yourself, substitute a positive statement. Do not even bother to say the negative statement.

Examine Negative Beliefs

Negative beliefs are the basis for negative feelings and behaviors. What are the core self-concept beliefs on which you operate your life? Some possibilities that may stem from early childhood are as follows:

- I am an unlovable person.
- I do things so poorly that nobody could like me.
- No matter how hard I try, things always turn out badly.
- Nobody likes me, so why should I try?
- I am unworthy of the love and attention of others.

When you treat yourself in an unloving way or behave in a way that depreciates yourself, ask "What must a person believe in order to behave in such a self-depreciating way?" Then turn the belief around to a positive statement that you repeat whenever you notice you are being unkind to yourself.

The beliefs that are the basis of your relationship with yourself are also the foundation for your beliefs about other people. This can be used to your advantage by changing your attitudes toward others and becoming more accepting, compassionate, and loving. As you release judgment of others, you may release judgment of yourself. A simple affirmation about others such as "Everyone does the best they can with what they have at any given time" allows you to let others be where they are without having to judge their actions. Such a statement does not mean that the person cannot grow and learn other ways of doing things; it merely says that they are doing the best they can. That affirmation can be extended to the self in stressful times: "I am doing the best I can with what I have right now."

"Go Fever"

We have known for years that specific patterns of behavior can adversely affect health. In other words the choice of a particular health behavior can be the determining factor in the development of a disease. The prime example is the well-known list of cardiovascular risk factors, which include smoking, lack of exercise, obesity, and high-fat diets. It has been clearly demonstrated that the consistent practice of one or more of these behaviors will increase susceptibility to heart disease.

It is possible that far more general behavioral tendencies can affect your health. Could it be that the way in which you generally interact with your environment may predispose you to stress and stress-related disease? The answer is a definite yes! Evidence strongly suggests that the manner in which you choose to interact with your surroundings can play a major role in determining whether you develop heart disease (Brown and Harris 1999, Eysenck 1995, Friedman 1996).

Two cardiologists, Meyer Friedman and Ray Rosenman, in the normal course of treating their patients, noticed some recurring behaviors among them, especially in relation to how they dealt with time. They noticed the extreme anxiousness of their patients in the waiting room and the constant focus of their conversations on time, work, and achievement. From their contact with coronary patients, Friedman and Rosenman in the late 1950s formulated a construct of action-emotion behavior patterns that seemed to embody the coronary-prone individual (1974). They referred to this construct as the *Type A personality* and included in it the following characteristics:

1. An intense sense of time urgency; a tendency to race against the clock; the need to do more and obtain more in the shortest possible time.
2. An aggressive personality that at times evolves into hostility; high motivation, yet very easy loss of temper; a high sense of competitiveness, often with the desire to make a contest out of everything; the inability to "play for fun."
3. An intense achievement motive, yet without properly defined goals.
4. Polyphasic behavior—that is, the involvement in several different tasks at the same time.

During a series of impressive research studies known as the Western Collaborative Studies, the Type A behavior pattern was shown to precede the development of coronary heart disease in 72 to 85 percent of the 3411 men tested. These results strongly suggest that Type A action-emotion behavior patterns may be predictive of the eventual onset of heart disease.

Since the pioneering studies of Friedman and Rosenman, a wealth of research data on the Type A behavior pattern has emerged. Physiologically oriented research has found Type A people to be more reactive in their sympathetic-nervous-system response when challenged or confronted by their environment than individuals who possess none of the type A characteristics (Cooper 1995, Siegman and Dembroski 1989, Williams and Williams 1994). This sympathetic overresponsiveness has been suggested as the key pathogenic process leading to increased cardiovascular risk. By-products of chronic sympathetic activation include elevated serum-cholesterol levels, decreased vascular flexibility, increased blood pressure, and increased cardiac output—all of which, when chronic, can contribute to cardiovascular disease.

Research by numerous authors aimed at refining the Type A pattern and defining its specific pathogenic components has led us to believe that the anger/hostility component may be the most toxic, pathogenic constituent in the entire Type A constellation (Williams and Williams 1994). Burg's (1995) review of anger, hostility, and heart disease develops a cogent argument for the disease-causing potential of anger and hostility. In a fascinating longitudinal study of midlife women, Adams (1994) found that hostility was correlated negatively with general health. Thus, this study extends the hostility research beyond heart disease.

Another interpretation of the results of this research is that individuals who are chronically and globally cynical may be Type A's who are at highest risk for heart disease. There is also some evidence that the time-urgent characteristic may be pathogenic as well, but the hostility trait seems to be the most pathogenic because of its high association with secretion of testosterone. Testosterone release is associated with atherosclerosis.

Thus, we have come far since the initial discovery in the late 1950s of the Type A pattern. Instead of Friedman and Rosenman's four-component construct, we now believe anger, hostility, and perhaps time-urgency are the major pathogenic factors of the pattern. Also, whereas we once believed that Type A was pathogenic for men only, we now believe it can be pathogenic for women as well. Finally, we can see that the Type A pattern includes not only adults but adolescents and preschoolers as well (Siegman and Dembroski 1989).

What makes the Type A person behave in such a manner? Studies on both male and female twins suggest that there may be some genetic involvement, but other research (Brown and Harris 1999) points us more toward sociocultural origins. Parental expectations and high standards with frequent urging and criticism of actions, as well as an intensely competitive atmosphere, may all be involved.

Cultural influences in general must be considered important contributors, especially our culture's work ethic, which motivates individuals toward hard work and achievement and rewards them for it. As a society we seem to have developed a chronic case of "Go Fever." However, one can be a hard worker without being hard driving and competitive. So it is not only the underlying values of the culture that are important but also how that culture's members perceive the methods for achieving what they value.

This idea points to an interesting phenomenon about the Type A behavior pattern: Those who exhibit it feel comfortable with it, value it, and reinforce it. They describe themselves as challenged and eager to meet the competition. They are happy with their work and wish they had more time to do more work. Type A individuals are confident and do not fear losing the struggle with life and work tasks. They are aggressive, ambitious, and competitive, are not fearful or anxious, and do not as a rule suffer neurotic states. On the contrary, they usually strive to control their environment and exert power over other people. Generally, they view their behavior as positive, and they receive rewards through their behavior. Thus, not only does society condition the behavior pattern, but it reinforces it as well. The Type A behavior pattern can exist only in an environment that stimulates it and allows it to function. Our fast-moving, competitive society does not lack challenges for those who would seek them out.

Self-Assessment Exercise 3 is a broad-ranged attempt at sampling the Type A behavior pattern. We emphasized the dimensions of anger/hostility (items 3, 4, 6, and 7) and time urgency (items 1, 2, 5, 8, 9, and 10). A total score in excess of 24 may indicate presence of the Type A pattern (although this assessment does not measure cardiovascular risk). You may wish to take a more careful look at the anger/hostility items, for characteristics similar to these may be at the core of the Type A pattern.

SELF-ASSESSMENT EXERCISE 3

Place your answer to the following questions in the space provided before each number.

_____ 1. I have no patience with tardiness.
        a. almost always   c. seldom
        b. often   d. almost never

_____ 2. I hate to wait in lines.
        a. almost always   c. seldom
        b. often   d. almost never

_____ 3. People tell me that I tend to get irritated too easily.
        a. almost always   c. seldom
        b. often   d. almost never

_____ 4. Whenever possible, I try to make my activities competitive.
        a. almost always   c. seldom
        b. often   d. almost never

_____ 5. I feel guilty for taking time off from work that needs to be done.
        a. almost always   c. seldom
        b. often   d. almost never

_____ 6. People tell me I'm a poor loser.
        a. almost always   c. seldom
        b. often   d. almost never

_____ 7. I tend to lose my temper or get irritable when I'm under a lot of pressure.
        a. almost always   c. seldom
        b. often   d. almost never

_____ 8. I tend to race against the clock.
        a. almost always   c. seldom
        b. often   d. almost never

_____ 9. I hate to wait for or depend on others in order to do what I want to do.
        a. almost always   c. seldom
        b. often   d. almost never

_____10. I catch myself rushing when there is no real need to do so.
        a. almost always   c. seldom
        b. often   d. almost never

_____   Total Score

Scoring: (a) = 4 points
           (b) = 3 points
           (c) = 2 points
           (d) = 1 point

Place your total score in the space provided and read the section "Go Fever."

Evidence points to the Type A behavior pattern as being a learned behavior. As such, it can be unlearned or at least modified. Friedman and Rosenman emphasized that Type A individuals want to avoid heart disease, not change their lifestyle. When realizing that a lifestyle change is indicated, the Type A who is trying to modify that behavior may quit in frustration. If you are a Type A person, that fact will be the hardest for you to face, but once you realize it, change can successfully occur. Changing Type A behavior does not mean giving up the desire to achieve or excel. It does mean using behaviors that are more healthfully appropriate.

Exercises

The following techniques are directed toward the four basic characteristics of the Type A personality: time urgency, anger-hostility, lack of planning, and polyphasic behavior. All of these contribute to stress and ultimately to stress-related disorders.

Practice Concentration

Polyphasic thinking and behavior goes on because you allow it to go on. Time may be better spent by concentrating completely on one task, finishing it, and then going on to the next.

1. Read material that makes you concentrate—something with difficult concepts rather than simple ones.
2. When working on one plan and another pops into your mind, say "Stop it," and go back to the original plan.
3. Practice meditation, detailed visualization, progressive muscle relaxation, or other relaxation-training techniques in which you must focus on one thing at a time.
4. If a good idea about something else pops up in the middle of another project, and you can't "stop it," jot it down, and immediately go back to the original project.

   Learn anger management as described in Chapter 4.

   Reduce negative self-talk

   Reduce negative self-talk using the technique presented in the previous category on self-concept within this chapter.

Planning

Rushing into tasks without having adequately planned them results in stress that is highly preventable. The remedy is the Goal Path Model given here:

Step 1. Define the task:
      Reasons for doing the task:
Step 2. Can the task be broken down into subtasks?
      NO   YES
      List each subtask and complete the rest of this form for each subtask.

Step 3. Evaluation or proofs of success (how will you know when you have succeeded with the task?). List proofs:

Step 4. What personnel or help will be needed? List:
What are possible resources for personnel?
Estimate costs and obstacles for getting personnel:

Step 5. What materials will be needed? List:
What are possible resources for materials?
Estimate costs and obstacles for getting materials:

Step 6. Estimate time required for each task in Step 2:

Step 7. Hypothesize all possible obstacles or blocks to success:

Step 8. For each obstacle, go back and develop at least one contingency plan:

Step 9. Evaluate your contingency plan:

Step 10. Begin.

Examine Attachment Involvement

Attachment means that the outcome of a behavior or a task will have a significant effect on the individual. You know you are too attached to the outcome when you ask yourself, "What will others think of me if I fail, if I don't do what they want, if the project I'm completing isn't on time?" Extreme attachment involvement is often based on rewards from the system or from one specific person rather than from completing the job for the internal reward of a job well done. The "system," schools and jobs, usually reward Type A behavior, and the Type A individual lives on those rewards. As long as the external rewards are the motivators for action, those who give out the rewards have control over the person seeking the rewards. Changing Type A behavior calls for gradual change to an internal reward system—that is, defining success according to individual outcomes, not outcomes set by outside institutions, family, or friends.

A basic technique here is to ask yourself, "Am I following a path with heart?" If so, the path will be more exciting than stressful. And if it is not a path with heart, try detaching, step back, and view stressful situations with objectivity:

- Am I the only one who can do this?
- Can I be the sole cause of failure at this task?
- Am I verifying others' reactions to me?
- Am I competing rather than cooperating?
- If I were an objective outsider, how would I view this situation?

The Reality Check presented in the category on control later in this chapter and the Goal Path Model discussed on the two previous pages may be helpful in reducing extreme attachment.

Anxiety

Anxiety is a basic component of stress. As we discuss it here, anxiety is not only a symptom or manifestation of stress but also a cause of further stress. Based on the observations of people who suffer from chronic anxiety and seem to complain of stress-related disorders, we have identified another behavior pattern that appears to create excessive, chronic stress. If you are one of these people, you suffer from anxiety far more than most people because your reaction to a stressor results in a form of anxiety that seems to perpetuate itself. Therefore, the characteristic that makes you different from other people lies in the feedback mechanisms involved in the anxiety reaction. Most people experience anxious moments that quickly end when the stressor is removed. The anxious-reactive individual experiences stress that seems to persist, or increase, even after the stressor is gone.

Anxiety may be thought of as fear, and in effect the two words may be used synonymously. The anxiety-reaction process begins when an individual perceives a stimulus (person, place, or thing) as challenging or threatening. This perception occurs in the higher (neocortical) regions of the brain and entails interpretation, or assignment of meaning to the stimulus, which makes the individual insecure or perhaps apprehensive. These feelings of insecurity are transformed into physiological arousal of the endocrines and sympathetic nervous system. So now not only are the thought processes aroused, but the bodily processes are also. Fortunately, this hyperaroused condition usually subsides shortly after the stimulus has been removed.

Most of us suffer from this form of arousal. It is quite common in this society to be occasionally faced with things that make us insecure and result in generalized anxiety. Ordinarily, the anxiety reaction represents no major threat to mental or physical health. Yet, the more severe form mentioned earlier does seem to represent a significant challenge to health and well-being by increasing the stress response.

This self-perpetuating anxiety reaction, which persists or increases even after the original stimulus has been removed, means that the anxious individual suffers from a feedback "loop" that continues the anxiety reaction. The basis of this anxiety feedback loop is as follows: Any arousal response to some perceived stressor can eventually assume the role of a stressor itself and, in turn, cause further arousal.

The feedback messages that further increase arousal can take three forms: cognitive, visceral (smooth muscle), and musculoskeletal (striated muscle). The first and perhaps most volatile feedback during stress reaches the body in the form of thoughts (cognitions) concerning the nature of the stressor and the possible outcomes. Fear-laden thoughts that follow the stressor are capable of inducing visceral arousal by way of the autonomic nervous system, and further thoughts may increase the musculoskeletal reaction of a stress response. These cognitions are perhaps the most harmful of the three feedback forms. Many individuals engage in what may be called "catastrophizing"; that is, they always perceive the stressor event as far worse than it really is. The catastrophizer often views all psychosocial stress in terms of life-or-death urgency. This tendency to consistently overreact may result in severe mental and physical incapacitation and trauma during a stress reaction and may increase the likelihood of psychosomatic disease. Items 1, 2, 5, and 7 in Self-Assessment Exercise 4 concern catastrophizing tendencies. How did you score on them?

Other sufferers from cognitive feedback are those who relive any and all crises over and over in their mind for days or weeks after an incident. These "relivers" suffer from distress every time they relive the incident. Do you tend to relive stressful events? Items 3, 4, 8, and 10 in Self-Assessment Exercise 4 deal with that aspect. The

SELF-ASSESSMENT EXERCISE 4

Choose the response that best summarizes how you usually react during anxious moments, and place the letter of that response in the space provided.
When I'm anxious I . . .

_____ **1.** tend to imagine all of the worst possible things happening to me as a result of whatever "crisis" made me anxious to begin with.
        a. almost always   c. seldom
        b. often   d. almost never

_____ **2.** do everything I can to resolve the problem immediately; if I don't, I'll go crazy worrying about it later.
        a. almost always   c. seldom
        b. often   d. almost never

_____ **3.** will relive the crisis over and over again in my mind even though it may be over and resolved.
        a. almost always   c. seldom
        b. often   d. almost never

_____ **4.** will be able to clearly picture the crisis in my mind hours or even days after it's over.
        a. almost always   c. seldom
        b. often   d. almost never

_____ **5.** get the feeling that I'm losing control.
        a. almost always   c. seldom
        b. often   d. almost never

_____ **6.** feel my stomach sinking, my mouth getting dry, or my heart pounding.
        a. almost always   c. seldom
        b. often   d. almost never

_____ **7.** tend to make "mountains out of molehills."
        a. almost always   c. seldom
        b. often   d. almost never

_____ **8.** have trouble falling asleep at night.
        a. almost always   c. seldom
        b. often   d. almost never

_____ **9.** have difficulty in speaking or notice my hands and fingers trembling.
        a. almost always   c. seldom
        b. often   d. almost never

_____**10.** notice my thoughts "racing."
        a. almost always   c. seldom
        b. often   d. almost never

_____   Total Score

Scoring: (a) = 4 points
          (b) = 3 points
          (c) = 2 points
          (d) = 1 point

Total your score, and read the section "The Anxious-Reactive Personality."

"catastrophizer" and the "reliver" are forms of the anxiety characterized by prolonged feedback about the stressful event. This mechanism is depicted in Figure 6.3.

The second form of feedback involved in anxious behavior and the stress reaction is visceral, or smooth-muscle, activity. This involves the heart, stomach, gastrointestinal tract, and so on. The awareness of smooth-muscle activity, such as heart pounding or stomach gurgling, can increase stressful thought processes. In this way, visceral awareness can perpetuate further visceral activity. How responsive are your visceral mechanisms? Item 6 in Self-Assessment Exercise 4 concerns this issue.

Finally, anxiety feedback can occur in the musculoskeletal system. This involves overt movement of the striated muscles—those muscles attached to tendons and bones. In our own observations and research with public-speaking students, we have found that the awareness of trembling hands, awkward speech, or muscle tension can increase visceral activity in the form of heart rate. Increased musculoskeletal activity has been found to lead to further increases in the same system. Item 9 in Self-Assessment Exercise 4 deals with how reactive this system is during stress. Figure 6.4 is a diagram of the anxiety feedback loop at work in the visceral and musculoskeletal reactions.

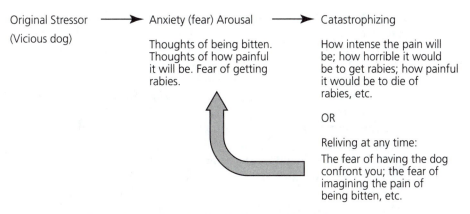

FIGURE 6.3   Cognitive Activity in the Anxiety Feedback Loop

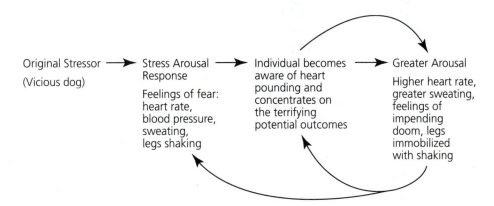

FIGURE 6.4   Visceral and Musculoskeletal Activity in the Anxiety Feedback Loop

In summary, the anxious individual is hypersensitive to stress reactions, which may occur on cognitive, visceral, and/or musculoskeletal levels. Once these reactions have been perceived by the individual, they form an automatic feedback loop that perpetuates and in some cases worsens the severity of the stress reaction. Perhaps the most severe form of this anxiety feedback is found in the catastrophizing individual, who consistently perceives problems (stressors) in the worst possible context. For these people stress is a constant companion, affecting their daily behavior; catastrophizers are vulnerable to incapacitation from the slightest stressor and also to stress-related disease.

A total score of 25 to 40 in Self-Assessment Exercise 4 would indicate a high degree of anxiety reactivity. A score of 20 to 24 is average, and a score below 20 indicates low reactivity.

Exercises

Thought Stopping

Thought stopping is a technique whereby an individual intentionally breaks the anxious cycle by abruptly leaving the obsessional thoughts. This can be done by two different methods. The more traditional technique of thought stopping involves shouting "STOP!" as soon as you become aware of the anxious reliving or catastrophizing. At first the word may be shouted to yourself. If this is not forceful enough, shouting it aloud will successfully destroy the anxious cycle. You may then attend to other less-stressful thoughts.

Another form of thought stopping is to switch abruptly to a pleasing, relaxing image or scene in your "mind's eye" as soon as you become aware of the anxious cycle. The scene should be the same one each time and should be a place, real or imagined, that you find aesthetically pleasing and relaxing. After dwelling on this place for thirty to sixty seconds, slowly reoccupy your mind with real-world demands. If no such relaxing image exists for you, counting backward from five to one will also work. Simply picture the numbers in your mind as large and bright images. By the time one is reached, the cycle will be broken, and you can begin thinking of other thoughts. If the cycle starts again, break it in the same manner. Continue doing so until the cycle remains broken, no matter how many thought-stopping maneuvers are necessary.

Other techniques were discussed in the fear emotion section of chapter 4.

Stress and the Need for Control

Noted psychologist Albert Bandura (1997) states that it is mainly perceived inefficacy in coping with potentially aversive events that makes them fearsome. To the extent that one can prevent, terminate, or reduce the severity of aversive events, we have little reason to fear them. In other words, we could argue that the most powerful stressor of all is real or imagined loss of control. Indeed, what may contribute to all of the

SELF-ASSESSMENT EXERCISE 5

Answer each question, and place the letter of your response in the space to the left.

_____ 1. How often do you find yourself feeling helpless or hopeless?
   a. almost never   c. often
   b. seldom   d. almost always

_____ 2. How often do you find yourself in a situation that seems out of control?
   a. almost never   c. often
   b. seldom   d. almost always

_____ 3. How often do you find yourself needing to have your life well planned and organized?
   a. almost never   c. often
   b. seldom   d. almost always

_____ 4. How often do you find yourself feeling sad or depressed?
   a. almost never   c. often
   b. seldom   d. almost always

_____ 5. How often do you find yourself fearful of losing control over your life?
   a. almost never   c. often
   b. seldom   d. almost always

_____ 6. How often do you find yourself feeling insecure?
   a. almost never   c. often
   b. seldom   d. almost always

_____ 7. How often do you find yourself needing to control the people around you?
   a. almost never   c. often
   b. seldom   d. almost always

_____ 8. How often do you find yourself needing to control your environment?
   a. almost never   c. often
   b. seldom   d. almost always

_____ 9. How often do you feel the need to have your daily activities highly structured?
   a. almost never   c. often
   b. seldom   d. almost always

_____ 10. How often do you feel secure?
   a. almost never   c. often
   b. seldom   d. almost always

_____   Total Score

Scoring: Items 1 to 9: (a) = 1 point; (b) = 2 points
         (c) = 3 points; (d) = 4 points
         Item 10: (a) = 4 points, (b) = 3 points
         (c) = 2 points, (d) = 1 point

psychosocial and personality stressors examined in this chapter is a real or imagined loss of control over one's life. Consider these stressors:

- Lifestyle/environment change
- Frustration
- Overload
- Underload
- Low self-esteem
- Type A behavior (anger/hostility/cynicism, time-urgency)
- Anxious reactivity

Contributing to each is clearly a real or imagined loss of control.

Richard Lazarus (1998) theorized many years ago that the more we perceive ourselves in control of a situation, the less severe the stress reaction will be. This conclusion certainly suggests that feelings of hopelessness and helplessness may be the fundamental cause of excessive stress. This point was clearly demonstrated during World War II. Psychiatrists observed that soldiers who could return enemy fire suffered fewer mental disorders than those who could not return fire but simply had to take shelter and hope that they would not be harmed. Similarly, it has been shown that just the expectation of control over stressors can reduce stress (Fischer 1995, Steptoe and Appels 1992).

Some researchers feel that the core of the Type A behavior pattern may be the need for control (Friedman 1996). Type A individuals' manifestation of competitiveness, time-urgency, hostility, and low tolerance for frustration may all be seen as conscious expressions of a need to control themselves and their environment. In an attempt to test this hypothesis, Dembroski, MacDougall, and Musante (1984) found that the need to control significantly correlated with the Type A pattern. Furthermore, they found evidence that autonomic-nervous-system arousal may create a psychological discomfort that could increase the need to exert control. On the positive side, such researchers as Lazarus (1998), Kobasa (1979), Bandura (1997), Cooper (1995), and Nuernberger (1997) all offer considerable evidence that a real or imagined sense of control over self or environment is a powerful stress-reducing mechanism. Classic studies of thirty years ago demonstrated that even animals (rats) that were given control over electric shock contingencies developed fewer ulcers than rats that had no control over the shocks.

It is clear that perceptions of personal control, that is, the perception that one can significantly alter events, figures prominently in most theories of how people respond to adversity, illness, and stress (Bremer 1995, Fitzgerald et al. 1993, Steptoe and Appels 1992). A most fascinating demonstration of the influence of perceived control over physiology comes from David Barlow's laboratory. The research team administered 5.5 percent carbon dioxide (CO_2) to two groups of ten panic patients. One group was falsely informed that they could control the CO_2 levels, while the second group was not given that expectation. The group that falsely believed they had control over the CO_2 had significantly fewer symptoms of anxiety and panic. This study (Barlow 1988) once again demonstrates the power of the feeling of control, even if it is an illusion. Atchley (1999) stresses the importance of resilience, setting goals,

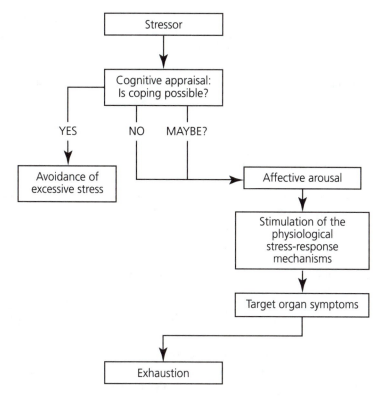

FIGURE 6.5   Control and Stress

self-confidence, and control in healthy adjustment to the aging process. Figure 6.5 depicts the self-efficacy and stress-control process.

Now go back and examine your responses to Self-Assessment Exercise 5. Total scores in excess of 24 may indicate vulnerability to excessive stress due to feelings of impotency, for example, a sense of lack of control. Items 3, 5, 7, 8, and 9 indicate a need to control; items 1, 2, 4, 6, and 10 indicate feelings of loss of control.

Exercises

Keep a Journal

Whenever you experience the frustration of not being able to control all the things and people around you or you feel that parts of your life are out of control, write your experiences in a journal. Just expressing your feelings about the situation will help alleviate stress.

Journaling can be an effective way of working out stressful problems. Just writing down thoughts and feelings rather than keeping them unsaid is helpful in releasing emotions (Desalvo 1999). Journaling can be as simple as "keeping a diary" of daily stressors or as involved as writing down answers to a group of formal, leading questions. Ira Progoff (1992) has offered guidance in journaling for many years through books and workshops. Through the use of his techniques, we can look into the unconscious mind and unlock some of the motivations that create many of our stressful situations.

Calm Yourself

When your body is experiencing a state of stress arousal, you are likely to interpret the symptoms as a sign that you are losing control. One way you might begin to exert more control over your environment is to first regain control over your body. Several excellent breathing exercises are presented in Chapter 12.

Reality Check

With the Reality Check, when life seems out of control, take the following steps:

1. Measure in numbers the difficulty of the situation. Get specific if you cannot assess the difficulties in numbers, and give them quantitative ratings on a scale of one to ten. This causes the mind to think rationally instead of in terms of feelings.
2. Rate your ability to do the job. Have you ever done this job or one like it before? How did you do? What resources do you have that have helped in the past? What new resources have you developed since that time that would help in this situation?
3. Examine the consequences. What is the worst thing that could happen? What is the real likelihood (probability) of that actually happening? Rate this on a scale of one to ten.
4. Release the irrational; develop an action plan for the rational.

Let Go of Judgments

If you can internalize that you are the only one responsible for your life, you must extend that to others around you. One person cannot make others do what they do not wish to do. Moreover, one individual does not have the right to manipulate the lives of others. The simple technique here is to say to yourself whenever you begin to judge others: "They are doing the best they can for themselves at this time."

Cognitive Restructuring

Cognitive restructuring refers to changing the meaning or your interpretation of the environmental stressors around you. Therapists such as Albert Ellis (1994, 1998, 1999) and Aaron Beck (1999), and Beck and Beck (1995) argue strongly that the environment is not what causes most people stress, but rather it is their interpretations that actually cause the stress response to be triggered. According to Beck (1999):

ENVIRONMENTAL   COGNITIVE MEANING   EMOTIONS
STIMULUS $\longrightarrow$ (INTERPRETATION) $\longrightarrow$ AND STRESS

The source, then, of dysfunctional emotions and excessive stress is in reality-irrational or maladaptive thoughts (ideation). Cognitive restructuring entails first identifying and then correcting these maladaptive thoughts.

Some of the most common maladaptive, incorrect, or irrational interpretations of environmental events are listed here (based on the work of Ellis and Beck) along with their cognitive solutions/reinterpretations:

Problem: The tendency to jump to a specific conclusion without adequate confirmation (overgeneralization).

Solution: Search for more evidence that the conclusion is correct. If so, and a problem exists, implement social engineering or problem-solving techniques.

Problem: The tendency to blame oneself for problems when little or no evidence exists for such a conclusion.

Solution: Search for other possible explanations to explain the problem.

Problem: The tendency to see things as "all or none," "good or bad," that is, the tendency to see only extremes.

Solution: Begin to search for the "gray" areas, the in-between states. See that few things are all good or all bad.

Problem: The tendency to catastrophize about unpleasant events and to "make mountains out of molehills."

Solution: Assess the realistic chances of the catastrophe actually occurring. If chances are high, then begin social engineering or problem-solving strategies. If chances are low, ask yourself, "Couldn't I be using this energy in a better way other than wasting it in worry?"

Problem: The tendency to be limited in problem-solving alternatives, that is, an inability to see potential solutions.

Solution: Practice exercises in creative, nontraditional problem solving.

These are but a few of the major maladaptive cognitive patterns that often lead to excessive stress. Beck and Beck's book Cognitive Therapy: Basics and Beyond (1999) is an excellent guide to such problems, as is Ellis and MacLaren's Rational Emotive Behavior Therapy (1998).

In sum, by controlling your body's response to stressors through breathing exercises and by controlling your attitudes through exercises such as cognitive restructuring, you will gain far more control over stress, over health, over life. You will find that at the same time you will become far less vulnerable to a dysfunctional need for control.

Examine Beliefs

Often the less we trust ourselves, the more we try to control others. As in the other discussions regarding beliefs in this chapter, people with a need to control the people and events around them must look at the irrational or negative belief system that is driving them. Some possible beliefs are

- Everything will fall apart if I do not maintain control.
- The only way people will need me is if I am in control.
- No one who is not as bright or talented as I am has the right to be in control.
- If I don't control others, they will try to control me.
- Power is control.

Turn negative or irrational beliefs into positive ones; continue to affirm these positive beliefs by using them as the basis for noncontrolling behavior.

SOURCES CITED

Adams, S. H. (1994). *Role of hostility in women's health during mid-life.* Health Psychology, 13, 448–95.

Alberti, R., and Emmons, M. (1995). *Your perfect right.* New York: Impact.

Atchley, R. C. (1999). *Continuity and adaptation in aging.* Baltimore: Johns Hopkins University Press.

Bandura, A. (1997). *Self-efficacy in changing societies.* Cambridge: Cambridge University Press.

Bandura, A. (1997). *Self-efficacy: The exercise of control.* New York: W. H. Freeman.

Barlow, D. H. (1988). *Anxiety and its disorders.* New York: Guilford.

Beck, A. T. (1999). *Cognitive therapy of personality disorders.* New York: Guilford Press.

Beck, J., and Beck, A.T. (1995). *Cognitive therapy: Basics and beyond.* New York: Guilford Press.

Bremer, B. A. (1995). *Absence of control over health and the psychological adjustment to end-stage renal disease.* Annals of Behavioral Medicine, 17, 227–33.

Brown, G., and Harris, T., eds. (1999). *Life events and illness.* New York: Guilford Press.

Burg, M. M. (1995). *Anger, hostility and coronary heart disease: A review.* Mind/Body Medicine, 1, 159–72.

Cooper, C. ed. (1995). *Handbook of stress, medicine, and health.* Boca Raton, FL: CRC Press.

Dembroski, T., MacDougall, J., and Musante, L. (1984). *Desirability of control versus locus of control.* Health Psychology, 3, 12–26.

Desalvo, L. (1999). *Writing as a way of healing.* San Francisco: HarperSanFrancisco.

Dusek, D., and Girdano, D. (1995). *Emotional risk factors.* Winter Park, CO: Paradox.

Ellis, A. (1994). Anger: *How to live with it and without it.* New York: Citadel.

Ellis, A. (1998). How to control your anxiety before it controls you. New York: Citadel.

Ellis, A. (1999). *How to make yourself happy and remarkably less disturbable.* New York: Citadel.

Ellis, A., and MacLaren, C. (1998). *Rational emotive behavior therapy.* New York: Springer.

Engler, B. (1999). *Personality theories.* New York: Houghton Mifflin College.

Eysenck, H. (1995) Personality and cancer. In *Handbook of stress, medicine, and health,* ed. C. Cary. Boca Raton, FL: CRC Press.

Fisher, R. (1995). Getting ready to negotiate. New York: Penquin.

Fitzgerald, T. E., Tennen, H., Affleck, G., and Pransky, G. (1993). *The relative importance of dispositional optimism and control appraisals in quality of life after coronary artery bypass surgery.* Journal of Behavioral Medicine, 16, 25–43.

Friedman, M. (1996). *Type A behavior: Its diagnosis and treatment.* New York: Plenum.

Friedman, M., and Rosenman, R. (1974). *Type A behavior and your heart.* New York: Knopf.

Goleman, D. (1998). *Working with emotional intelligence.* New York: Bantam.

Ingram, L. (1998). *Managing and coping with anger.* London: Royal House.

Jones, R. (1977). *Self-fulfilling prophecies.* Hillsdale, NJ: Erlbaum.

Kobasa, S. C. (1979). *Stressful life events, personality, and health.* Journal of Personality and Social Psychology, 37, 1–11.

Lazarus, R. S. (1998). *Fifty Years of the research and history of R. S. Lazarus.* Hillsdale, NJ: Lawrence Erlbaum.

Nuernberger, P. (1997). *The quest for personal power.* New York: Perigee.

Progoff, I. (1992). *At a journal workshop: Writing to access the power of the unconscious and evoke creative potential.* New York: J. P. Tarcher.

Seligman, M. (1992). *Helplessness.* San Francisco: W. H. Freeman.

Siegel, B. S. (1990). *Love, medicine and miracles.* New York: Harper and Row.

Siegel, B. S. (1999). *Prescriptions for living.* New York: Harperperennial.

Siegman, A.W., and Dembroski, T. M., eds. (1989). *In search of coronary-prone behavior.* Hillsdale, NJ: Lawrence Erlbaum.

Steptoe, A., and Apples, A. O. eds (1992) Stress, personal control and health. New York: John Wiley and Sons.

Vargiu, J. (1977). *Subpersonalities.* Synthesis, 1, 51–90.

Williams, R., and Williams, V. (1994). *Anger kills.* New York: Harperperennial Library.

CHAPTER

7

Demands and Expectations

Stressors originate in the complex interaction between socialization and perception. That is, they are sociological events we may perceive as undesirable on the basis of our experiences or other learning processes. People and our relationship to them, along with our perception of the relationships, construct a fascinating mosaic that greatly affects our stress, health, and happiness. This chapter examines the stressful impact of the expectations that society in general, and people in particular, have on all of us.

Five life processes appear to have strong connections with stress; they are as follows: (1) change and our relationship to our ever-changing life, (2) overload, or expectations accelerating out of control as we attempt to keep up with the fast-moving people and events in our lives, (3) frustration, or our inability to gain satisfaction from the people, events, and institutions in our lives, (4) boredom and loneliness, the failure of our relationships, and (5) the relationship interdynamic itself. We will examine these potential sources of distress and look at examples of how each touches our daily lives. Before you read each section, be sure to complete the self-assessment exercise that precedes it. These exercises help clarify the material that follows. Each section is followed by several effective stress management tools for you to try if you are vulnerable to any of these stressors.

Change

We are simultaneously experiencing a youth revolution, a racial revolution, a sexual revolution, a colonial revolution, an economic revolution, and the most rapid and deep-going technological revolution in history. This description of the massive process of change was true in 1970 and is even more in evidence today. "Era of change" could be the single most descriptive phrase for the twentieth century. It appears that the 21st century can see only continued change, and at an even faster rate!

Most of us have been reared with the belief that change is good and desirable, as it usually denotes an easier and more productive life. However, in his book, *Future Shock*, Alvin Toffler suggested that even though change is a necessary element in societal behavior, if it is too intense or too massive, the participants may cease reaping its rewards and begin realizing how devastating it can be. Although Toffler spoke somewhat as a philosopher and social critic, the scientific literature strongly supports his contentions.

Adaptive stress occurs when life situations demand that change occur. In the Western world, change is seen as "the end" of a period of stability or security of some kind and is therefore related to fear. Even when change is desired, movement from the old situation in which comfort and security have been established is somewhat stressful. The Eastern concept of change is that it is the only constant and is to be expected, not feared. In our society, in which change occurs quickly, there is little emphasis on the transition between the old and the new. Cultural anthropologist Angeles Arrien (1994) reminds us to look at a culture's literature to find what is most and least important to that culture. She then points out that in the United States, very little literature on transformation and transition exists. There are few major rites of passage and few ceremonies that honor the change process. The new is prized and the old is discarded. In this culture there is an expectation that we should make changes quickly and get on to the next item.

Birth and death are excellent examples of the "instant change" mentality. After a woman gives birth, she is expected to get right back into her predelivery routine. Likewise, upon the death of a loved one, the bereaved may show their grief perhaps through the time of the funeral rites but are then expected to get back to the usual lifestyle.

Your health, and even your very survival, are based largely on your body's ability to maintain a healthy balance of mental and physical processes. This equilibrium is called *homeostasis*. It has been suggested that excessive change is harmful to health because it tends to destroy homeostasis and thereby force the body to restore homeostasis through adaptation.

Homeostasis: equilibrium in the internal functions of the body.
Adaptation: the body's tendency to fight to restore homeostasis in the face of forces that upset this natural bodily balance.

In the early 1960s, Thomas H. Holmes and Richard H. Rahe attempted to discover whether change had major effects on human health. Generic change—that is, change having either positive or negative consequences—was the focus of their research. Based on earlier work by Adolph Meyer with "life charts" (paper-and-pencil tools for creating a medical biography), Holmes and Rahe compiled a list of positive and negative life events that seemed to contribute to the stress reaction. From these efforts emerged the Social Readjustment Rating Scale (SRRS), first published by Holmes and Rahe in 1968. This scale originally listed forty-three life events, and each carried a weighting indicating the amount of stress to be attributed to it. The weightings were determined by the sample populations they tested, and the weighting units were called life change units (LCUs). The most highly weighted life event was the death of a spouse (100 LCUs), and the lowest-weighted event was a minor violation of the law (11 LCUs). Interestingly enough, outstanding personal achievement was weighted with 28 LCU, only one point less than trouble with in-laws! This points to one of the more important aspects of this study of life events: It concentrated on generic change, a force that causes stress through the destruction of homeostasis.

SELF-ASSESSMENT EXERCISE 6

The following are events that occur in the life of a college student. Check each event that has happened to you during the last twelve months.

Life Event	Point Value
_____ Death of a close family member	100
_____ Jail term	80
_____ Final year or first year of college	63
_____ Pregnancy (to you or caused by you)	60
_____ Severe personal illness or injury	53
_____ Marriage	50
_____ Any interpersonal problems	45
_____ Financial difficulties	40
_____ Death of a close friend	40
_____ Arguments with your roommate (more than every other day)	40
_____ Major disagreements with your family	40
_____ Major change in personal habits	30
_____ Change in living environment	30
_____ Beginning or ending a job	30
_____ Problems with your boss or professor	25
_____ Outstanding personal achievement	25
_____ Failure in a course	25
_____ Final exams	20
_____ Increased or decreased dating	20
_____ Change in working conditions	20
_____ Change in your academic major	20
_____ Change in your sleeping habits	18
_____ Several-day vacation	15
_____ Change in eating habits	15
_____ Family reunion	15
_____ Change in recreational activities	15
_____ Minor illness or injury	15
_____ Minor violations of the law	11

Score: _____

Add up the point values for all the items you checked. Then read the section "Change" to interpret your score.

Remember, change, or the disruption of homeostasis, produces stress and adaptation, whether the event is desirable or undesirable. Negative or distressful events are usually the most harmful, for they are more disruptive for a longer period. They have a secondary effect in that they stimulate fear, self-doubt, catastrophic imaginings, and other negative thoughts that linger in the mind. However, positive events can likewise be stressful in that they also initiate change that necessitates adaptation. Usually, though, positive change does not produce the secondary effect of the negative event and thus is given fewer points in the weighting of life events.

One question that always arises in weighting life events is "Doesn't a specific event exert differing amounts of stress on different individuals?" Technically, the answer is yes because everyone's perception of the events in their lives differs. How you perceive an event in your life is tempered by your past experiences. For example, knowing what to expect is a great help in overcoming stress. Someone who has not lived through an event will anticipate the event as being more stressful than someone who has already experienced it. Novelty is always stress arousing, but that new situation becomes tempered through subsequent experiences. Nevertheless, some events are stressful no matter how many times you experience them, and as such they are only minimally less stressful through experience.

Consider moving, for example. The first move is the most difficult, and you become more efficient with experience, but each move still requires much adaptation. If you own a house, the process of finding a realtor, negotiating prices, being displaced during showings, trying to live in a perpetually clean house for weeks or months, finding a new residence, securing new loans, and countless other details is a source of constant stress. Packing, accumulating records, taking care of making the move itself, and finding a new physician and dentist and new stores, schools, and friends are additional stressors. Thus, even if the move is to a better job in a nicer place, and even if moves have been made before, moving still causes much change and much adaptation. Moving is therefore considered a stressful event.

With this concept of generic change as a stressor in mind, Rahe and Holmes amassed data from their Social Readjustment Rating Scale. The SRRS is administered by asking respondents to indicate how many of the items they have experienced over the past twelve months. A total LCU score is then obtained by adding up the LCUs for all of the items that have been checked. This scale has proved to be a remarkable predictor of physical and mental illness for a two-year period after the accumulation of the stressors. This scale has also been modified and designed for various populations, such as college students, and Lazarus (1998) also designed a "hassle scale" that was made up of smaller daily-life stressors such as concerns about body weight or not getting enough sleep.

An important concept here is susceptibility. A high score does not mean that the individual will definitely become ill. It means that the individual is more susceptible to illness than those with lower scores. There are many intervening variables, the most important of which might be the stress intervention techniques the individual currently practices.

If you have not yet done so, go back and add up your score on Self-Assessment Exercise 6. If your total score for the year was under 150 points, your level of stress, based on life change, is low. If your total was between 150 and 300, your stress level is moderate; you should minimize other changes in your life at this time. If your total was more than 300, your life-change level of stress is high; you should minimize any other changes in your life, and work more vigorously at instituting some of the stress intervention techniques presented later in this book.

Now that you have determined your life-change score, let us see how life change may lead to illness. Remember that change, whether favorable or unfavorable, requires adaptation. Change disturbs the equilibrium, inducing a temporary destruction of homeostasis. Such disequilibrium is met by the body with attempts to restore homeostasis. Selye (1976) points out that adaptation stresses the body by requiring a concerted effort on its part to restore balance. This effort to restore homeostasis requires adaptive energy, and, unfortunately, adaptive energy will eventually diminish if the disequilibrium becomes highly intense or chronic. When a person's adaptive energy is drained, dysfunction can occur on a localized, or specific, level. When the body is totally depleted of adaptive energy, general bodily exhaustion may result in death.

That excessively intense disequilibrium (change) can result in death is supported by the studies of George Engel (1977), who found that over 250 cases of sudden death usually occurred within minutes or hours of a major event in the person's life. Of added interest is the fact that most of these people were in good or fair health before they died. Engel looked for patterns to the sudden-death phenomenon, and his investigations supported Holmes and Rahe's contention that favorable as well as unfavorable change can be stressful. Although the leading category of sudden deaths was those deaths preceded by some "traumatic disruption of a close human relationship," another major category consisted of people who died suddenly during moments of great triumph or personal satisfaction. Engel noted the example of a fifty-five-year-old man who died during a joyous reunion with his eighty-eight-year-old father after a twenty-year separation. The father then died as well. Paul Rosch, M.D., states that stress is clearly a major culprit in sudden death, the leading cause of mortality in the world (1998).

Richard Lazarus (1998) proposes that stress usually depends less on life events than on the cognitive processes involved in the individual's perception of those events. He notes that although life events can indeed predict illness, some individuals with high life-change scores simply do not get ill. Conversely, many individuals have low life-change scores but do get ill. These noteworthy observations led Richard Rahe to suggest that future research focus on moderating variables such as factors that allow people to tolerate high levels of change without suffering illness. Rahe (1979, 3) states:

> [T]he qualities of life change events are qualities of the individual rather than aspects of the environment. It should be clear to investigators that when they gather sentiments of upsettingness, desirability . . . and what have you, they are measuring a variety of subjective responses to the environment which confound objective estimates of life change.

What are some of the factors that seem to moderate the process whereby life events lead to illness?

Control

Albert Bandura argues that it is mainly perceived inefficacy in coping with potentially aversive events that makes them fearsome. To the extent that one can prevent, stop, or diminish the severity of stressful events, there is little reason to fear them (1997). In other words, situations in which we perceive ourselves as being helpless or trapped or feeling out of control will be far more stressful than situations over which we believe we have some control.

Challenge

Suzanne Kobasa (1979) identifies the personality factor of "change as perceived challenge," meaning that one tends to believe that change is a normal process of living and can be an incentive for personal growth.

Commitment

Kobasa (1979) and Maddi (1996) also identify the personality factor of commitment, or the tendency to involve oneself in life experiences, rather than to be alienated or threatened by them or to passively observe them. Kobasa and her colleagues have called these three moderating factors *hardiness*. Hardiness seems to be a powerful force that protects us from the potentially harmful effects of high life-change. For years Kobasa's work was the major investigation into the concept of hardiness, or stress resistance. More recent investigations have extended the concept. Based on the Stress Resistance Project at Boston College, Ray Flannery Jr. has added to our insight regarding how people withstand the adverse effects of stress. Studying over 1200 men and women, Flannery (1993) was able to move beyond Kobasa's original findings. He describes stress-resistant individuals as having these eight specific characteristics:

1. take personal control in their lives
2. are task involved and focused
3. consume few dietary stimulants
4. exercise aerobically
5. practice relaxation exercises
6. seek social support systems
7. have a sense of humor
8. claim religious values

Another analysis of this notion of stress resistance comes from Ken Pelletier (1994). Pelletier conducted a five-year investigation of fifty-one prominent individuals who showed an unusual ability to cope with stress and to grow in spite of it. A key finding was the discovery of an altruistic theme that was consistent among those interviewed. But the altruism discovered was not an inherently self-sacrificing altruism as we typically think of it. Rather it was an altruism that seemed to make these altruists healthier by engaging in the process of giving to others. Pelletier referred to it as "enlightened selfishness." An altruism through which one reaches for the deeper meaning of being human may be the most powerful stress buffer of all.

When changes must occur, three main elements are involved: (1) the present situation, (2) a picture of what the changed situation will be like, and (3) the transitional

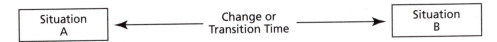

FIGURE 7.1   Components of Change

time between those two situations. What we call change is the transition time that it takes to get from situation A to situation B, as Figure 7.1 shows.

Adaptive stress may occur at various points in Figure 7.1. It may occur at point A, when an individual is asked or expected to change, and that person does not aspire to change. It may also occur at A, when an individual is tired of or bored in the present situation but doesn't know what else to do. It may occur when an individual no longer wants the old situation, aspires to a new situation, but doesn't know how to go about getting there. Then, once a new, attainable situation is desired and the individual steps into the transition area, there may be the stress of learning new skills, meeting new people, and so on. Even when the new situation is reached, adaptive stress may occur if the individual feels uncomfortable with the change. Regardless of the point at which one feels adaptive stress, there are techniques that can help resolve or eliminate the problem. The following exercises have been found to be helpful in adaptive-stress situations.

In summary, change can be a positive force for growth or a negative force that may lead to mental and/or physical deterioration. The key lies not so much in whether the change is positive or negative, a major life event or a minor hassle, but rather in how intense and chronic its impact is; and the impact of life changes will be as intense and chronic as you perceive and allow them to be.

Exercises

Establish Routines

If you are happy in your present situation but don't like surprises in your schedule, establish predictable patterns in your life. Write them down. For each routine, give ten minutes or more for transition time from one set of activities to another.

1. Establish daily routines at home, work, and school.
2. Establish a regular eating and physical-activity program.
3. Establish set sleep patterns.
4. Establish rest and relaxation times and places. You might establish certain hours of the week as a mental-health getaway. Make sure they are times when you engage in truly relaxing behavior. A vacation during which you travel is usually not free from adaptive stress, so do not count vacations as mental health days unless they are truly relaxing to you.

Avoid Change

If your Life Change Points in Self-Assessment Exercise 6 totaled over 300 and if you are in a position to choose whether or not change is going to occur in your life, avoid change at this time. Some individuals who are going through a great deal of life change choose to stop smoking or go on a diet while their anxiety levels are high. It is usually better to wait until life settles down to engage in new ventures.

Plan for Change

Adopting the belief that change is one of the constants in life can get one ready emotionally and psychologically for change. When change comes, it is expected. Some changes, such as a new boss entering the company or new professors or advisors in place of the old, can be small reminders that change is constant. Other changes, such as an unexpected death, may be much more serious but are also reminders that change constantly occurs.

An exercise for this technique is to say to yourself, "Change is constant," or "I expect things to be constantly changing," whenever you note any kind of change, even a bud turning into a flower or a sunny day being interrupted by storm clouds and rain.

A second exercise is to learn to say what you prefer without being addicted to the "old" way: For example, "I prefer to have Dr. Jones teach this class, but since she is gone, I'll take it from someone else."

Action Plan

This involves completely thinking through the process shown in Figure 7.1 and then committing to writing a specific plan of action for change. To do this, follow these steps:

1. Get a good picture of the present situation. Write or even draw it on a piece of paper.
2. Get a good picture of the situation as you would like it, making sure that it is a picture that you can achieve on your own. We are often confronted with divorced men or women whose ideal picture is of the partner returning and the two of them living happily ever after. Their real need is to paint a picture that they can achieve themselves. Once a realistic picture is clear in your mind, write or draw it on paper.
3. Prepare a detailed, sequential plan to get from your present situation to your ideal situation.
    a. Define the ideal situation so that it is clear in your mind.
    b. List the main subtasks in sequential order—what must be done first, second, and so on.
    c. Under each subtask, identify what resources (both people and materials) will be needed, what skills (new and old) will be necessary, what proof you will insist on in order to know that each subtask is complete, what may block your action at each subtask, and how to get around those blocks.
    d. Identify activities that must be ongoing throughout the transition period (for example, assertiveness training, relaxation training, or exercise program).
    e. On one large sheet of paper (or smaller ones taped together), diagram your transition process, using Figure 7.1 as a model. Draw each subtask as a stepping stone. When the path between situation A and situation B is familiar and active, it becomes less fearful and thus less stressful.

Frustration

Did you ever get uptight because the car in front of you was going too slowly? Have you ever stood in a long line and become antsy because it didn't move fast enough? If you've experienced these or similar situations, then you know what it is like to be frustrated.

Frustration: the thwarting or inhibiting of natural or desired behaviors and goals. Frustration occurs when we're blocked from doing something we want to do, whether that something is a behavior we wish to perform or a goal we wish to attain. Emotionally, we respond to frustration with feelings of anger and aggression and with the nervous and hormonal responses that accompany them. Frustration, then, causes the stress response, and in a highly technological, urban society this source of stress should be recognized so that it may be dealt with. Four major sources of everyday frustration in the urban and sub-urban society are overcrowding, discrimination, socioeconomic factors, and bureaucracy.

Overcrowding

As our cities slowly grow into mass urban corridors, or megalopolises, social scientists wonder about the effects of such increasing human density on the overall quality of life (Hollingsworth 1996). Unfortunately, reports on the impact of crowding on health and happiness are conflicting or at least inconclusive.

The essence of the confusion seems to lie in the definition of crowding: the space allotted per organism, or the sensation or perception of being crowded. The latter part of the definition makes the way we perceive a situation the determinant of whether crowding exists. Crowding, then, becomes a function not solely of space and people but also of an individual's perception or feeling of being crowded. Such a perception is highly relative. Three could be a crowd in one situation, and thirty-three might not be a crowd in a different situation. If you perceive yourself as being crowded (inhibited in your behavior or goal attainment by the presence of others), then overcrowding exists, and it is a stressor for you.

During the 1970s overcrowding was a topic of high interest as predictions on expanding populations filled the news. Many good studies were conducted that have been replicated since with similar interesting results. A review of experiments with animals has shown that crowding produces excessive stress-hormone secretion, excessive adrenalin secretion, atrophy of the thymus gland (which involves the immune system) and of secondary sexual characteristics, and elevated blood pressure. Researchers at the National Institute of Mental Health conclude that there is abundant evidence that among animals, at least, crowded living conditions and their immediate consequences impose a stress that can lead to abnormal behavior, reproductive failure, sickness, and even death.

This research on animals seems conclusive, but there is still doubt whether these findings apply to humans. The problem in research on humans is that a feeling of crowding depends on our perception, which is a function of complex sensory and thought processes in addition to the more basic lower-brain processes that we share with the so-called lower animals. In addition, this complex integration of perceptual processes may be different for different types of people or different ethnic groups. However, in general, research supports the theory that when individuals feel inhibited or frustrated due to overcrowding, the stress response results.

SELF-ASSESSMENT EXERCISE 7

Choose the most appropriate answer for each of the following ten statements, and write the letter of your response to the left of the question.
How often do you . . .

_____ **1.** feel stifled or held back in your personal or professional life?
         a. almost always   c. seldom
         b. often   d. almost never

_____ **2.** feel a need for greater accomplishment?
         a. almost always   c. seldom
         b. often   d. almost never

_____ **3.** feel as though your life needs guidance or direction?
         a. almost always   c. seldom
         b. often   d. almost never

_____ **4.** notice yourself growing impatient?
         a. almost always   c. seldom
         b. often   d. almost never

_____ **5.** feel you are in a "rut?"
         a. almost always   c. seldom
         b. often   d. almost never

_____ **6.** feel disillusioned?
         a. almost always   c. seldom
         b. often   d. almost never

_____ **7.** feel frustrated?
         a. almost always   c. seldom
         b. often   d. almost never

_____ **8.** feel disappointed?
         a. almost always   c. seldom
         b. often   d. almost never

_____ **9.** feel inferior?
         a. almost always   c. seldom
         b. often   d. almost never

_____ **10.** feel upset because things haven't gone according to plan?
         a. almost always   c. seldom
         b. often   d. almost never

_____   Total Score

Calculate your total score as follows:
a = 4 points
b = 3 points
c = 2 points
d = 1 point
Write your total score in the space provided, and read the section "Frustration."

Commuter stress, often seen as "road rage," is the mental and emotional stress derived from driving to and from work (Koslowsky et al. 1995). Early research was done by Tanner (1976) and Singer (1975) who studied train commuters in Stockholm and found that the first passengers on a commuter train experienced less stress than those who boarded the train after the halfway point. This was true even though the earlier boarders had to tolerate the crowding for twice as long. He concluded that the resultant stress was not a function of crowding alone, but came more from the later arrivals being inhibited from gaining a seat and from stowing their coats and briefcases. Koslowsky, Kluger, and Reich (1995) found similar results and added that the stress of crowding was exacerbated by the feeling of competition with other people in the crowd for places, seats, and so on. When shortness of time was added to the equation, stress became severe.

Finally, studies of crowding in penal institutions have found that inmates confined to cells with many other prisoners exhibit higher blood pressure than those in less crowded cells. Highly crowded cells create an atmosphere of insecurity and depersonalization that was more frustrating and inhibitive than the atmosphere in less crowded cells (Kinkade, Leone, and Semond 1995; Lester 1990; Tonry and Hamilton, 1995).

Discrimination

Discrimination may be the most widely destructive form of frustration-caused stress. Discrimination refers to unfavorable actions taken against others because of religion, race, social status, gender, sexual preference, physical characteristics, national origin, or even general lifestyle. Although it is widely denounced as inhumane, discrimination appears to be ingrained in much of our social fiber and has been the basis of many social and occupational attitudes and practices (Burnback 1998, Stith 1998, Welch and Gruhl 1998). Discrimination taken to its extreme in the form of "ethnic cleansing" has been responsible for the death and torture of millions in eastern Europe.

Prejudice and discrimination can stifle anything from simple day-to-day activities to long-range goals and dreams (Heilbroner 1993, Young-Bruehl 1998). The 1969 National Institute of Mental Health report suggests that prejudice and discrimination result in the retardation of intellectual functioning and a decreased probability of healthy personality development, particularly in children. The report indicts prejudice as a potential cause of increased violent tendencies and a general distrust of democratic institutions and systems. Finally, it concludes that prejudice harms the development of self-concept in children.

Reverse discrimination has appeared in the United States as a means of compensating for the discrimination injustices of the past. All the same, it too is discrimination and involves essentially the same stress reactions for those discriminated against. Therefore, reverse discrimination is just as harmful to health as the discriminatory practices it was designed to correct.

Socioeconomic Factors

Stress may also be caused by frustrating socioeconomic conditions. Inflation, unemployment, excessive taxation, and general economic recession or depression can create stress on massive social scales, as was apparent in the Great Depression of the 1930s. During periods of economic turmoil, ambitions may be shattered. Maintaining financial security may become a day-to-day endeavor. Sending one's children to college, retiring early, owning a house—all of these aspirations may be frustrated by financial insecurity. The stress of such realities can be as detrimental to the health of the frustrated individual as it is to his or her finances. It has been shown that mental disorders, suicide, crime, and disease increase significantly during socioeconomic hardship, and family and marital relationships seem to be strained as well.

The effects of poverty on those at the lowest socioeconomic levels may lead to personal insecurity. Many of those living at the poverty level have a sense of powerlessness and hopelessness, and many suffer from a general personality disorientation in which they believe their role in life is meaningless. Such conditions are clearly harmful to the health of these people and of society in general.

Bureaucracy

If you feel trapped in a job that is unrewarding or without a future, one possible explanation may be that you are caught in the tentacles of a massive bureaucracy. Large bureaucracies seem to promote stress from frustration. They are almost inherently frustrating because of their complexities, "red tape," and impersonal nature. They often dampen individual initiative and motivation and decrease job satisfaction. Today's workers demand greater job satisfaction than their predecessors, and jobs that offer self-esteem and education as part of the work functions are in high demand. Clearly, money is no longer the sole determinant of job satisfaction. The bureaucracy cannot seem to meet the job-satisfaction demands of today's new, enlightened workers.

Those served by bureaucracies are also victims of stress when they are frustrated by bureaucratic inefficiencies. The growth of the consumer movement may reflect, to some degree, the frustration and anger of those who feel at the mercy of corporate policies they neither understand nor agree with.

Overcrowding, prejudice and discrimination, socioeconomic conditions, and large bureaucratic structures are four major sources of frustration, or the inhibition of human behavior, in modern urban society. Such inhibition can produce stress reactions that are expressed in anger, aggression, increased sympathetic nervous activity, and increased mental trauma.

Now that you have reviewed some of the causes of frustrational stress, return to Self-Assessment Exercise 7. The highest score possible is 40, and the lowest is 10. The higher your score, the greater your perception of frustration and the more stressful frustration would appear to be for you. General guidelines are 25 to 40 = high frustration/ high stress; 20 to 24 = moderate frustration/moderate stress; 10 to 19 = low frustration/ low stress.

Burnout.   Because frustration is characteristically inhibitive or thwarting, it appears to be one of the major factors in a condition known as *burnout.* The other major factor is overload (to be discussed in the next section).

Burnout: a state of mental and/or physical exhaustion caused by excessive stress. Burnout is caused by excessively prolonged or excessively intense stress arousal (Burke and Richardsen 1995; Maslach and Leiter 1997; Schaufeli and Enzmann 1998). Two of the major causes of burnout are bureaucratic atmospheres and a continuously heavy workload. The three stages of burnout appear in Table 7.1.

TABLE 7.1   The Stages of Burnout

Stage 1: Stress Arousal (includes any two of the following symptoms)

1. Persistent irritability
2. Persistent anxiety
3. Periods of high blood pressure
4. Bruxism (grinding your teeth at night)
5. Insomnia
6. Forgetfulness
7. Heart palpitations
8. Unusual heart rhythms (skipped beats)
9. Inability to concentrate
10. Headaches

Stage 2: Energy Conservation (includes any two of the following)

1. Lateness for work
2. Procrastination
3. Needed three-day weekends
4. Decreased sexual desire
5. Persistent tiredness in the mornings
6. Turning work in late
7. Social withdrawal (from friends and/or family)
8. Cynical attitudes
9. Resentfulness
10. Increased alcohol consumption
11. Increased coffee, tea, or cola consumption
12. Apathy

Stage 3: Exhaustion (includes any two of the following)

1. Chronic sadness or depression
2. Chronic stomach or bowel problems
3. Chronic mental fatigue
4. Chronic physical fatigue
5. Chronic headaches
6. The desire to "drop out" of society
7. The desire to move away from friends, work, and perhaps even family
8. Perhaps the desire to commit suicide

Source: Everly 1985, 186. Occupational Stress Management. In G. Everly and R. Feldman, eds. *Occupational Health Promotion.* New York: Wiley.
Note: These stages usually occur sequentially, from Stage 1 to Stage 3, although the process can be stopped at any point

Fortunately, burnout is not permanent—it is reversible. Furthermore, it is preventable (Kompier and Cooper 1999). Relaxation, proper diet, and physical exercise not only help you recover from burnout but can prevent this problem from occurring in the first place. These topics are discussed in depth later in this book.

Frustration is a stressor because it is by definition inhibitive. Frustration impedes progress toward a desired goal or blocks desired behavior. The techniques given here present ways that action can be continued, even though you are being thwarted in some part of your life.

Exercises

Express Your Frustration

Until alternatives as satisfying and immediate as the original goal are found, it is helpful to express frustration either by talking with someone else or by writing thoughts down on paper. This helps release the stress buildup and may give insights about the situation.

Determine Your Real Outcomes

Using the Outcome Model (Girdano and Dusek 1988), follow each step from stating what you want to a concrete action plan. The steps are as follows.

What Do I Want? Although frustration is caused by blocks of progress, many blocks occur because we are not really sure what we want in the first place. If the outcome is not clear, the path is not direct, and we tend to wander off course, letting relatively minor obstacles block our path and cause frustration.

How Will Things Be Different and Better in My Life When I Get What I Want? This is the "heart" question. If the path does not have meaning in the first place, it is easy to surrender to frustration. If the outcome is stated in the positive, the human mind will work harder to achieve that outcome. Thinking of one's life in negative terms expands negative energy around the outcome, and the body automatically defends itself against negative events. The ego does not want to face negative inputs, so defenses are built up against the activity. Thus, sometimes the block that frustrates us is of our own creation so that we will not pursue activities that make us feel bad about ourselves.

What Will I Take as Proof That I Have Been Successful in Reaching My Outcome? Sometimes our frustrations and subsequent stress are the result of actually meeting our real goals but not knowing it. We have what we wanted but do not realize it. It is important to set up concrete and countable signposts that will indicate when we are nearing our goal and when we reach it.

What Are My Useful Resources? This will be specific to each project, although after several projects, common resources (especially positive personality traits) will begin to emerge. List all of your internal and external resources. Remember your family, friends, financial ability, and your inner resources that have gotten you to where you are now.

What Has Kept Me from Reaching This Outcome Before? If you have attempted to reach this outcome before or have tried for success in a similar endeavor, what stopped you? Past blocks will almost certainly be blocks in the future unless they are discovered and removed. Spending time analyzing and correcting blocks may be the single most effective frustration-management technique.

What Am I Willing to Do as a Plan of Action to Get to My Outcome? Although this is a specific project, you will probably use old successful patterns to help you get to this outcome. If your style works, find a way to adapt it to your new situation. If your old plan does not work, change it by increasing your resources and diminishing your blocks. Formulate a specific plan much like that used in the Goal Alternative System presented next.

Choose Alternatives

The following Goal Alternative System is designed to help you cope with frustrational stress by exploring alternatives to goals that have been directly inhibited or stifled.

THE GOAL ALTERNATIVE SYSTEM

Example: Tennis Playing

Step 1   What is the desired behavior or goal?   *Playing tennis*

Step 2   Is this goal immediately obtainable?

    NO   YES
    ↓   └──────► STOP! Why are you doing this exercise?

Step 3   What is (are) the obstacle(s) that keep(s) you from obtaining this goal? ◄──────────────────────┐

    Tennis elbow

Step 4   Can this obstacle be removed within a reasonable time period?

    NO   YES
    ↓   └──────► If any reasonable methods exist by which you may obtain your goal by removing the obstacle, do so. ───┘

Step 5   Consider your desired goal. Take some time and make a list of the specific rewards or desirable characteristics that make that goal desirable to you. Now go back and give each one of those desirable characteristics a score indicative of how important each one is to you. A score of 1 would be the lowest, 10 the highest. Do this very carefully; it is very important.

Rewards	Points
Being outdoors	8
Getting exercise	6
Fast action	5
Competition	5

Step 6 Are there any other reasonable ways to obtain those same rewards listed in Step 5?

YES	NO
List alternatives, then try them out:	If you have arrived at this point, it seems apparent that *all* of those desirable characteristics listed in Step 5 are currently unobtainable. Therefore, instead of feeling sorry for yourself, make a list of alternatives that *are possible* and that have at least some of the same desirable characteristics as the original goal. Select the behavior that results in the highest score possible. This alternative is your best one because it is most similar, based on the points assigned in Step 5, to your original behavior.

none
_____
_____
_____

Alternatives	Points
Fishing	8
Golf (outdoor exercise, competition)	16
_____	___

THE GOAL ALTERNATIVE SYSTEM

Blank Form

Step 1 What is the desired behavior or goal? _____

Step 2 Is this goal immediately obtainable?

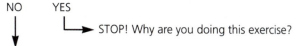

NO   YES

STOP! Why are you doing this exercise?

Step 3 What is (are) the obstacle(s) that keep(s) you from obtaining this goal?

_____
_____

Step 4 Can this obstacle be removed within a reasonable time period?

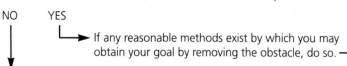

NO   YES

If any reasonable methods exist by which you may obtain your goal by removing the obstacle, do so.

Step 5 Consider your desired goal. Take some time and make a list of the specific rewards or desirable characteristics that make that goal desirable to you. Now go back and give each one of those desirable characteristics a score indicative of how important each one is to you. A score of 1 would be the lowest, 10 the highest. Do this very carefully; it is very important.

(continued)

THE GOAL ALTERNATIVE SYSTEM   (*Continued*)

Rewards   *Points*

_____   _____

_____   _____

_____   _____

_____   _____

Step 6   Are there any other reasonable ways to obtain those same rewards listed in Step 5?

YES	NO
List alternatives, then try them out:	If you have arrived at this point, it seems apparent that *all* of those desirable characteristics listed in Step 5 are currently unobtainable. Therefore, instead of feeling sorry for yourself, make a list of alternatives that *are possible* and that have at least some of the same desirable characteristics as the original goal. Select the behavior that results in the highest score possible. This alternative is your best one because it is most similar, based on the points assigned in Step 5, to your original behavior.
_____	
_____	
_____	
_____	

Alternatives   *Points*

_____   _____

_____   _____

_____   _____

Examine Beliefs

The beliefs that we hold regarding our relationship to the rest of the world have been formed very early in life and therefore are deeply ingrained. Old, buried beliefs are sometimes difficult to unearth so that we may look at their logic in light of our present development. Beliefs formed during childhood are based on the beliefs of significant others and also on the skills and knowledge that the child possessed. The beliefs that worked for a certain period of time may no longer be useful because the individual has new knowledge, skills, and experiences as an adult. The steps that can be used to examine beliefs are as follows:

Question

When frustration occurs, say to yourself, "What would a person have to believe in order to become frustrated in such a situation?"

Answers

Examine some possible answers to your questions. The beliefs listed here (Girdano and Dusek 1988) may provide a starting point.

- I must not change my beliefs, attitudes, or actions because they have gotten me this far.
- I must understand the universe before I can live happily in it.
- I will be seen as an inferior person unless I do well and win the approval of others.
- I cannot exist without sincere and constant love and approval from everyone who is in my life.
- I must be able to do at least one thing with thorough competence.
- Justice, fairness, and equality must prevail, or life is too unbearable.
- I must not experience or show negative emotions because they make me perform badly and others don't like them.
- I must control or change people who I consider dangerous.
- I must not question or doubt the beliefs that authorities hold. If I do, I should be punished.
- I should get what I want when I want it, regardless of what others think or do.
- Others must not unjustly criticize me.
- Others should not behave in a stupid or incompetent manner.
- Others will treat me the way I think I should be treated.

Turning Beliefs Around

After identifying the belief on which the frustration is based, turn the belief around so that it becomes positive. For example: "I cannot buy the computer I want because my father says it is an inferior machine and I could get a better price on a model that I don't really want. I identify that my frustration stems from my belief that my father knows what is best for me. I turn the belief around to 'I am the only one who knows what is best for me,' or 'I can choose to take the advice of others, especially when I honor their expertise, but I must make my own choices."

Take Action

Act on the positive belief. Continue to affirm that belief. Write it down on a card, and place the card in a conspicuous place in your house or car.

Behavioral Skills

Acting on new positive beliefs may call for the learning of new skills such as assertiveness. Telling others that they are no longer expected to control your behaviors may call for preparatory skills that you must be willing to learn.

Overload

Have you ever felt that the pressures of life were building up so that you could no longer meet their demands? Perhaps you felt as though there simply wasn't enough time in the day for you to accomplish all the things you needed to do. During this time you may have noticed a decline in your social life and more of a "self-centeredness." Perhaps you lost sleep and so became tired and irritable. You may even have become more susceptible to colds and flu. If any of these things sounds familiar, chances are you were a victim of overload.

Overload, which means the same as overstimulation, refers to the state in which the demands around you exceed your capacity to meet them. Some aspects of your life are placing excessive demands on you. When these demands exceed your ability to comply with them, you experience distress.

> *Overload:* a level of stimulation or demand that exceeds the capacity to process or comply with that input; overstimulation.

The four major factors in overload are (1) time pressures, (2) excessive responsibility or accountability, (3) lack of support, and (4) excessive expectations from yourself and those around you. Any one or a combination of these factors can result in stress from overload. Overload is one of the most pervasive stressors in modern society. It encompasses the city, the occupational environment, the school, and even the home.

Urban Overload

Visitors to large cities often comment on the unfriendly or impersonal ways of urban life in contrast with the more personal suburban or rural lifestyles. Many scientists are at a loss to explain an event such as the rape of a woman in a large city, witnessed by over a dozen people who made no attempts to help her. Such shocking lack of concern for the welfare of others and the blatant egocentric attitudes that seem to fester in many large cities are of concern to us all. The concept of overload was developed to explain the impersonal attitude of many urban dwellers. Several decades ago Milgram (1970) viewed the large urban center as a vast collection of potential stressors—

SELF-ASSESSMENT EXERCISE 8

Choose the most appropriate answer for each of the following ten statements, and write the letter of your response to the left of the question.

How often do you . . .

_____ 1. find yourself with insufficient time to do things you really enjoy?
   a. almost always   c. seldom
   b. often   d. almost never

_____ 2. wish you had more support/assistance?
   a. almost always   c. seldom
   b. often   d. almost never

_____ 3. lack sufficient time to complete your work most effectively?
   a. almost always   c. seldom
   b. often   d. almost never

_____ 4. have difficulty falling asleep because you have too much on your mind?
   a. almost always   c. seldom
   b. often   d. almost never

_____ 5. feel people simply expect too much from you?
   a. almost always   c. seldom
   b. often   d. almost never

_____ 6. feel overwhelmed?
   a. almost always   c. seldom
   b. often   d. almost never

_____ 7. become forgetful or indecisive because you have too much on your mind?
   a. almost always   c. seldom
   b. often   d. almost never

_____ 8. consider yourself to be in a high-pressure situation?
   a. almost always   c. seldom
   b. often   d. almost never

_____ 9. feel you have too much responsibility for one person?
   a. almost always   c. seldom
   b. often   d. almost never

_____10. feel exhausted at the end of the day?
   a. almost always   c. seldom
   b. often   d. almost never

_____   Total Score

Calculate your total score as follows:

a = 4 points
b = 3 points
c = 2 points
d = 1 point

Write your total score in the space provided, and read the section "Overload."

mass media, mass transportation, vast technological innovations, intense interpersonal stimulation, a deadline-oriented society, and excessive and diverse responsibilities. He suggested that lack of interpersonal concern is a defense mechanism by which urbanites cope with this bombardment of social stimuli. Impersonality protects urbanites' psychological well-being by shielding them from all but the most necessary environmental demands. In general, there appears to be growing concern over the quality of life in urban environments (Burton 1990, Elkin 1999).

Occupational Overload

Toward the end of the 1970s, predictions were that the forty-hour work week would fade into memory, and the remainder of the century would see workers with more and more free time. New disciplines such as leisure counseling were being developed to help people sort out how best to use this newfound free time. These predictions were not all wrong. The forty-hour week is indeed a thing of the past. It has been replaced with the forty-five-plus-hour work week. Demand for higher productivity (especially in high-tech industries) has made overload in the workplace a virtual certainty. Deadlines (time pressure); excessive responsibility and accountability; lack of managerial or subordinate support; and excessive role expectations from self, supervisor, and subordinates can all create overload. Task overload occurs when the work environment places demands that are beyond a person's resources. In our time- and money-oriented society, it is not surprising that many jobs are deemed more stressful than is healthy for employees. This is especially true in this age of increased organizational accountability. Think of the tasks that are creating (or have created) overload for you. Make a list of them for further reference as you read the intervention techniques presented later.

The effects of time pressure on workers have been known to researchers for almost a half century. Friedman, Rosenman, and Carroll (1958) studied tax accountants at the peak season (just prior to April 15). Analysis of blood samples revealed significant increases in serum cholesterol and blood-coagulation times. Both of these signs indicate excessive stress, which may eventually contribute to the development of heart disease.

Perhaps the best example of occupational task overload is seen in air-traffic controllers (ATCs). They are faced with a combination of excessive time pressures, life-and-death responsibility, often insufficient support (managerial and/or technical), and a virtually damning expectation for perfection from themselves and others. Research on these workers clearly demonstrates the stressful outcome of task overload. For example, at Chicago's O'Hare airport researchers found that ATCs were under greater stress than pilots flying ten-hour flights in simulators. This conclusion was reached by measuring secretions of the adrenal medullae and the adrenal cortex (the main stress hormones). Compared with telecommunication operators, ATCs showed considerably stronger stress reactions on the job, based on analysis of their blood. Research has revealed that ATCs are occupationally predisposed to certain stress-related diseases, the most significant of which is hypertension, followed by peptic ulcers, and finally diabetes.

These studies demonstrate the devastating effects of task overload as a stressor. The important point here is not that work is stressful but rather that certain intrinsic elements of a job task may be highly stressful if the occupational demands are hyper-stimulating and exceed an individual's resources (Repetti 1993).

Academic Overload

Overload doesn't stop in the urban milieu; it reaches into the classroom as well. Teachers are experiencing increased demands for accountability and are expected not only to contribute to the search for knowledge (research) and serve the community in a professional manner but also to excel in teaching skills. These demands are often coupled with sidelines such as advising, collecting milk money, and parent-student counseling—tasks upon which salary increase, promotion, and/or tenure often depend (Cooper 1995).

The academic environment is also becoming increasingly stressful for students. This society's demand for higher education has created a highly competitive academic environment reaching back even to the primary grades. Children are pressured to do well academically to ensure college admission. Once in college, the student is exposed to the possibility of graduate or professional schooling, but many graduate and professional schools demand "honors status" for a student to even be considered for admission. Added to the grade battle are admissions tests, which are stressors in themselves. Little wonder that test anxiety is becoming a major problem in the academic world. Test anxiety may lead to inaccurately low evaluations of a student's scholastic achievement or potential.

For many students the academic grind has led to dropping out of school, poor self-concept, and more severe mental disturbances (the most severe of which has been suicide). In response to the growing pressures of education, many schools have increased their funding for counseling and mental health services; this is especially true in higher education. Schools have initiated programs to help students learn to study, reduce test anxiety, and generally improve coping skills.

Domestic Overload

The home has always been a potential source of overload stress. The small, comparatively low-cost "first home" of many couples with children is easily outgrown, and space is at a premium. In addition to perceived crowding, a multiplicity of electronic gadgets around the home—televisions, radios, CD players, and VCRs—contribute to overload stress. Never-ending home repair, yard work, and everyday household chores round out a picture of the home as an overload stressor. Unfortunately, it seems that no matter where you go or what you do, you become a prime candidate for this society's far-reaching stressor: overload.

Overload is not only imposed by the outside, it is often self-initiated. The Internet and television have influenced a heightened susceptibility to advertising. Buying the latest stuff, which keeps getting better and faster and more convenient has increased consumerism and fueled the fast-growing economy experienced in the 1990s. Wanting more and more demands more money, which of course comes from more work and more self-imposed overload. In the old mining communities in

Appalachia, workers would have to buy all of their goods from the company store. At the end of a hard week's work, they often owed the company instead of walking away with money. As the song went, "another day older and deeper in debt." Today the company is consumer economy fueled by advertising that keeps the people working harder to buy the latest, fastest, trendy (often unnecessary) items. The cost? Excessive stress, stress-related illness, and overall less satisfaction with life.

Self-Assessment Exercise 8 was designed to assess your level of stress due to overload. Total your points and see how stressed you are by overload. Roughly speaking, a total of 25 to 40 indicates a high stress level, one that could be psychologically and physiologically debilitating. As mentioned in the last section, overload is one of two major factors in burnout. You suffer from overload when faced with excessive demands to the point where your stress response is aroused. Overload is a function of four major factors: (1) time pressure, (2) excessive responsibility or accountability, (3) lack of support, and (4) excessive expectations imposed by yourself or by others. Consider the following techniques for alleviating the stress of overload.

Exercises

Express Your Feelings

Talk with someone or write down your feelings on paper. Do not allow your emotions to get bottled up. For detailed instruction, see the suggestions regarding assertiveness in Chapter 6.

Negotiate

If you perceive that your feelings of overload are being brought on by a person, negotiate with that person to reduce the load or the deadline.

Some sound rules of negotiation include the following (Fisher, Ury, and Patton 1991):

1. Focus on the benefits that will come from your position, such as value, results, and recognition rather than standing for or against certain positions, such as time or price.
2. Separate the personal relationships from the problem you are negotiating.
3. Handle emotions as legitimate but unrelated to the substance.
4. Let people blow off steam and do not take it personally.
5. To be understood, speak purposefully. Speak about yourself, not about "them," which promotes defensiveness.
6. Build a relationship so that you may prevent future negotiation problems.
7. Focus on common elements, values, and interests rather than differences.
8. Invent options for mutual gain. Brainstorm for new ideas.
9. If they are more powerful, recast an attack on yourself as an attack on the problem.

Manage Time

Working under a deadline is the most obvious form of time overload, but much of this stress can be controlled by effective time management. When the task seems too formidable, follow these steps to set priorities and schedule tasks into a workable, efficient order:

Step 1. Establish long-term goals (one, five, ten years or more) and develop a plan of action.

Step 2. Establish intermediate goals or priorities (three or six months), and develop a plan of action.

Step 3. Develop a weekly habit of setting short-term priorities and an action plan for the coming week. Once you have completed the weekly plan, use the same steps to plan for your intermediate and long-term goals.

Remember to get the important tasks done before taking care of less important ones that might be easier but that fill up your valuable time. Sometimes a less important task can be dropped off the list completely as it loses its importance. You'll be glad you didn't waste your time doing that one! As you list and prioritize your tasks, be aware of tasks that might best be delegated to the helpers around you. If you must be a perfectionist, be selective about it. It is reasonable to shoot at perfection on your A tasks and maybe some Bs, but don't get side-tracked by doing your low-priority tasks perfectly. Your helpers may not do the job exactly as you would, but while they are getting it done, you have time to accomplish your top priorities. If you find yourself overwhelmed by a monster task, break it into parts. Chapters are easier to write than novels. Learn to say no to free up your time. People will learn to respect your time as you learn to manage it. Remember that the object is to get where you want while also staying happy and healthy. Be sure to schedule play time and relaxation time: Not only do these times reward you, but they also reenergize you. The busiest, most hectic times are the those when planning can be most beneficial even though you must take time out to do it. As you are planning and doing your tasks, remind yourself that although some tasks are unpleasant, most are enjoyable and rewarding. If not, you may want to rethink your long-term goals. If joy is the end, then joy must be the means.

Use these steps to plan the coming week:

1. Make a list of things to do this week.
2. Prioritize your "things to do" by assigning them to one of the following categories:
   A. Top priority tasks that must be completed by the end of this week. (What is top priority for you? Decide what is important in order to accomplish your medium- and long-term goals!)
   B. Medium priority tasks without urgent deadlines.
   C. Tasks that really can wait.

3. Estimate and record the time required to complete each task—be realistic. Then increase each of the time estimates by 10 to 15 percent. This provides some cushion for error or for unexpected problems.

A	B	C
_____	_____	_____
_____	_____	_____
_____	_____	_____
_____	_____	_____
_____	_____	_____

4. Transfer your "things to do" to a weekly calendar in this manner:
   A. First, place all "A" tasks in the best time slots for you.
   B. If there is time available, add B tasks.
   C. List C tasks at the bottom of your calendar, and when all A and B tasks are taken care of, do a C task or two.

Say What You Want

When you feel that someone is imposing more work or responsibility on you than is appropriate at the time, tell that person that the timing is inappropriate. If you do not wish to do a task, say no. Ask for help from others. Sit down and objectively look at your load in relation to those around you. If you get up and make breakfast for everyone before you go to work, cook dinner, straighten the house, and put everybody to bed after you come home from work, and do the laundry on your day off, look at the responsibilities of everyone else in the household. If the responsibilities are out of balance and the expertise of others is sufficient to carry out some of your duties, ask for a family meeting. Discuss the inequities and reassign some of the duties.

Delegate

As in the preceding technique, duties can be shared when you learn to delegate some of the tasks and responsibilities. This is more than asking for what you want; it is giving up some control over how things will be done by completely giving a task to someone else. The connotation of delegation is that you are in a position of authority and that others are there to help you complete certain tasks. Be thoughtful when you delegate, and take into consideration the workload of others so that you do not overload them. Also, when you give a task to someone else, either give them detailed instructions or give them the authority to do their way.

Expectation History

Where did your levels of expectation originate? What kind of expectations did you learn from your mother and father? What do (did) your parents and other significant people in your life expect from you? from themselves? from others? What is a reasonable expectation level? There is an old equation:

Happiness = What you get ÷ What you expect

If you get $100 but you expected $1000, your quotient is less than 1. If you get $100 but expected that amount or less, the quotient is 1 or more. When unrealistically high expectations are set, they result in overload stress. When expectations are kept to a minimum and are realistically set, they result in foundational goals rather than system overload.

Examine Beliefs

Using the discussion on beliefs given in the previous section on frustration, think about your long-held beliefs regarding what you expect from others, which is a good reflection of what you expect from yourself. If others cannot please you with their performance, you probably cannot please yourself with your performance. Some of the negative beliefs that may arise here are as follows:

- Work is not done until it is done perfectly.
- I must always perform at the 90-percent level of effectiveness, creativity, and intellectual excellence, or I will be considered a sloppy person.
- Others cannot do the job as well as I can.
- If you want it done right, you have to do it yourself.
- The world has no room for a person who performs at less than maximum effort all the time.

When you find that you hold negative beliefs about perfection and expectations, reverse that belief and continue to affirm it until it is the basis for your expectations. Example: "I must perform with perfection, or I will not be accepted (loved) by others." This belief might be turned around to: "I will do the best I can within reason. Pleasing myself is more important than pleasing others."

Decision Making and Problem Solving

There are a few events in our lives that are almost guaranteed to cause stress, and one such event is making a decision. Making decisions encompasses the stress of change and the stress of overload exacerbated by the fear of making the wrong choice. Making decisions can be so stressful and anxiety producing that many people make a lifestyle out of avoiding making choices and putting off the ones they do until the last possible minute. That is why there are so many undeclared majors among college juniors and even seniors. The stress risk in decision making is most pronounced when one becomes obsessed with the details of decision making and insists that one must always find the "right answer." During a crisis, the ability to handle difficult tasks requiring intensely focused attention is decreased.

Traditional decision-making theory says that the decision maker should do the following:

1. Thoroughly examine a wide range of alternatives.
2. Take into account the full range of objectives to be fulfilled and the values implicated by the choice.
3. Carefully weigh both the costs or drawbacks and benefits of the alternatives.
4. Intensively search for new information relevant to alternatives.
5. Conscientiously take account of any new information or expert judgment that may or may not support previously held preferences.
6. Reexamine positive and negative consequences.
7. Make detailed provisions for implementing the chosen course of action with a contingency plan for dealing with known risks. (Janis and Mann 1976)

In real life the process goes more like this:

The consideration of the problem and potential solutions is time and pressure dependent. In other words, the hunt for the best solution loses intensity when you uncover an acceptable solution. An increase in stress caused by time constraints or worry over being wrong leads to premature closure. The greater the stress, the greater the tendency to make a premature choice of alternatives for a correct response. The greater the stress, the greater the likelihood that a decision-maker will choose a risky alternative (Russo 1990).

Prejudiced feelings or subconscious preferences guide the "full range" of objectives, which systematically eliminates alternatives as they emerge instead of bringing all facts to the table and scrutinizing them. Key factors are enhanced or inhibited, and alternatives are prematurely colored for choice or rejection at this stage. The greater the stress, the greater both the distortion in perception of threat and poor judgment. Under increasing stress, productive thoughts decrease and distracting thoughts increase.

Focused problem solving includes seeking preliminary information and then more information and input from others. Problem-solving action includes making alternatives, taking specific action, and learning new skills, especially how to negotiate a compromise

The emotional focus is on affective regulation, or control of emotion. This is often done with suppression—trying not to think about it, denying feelings, and withholding immediate action; by resigned acceptance—waiting for time to solve the problem, submitting to fate; or using emotional discharge—letting off steam, crying, smoking, overeating, or acting out.

Here are some known patterns of decision making: (1) unconflicted inertia—complacently continuing the status quo and ignoring the risk of deciding (2) unconflicted change—uncritically adopting whatever is suggested with preparation for setbacks; accepting reality; redefining the situation to find something good, (i.e., things could be worse); (3) defensive avoidance—doing nothing, denying fear, anxiety, trying to forget the whole situation, and engaging in fantasy rather than thinking about the problem; (4) hypervigilance—panic, searching for a way out, shifting back and forth between alternatives, taking almost anything for relief, cognitive construction, repetitive thinking, and emotional excitement; (5) vigilance—searching for relevant information, assimilating it in an unbiased manner, appraising, looking at alternatives, and deciding. (Clemen 1996, Golub 1996, Wheeler and Janis 1980).

The goal is to select the best solution from among the alternatives you have considered while at the same time controlling excess stress that is detrimental to good decision making and to your health (Keeney 1996). You can usually eliminate poor solutions by recognizing they won't work or require skills and resources you don't now have. Other choices can be eliminated because they might involve too high a price— some kind of potential disaster.

Even more important to the discussion of decision making as a stressor is the impact the process has on health. The philosophical take on decisions is to accept the best choice and stop obsessing about the decision. Let go of the unselected options. After making a decision, it takes a little time to reprogram your thinking and to fully commit yourself to the chosen course of action. It may be helpful, especially where the decision is hard to make, to remember that in many cases there is very little difference among the alternative solutions. Give up the notion of finding the one right answer. All your options will probably work out about equally well. We are faced with decisions every day even though most of them are minor. On even the major ones you cannot "should have" yourself to death. Just get on with making your decision work for you. Although you cannot do everything right, you can make something right out of everything you do.

Exercise

Write down the pros and cons for each alternative choice, and assign a weight (0 to + 10) to each pro and each con (0 to –10), indicating how important that factor is. By adding up the pros and cons separately, you get a total score for each alternative. Next, compare the totals for each alternative course of action. This should usually reveal the best choice. This is a cost/benefit analysis that involves weighing the eventual effectiveness of the solution in solving the problem.

This process is used mostly with big decisions and should save your emotional well-being during and after the decision. Unfortunately, many decisions become exceedingly complex, either because there are several alternatives or many pros and cons to consider. Moreover, the weight you would assign a pro or a con will probably vary from time to time and may actually be prejudiced by feelings one way or the other. Indeed, optimists tend to over emphasize the opportunities in certain choices, whereas pessimists exaggerate the possible dangers of certain alternatives. Usually, if the decision is a major one, you need to weigh the pros and cons, and get a second opinion to double-check your judgments. With the ever-increasing reliance on computers, it is not surprising that computer-supported decision models are becoming popular. Even though complex data can be handled with computer assistance, defining issues and selecting responses are still subject to human bias (Smith 1998).

Boredom and Loneliness

The idea that overstimulation of your mental and emotional processes can result in stress and ill health probably did not surprise you. But now consider the notion that understimulation of these very same processes can result in the same stress response and the same deterioration of your health. We call this state *deprivational stress.*

> *Deprivational Stress:* the psychophysiological stress response caused by states of boredom and/or loneliness.

Deprivational stress was defined over fifty years ago as "the internal bodily reaction to cognitive understimulation"—that is, our body's response to boredom (monotonous, unchallenging tasks) and loneliness (emotional deprivation) (Galdston 1954, 45). Nothing has changed since then to alter the perception of monotony. In affluent societies, advanced technology relieves humans of many tasks, but the human time and interest in those tasks are often replaced with the boredom of watching a machine do the work. Highly repetitive or insufficiently challenging tasks can result in distress. There is certainly nothing wrong with having machines do monotonous work provided you can find more stimulating things to do with the time.

Even with hundreds of channels on TV, video games, and the Internet, boredom appears to prey quite heavily on adolescents. Some psychologists suggest that as many as 20 percent of adolescents in the United States are psychologically handicapped by boredom and depression. Such a handicap may lead to loss of self-esteem and eventually to self-destructive behaviors such as drug abuse and even suicide, one of the leading causes of adolescent death. As a result, billions of dollars are spent each year on entertainment and diversions for adolescents. All of these signs appear to indicate that massive technological advances are serving to bore many Americans to death! The critical factor seems to be how creative, active, or challenging an activity is. Without these factors, no matter how much time is spent in the activity, it is still boring.

Loneliness can also be a devastating stressor. Children who are not given adequate, caring attention are known to suffer from stimulus deprivation. Such emotionally deprived children may suffer a decreased production of growth hormones and subsequent retardation of growth and development. But when these children are placed in an emotionally supportive environment, their growth returns to normal. Nevertheless, psychological scars may persist for a lifetime.

For the major causes of death in the United States (heart disease, cancer, and automobile accidents), mortality is higher among single, widowed, and divorced individuals of all races and both sexes than among married individuals; and interpersonal unhappiness, the lack of love, and human loneliness appear to be the root of physical problems (Bruno 1997, Sanders 1998).

How well do you tolerate deprivational stress? Self-Assessment Exercise 9 was designed to help you find out. If your score is 25 to 40, you are vulnerable to deprivational stress; you seem to need stimulation to avoid stress. If your score is 20 to 24, you are average. If your score is 10 to 19, you have a high tolerance for low stimulation.

SELF-ASSESSMENT EXERCISE 9

Choose the most appropriate answer for each of the following ten statements, and write the letter of your response to the left of the question.
How often do you . . .

_____ **1.** feel that your work is not stimulating enough?
     a. almost always   c. seldom
     b. often   d. almost never

_____ **2.** lose interest in your daily activities?
     a. almost always   c. seldom
     b. often   d. almost never

_____ **3.** become restless during your daily routine?
     a. almost always   c. seldom
     b. often   d. almost never

_____ **4.** feel "insulted" by the simplicity of your work?
     a. almost always   c. seldom
     b. often   d. almost never

_____ **5.** wish your life were more exciting?
     a. almost always   c. seldom
     b. often   d. almost never

_____ **6.** become anxious from a lack of stimulation?
     a. almost always   c. seldom
     b. often   d. almost never

_____ **7.** become bored?
     a. almost always   c. seldom
     b. often   d. almost never

_____ **8.** feel that your usual activities aren't challenging enough?
     a. almost always   c. seldom
     b. often   d. almost never

_____ **9.** daydream during your work?
     a. almost always   c. seldom
     b. often   d. almost never

_____ **10.** feel lonely?
     a. almost always   c. seldom
     b. often   d. almost never

_____ Total Score

Calculate your total score as follows:
a = 4 points
b = 3 points
c = 2 points
d = 1 point
Write your total score in the space provided, and read the section "Boredom and Loneliness"

As overload is a stressor because of excessive stimulation, deprivation or boredom is one because of insufficient stimulation. Like all of the stressors discussed here, deprivation is an idiosyncratic and relative phenomenon. In general, deprivation is alleviated by increasing the level of stimulation. The techniques given here present various ways of increasing stimulation and interaction.

Exercises

Keep a Journal

Writing your feelings about loneliness, boredom, or lack of involvement helps alleviate deprivational stress in two ways: (1) It is an active process that may also include creativity, and (2) the expression of negative emotions helps to release these feelings.

Physical Activity

Become active in a preset or self-originated activity program. Larger cities have YMCAs offering activity courses for small fees. Also available are spas and health clubs, although these are usually more expensive. Every college has a physical education department and campus recreation. Collect catalogs and/or call these establishments to compile a list of possible activities, and then choose one or two that you have always wanted to do. Joining activity classes is also a very good way to meet people with interests similar to yours.

If you have the expertise and desire to set up your own activity program, sit down and plan how you will carry it out for the first month. (A plan for starting a physical activity program is presented in Chapter 17). Write your activity plan on a calendar. Also, try to get a friend to join you; motivation is usually enhanced by performing activities with others.

Join a Social Group

Using the references to institutions that offer physical activities, obtain information from them regarding other activities such as men's or women's support groups, single-parent groups, reading groups, and so forth. Your city may have a formal listing of social-support groups available in the community. If you have a special interest but there is no established group, consider starting such a group by placing a notice in your apartment building or dorm or by placing an advertisement in the local paper.

Ask for Human Contact

This technique calls for learning assertiveness skills discussed in the self-concept section in Chapter 6. Please read that section.

Examine Beliefs

What would a person have to believe to remain unhappily in isolation or boredom?
Possible negative beliefs:

- I do not deserve the company of fun and interesting people.
- I cannot disclose who I am to others, or they won't like me.
- People will only hurt me and take advantage of me.
- It takes too much effort to make friends.
- I am perfectly happy being by myself.
- If I do make friends, they will just abandon me.

As in past discussions of beliefs, the technique here is to not only examine the
negative beliefs that keep you in isolation or boredom but also to turn the belief into
a positive statement and begin to live by the new belief. Example: "It takes too much
effort to find something exciting to do." This belief can be turned around to: "Getting
involved in activities I really like to do is becoming easier and easier."

SOURCES CITED

Arrien, A. (1994). *The fourfold way.* San Francisco: HarperCollins.

Bandura, A. (1997). *Self-efficacy: The exercise of control.* New York: W. H. Freeman.

Bruno, F. (1997). *Conquer loneliness.* Foster City, CA: IDG Books Worldwide.

Burke, R., and Richardsen, A. (1995). Stress, burnout, and health. In *Handbook of stress,* ed. C. Cooper,
Boca Raton, FL: CRC Press.

Burnbach, J. (1998). *Job discrimination.* Ojai, CA: Voir Dire Press.

Burton, I. (1990). *Factors in urban stress.* Journal of Sociology and Social Welfare, 17, 79–92.

Clemen, R. (1996). *Making hard decisions.* Pacific Grove, CA: Duxbury Press.

Cooper, C. (1995). *Life at the chalkface: Identifying and measuring teacher stress.* British Journal of Education Psychology, 65, 69–71.

Davidson, J. (1991). *Clinical efficacy shown in pharmacologic treatment of post-traumatic stress disorder.*
Psychiatric Times (September), 62–63.

Dusek, D., and Girdano, D. (1995). *Emotional risk factors.* Winter Park, CO: Paradox.

Elkin, A. (1999). *Urban ease: Stress-free living in the big city.* New York: Plume.

Engel, G. (1977). *Emotional stress and sudden death.* Psychology Today, 1, 114–18, 153–54.

Engel, G. (1989). *A clinical guide to the treatment of the human stress response.* New York: Plenum.

Engel, G. (1991). Neurophysiological considerations in the treatment of PTSD: A neurocognitive
perspective. In *International handbook for traumatic stress syndrome,* ed. J. Wilson and B. Raphael.
New York: Plenum, 356.

Fisher, R. (1995). *Getting ready to negotiate.* New York: Penguin.

Fisher, R., Ury, W., and Patton, B. (1991). *Getting to yes: Negotiating without giving in,* 2d ed. New
York: Penguin.

Flannery, R. B. (1993). *Becoming stress resistant.* New York: Continuum.

Friedman, M., Rosenman, R., and Carroll, V. (1958). *Changes in the serum cholesterol and blood clotting
time in men subjected to cyclic variation of occupational stress.* Circulation, 18, 852–61.

Galdston, I. (1954). *Beyond the germ theory.* New York: Health Educational Council.

Girdano, D., and Dusek D. (1988). *Changing health behavior.* Scottsdale, AZ: Gorsuch.

Golub, A. (1996). *Decision analysis: An integrated approach.* New York: John Wiley and Sons.

Heilbroner, R. (1993). Stereotypes, prejudice and discrimination. In *Experiencing race, class, and gender in the United States*, ed. V. Cyrus. Mountain View, CA: Mayfield, 144–45.

Hollingsworth, W. G. (1996). *Ending the explosion.* Santa Ana, CA: Seven Locks Press.

Holm, J., and Holroyd, K. (1992). *The daily hassles scale revised.* Behavioral Assessment, 14, 465–82.

Holmes, T. H., and Rahe, R. H. (1968). *The social readjustment rating scale.* Journal of Psychosomatic Research, 11, 213–18.

Janis, I. L., and Mann, L. (1976). *Decision-making.* Riverside, NJ: Free Press.

Keeney, R. (1996). *Value-focused thinking.* Boston: Harvard University Press.

Kinkade, P., Leone, M., and Semond, S., (1995). *The consequences of jail crowding.* Crime and Delinquency, 41, 150–61.

Kobasa, S. C. (1979). *Stressful life events, personality, and health.* Journal of Personality and Social Psychology, 37, 1–11.

Kohn, P. M., and Macdonald, J. E. (1992). *The survey of recent life experiences.* Journal of Behavioral Medicine, 15, 221–36.

Kompier, M., and Cooper, C. (1999). *Preventing stress, improving productivity.* New York: Routledge.

Koslowsky, M., Kluger, A., and Reich, M., eds. (1995). *Commuting stress: Causes, effects, and methods of coping.* New York: Plenum.

Lazarus, R. S. (1998). *Fifty Years of the research and history of R. S. Lazarus.* Hillsdale, NJ: Lawrence Erlbaum.

Lester, D. (1990). *Overcrowding in prisons and rates of suicide and homicide.* Perceptual and Motor Skills, 70, 274.

Lynch, J. J. (1977). *The broken heart: The medical consequences of loneliness.* New York: Basic Books.

Maddi, S.R. (1996). Personality theories: A comparative analysis. New York: Brooks/Cole.

Maslach, C. and Leiter, M. (1997). *The truth about burnout.* New York: Jossey-Bass.

Milgram, S. (1970). *The experience of living in cities.* Science, 165, 1461–68.

Pelletier, K. R. (1994). *Sound mind, sound body.* New York: Simon and Schuster.

Rahe, R. H. (1967). *Life crisis and health change* (Report No. 67-4). U.S. Navy Bureau of Medicine and Surgery.

Rahe, R. H. (1979). *Life change events and mental illness: An overview.* Journal of Human Stress, 5, 2–10.

Repetti, R. (1993). The effects of working and the social environment at work on health. In *Handbook of stress*, ed. L. Goldberger and S. Breznitz. New York: Free Press, 368–85.

Rosch, P. J. (1998). *Measuring job stress.* American Journal of Health Promotion, 11(6), 400–401.

Rubin, T. I. (1986). *Overcoming indecisiveness.* New York: Avon.

Russo, J. E. (1990). *Decision traps.* New York: Fireside.

Sanders, J. (1998). *Facing loneliness.* New York: Discovery House.

Schaufeli, W., and Enzmann, D. (1998). *The burnout companion to study and practice: A critical analysis.* New York: Taylor and Francis.

Selye, H. (1976). *The stress of life.* New York: McGraw-Hill.

Singer, J. (1975). *Commuter stress.* Science Digest (August), 18–19.

Smith, C. L. (1998). *Computer-supported decision making: Meeting the decision demands of modern organizations.* Norwood, NJ: Ablex.

Stith, A. (1998). *Breaking the glass ceiling: Sexism and racism in corporate America.* New York: Warwich.

Tanner, O. (1976). *Stress.* New York: Time-Life.

Toffler, A. (1970). *Future shock.* New York: Random House.

Tonry, M. and Hamilton, K., eds. (1995). *Intermediate sanctions in overcrowded times.* Chicago: Northeastern University Press.

Welch, S., and Gruhl, J. (1998). *Affirmative action and minority enrollments in medical and law schools.* Ann Arbor: University of Michigan Press.

Wheeler, D. D., and Janis, I. L. (1980). *A practical guide for making decisions.* New York: The Free Press.

Young-Bruehl, E. (1998). *The anatomy of prejudices.* Boston: Harvard University Press.

CHAPTER

8

Stress and the Human Environment Interaction

Human relationships may be responsible for most of our excess stress, but there is also a great potential for excess stress arising from our relationship with the environment. This type of stressor acts through an innate biological mechanism and is less colored by our higher perception and thought. Five classes of environmental stimuli that may play a role in distress are (1) body rhythms, (2) eating and drinking habits, (3) drugs, including alcohol and nicotine, (4) noise pollution, and (5) changes in climate and altitude. We discuss each of these in this chapter.

Time and Body Rhythms

Time has always been recognized as a major stressor. Most people think of deadlines as the only cause of time-related stress. There are, however, other stressful aspects of time. The natural world also runs on time. Solar or light time, lunar time, and seasonal time are but a few examples. The human body also runs on time–temperature time, metabolic time, energy time, and hormonal time (Toates 1998). As social, cultural, and technological beings, we have arrogantly ignored our biological time or rhythm for the sake of convenience and conformity. However, we need to synchronize work and recreation schedules with what is socially and economically efficient. Therefore, we utilize artificial light, and we speed through time zones. All of these things affect the body's natural tempo and rhythm. Undue irritability, emotional instability, and increased susceptibility to illness are the price we pay from being out of phase with the body.

Through the pineal gland the body has a system of adapting to various environmental lighting situations. This is important not only for adapting to the changing seasons but also for adapting to socially imposed environmental changes such as lighting, travel, and shift work. The industrial revolution, maximal production, efficiency, war, and around-the-clock police, fire, and medical attention have all prompted the shift- or night-work concept. The studies conducted on shift workers have shown an increase in accidents between two and four in the morning, accompanied by a decrease in work performance, and police officers are more apt to sleep on duty during these hours. Airline pilots exhibit their quickest reaction time and best psychomotor coordination between two and four in the afternoon and their poorest performance between two and four in the morning. Radar operators are more likely to make errors and have a harder time staying awake during the hours they would normally be asleep. (Have you ever wondered why the airlines offer reduced rates for overnight flights?)

It is not that the body cannot adjust to changes in lighting or time zones; rather, it cannot make the necessary adjustment in the short time usually allowed (Shiftwork Alert Editors 1998). For example, a night worker's body temperature cycle would be expected to be opposite that of a day worker's; yet it usually is not unless the night-shift schedule is maintained for several weeks—long enough for the body to adapt to a new schedule. In many companies a worker may rotate shifts each week, one week working nights and the next week working days. Such rotation does not allow the worker adequate time to adapt.

The recent interest in jet lag has spurred several studies that have found a syndrome of symptoms: headache, gastrointestinal problems including loss of appetite, increased sweating, blurred vision, and alteration of sleep patterns (nightmares, insomnia), with the addition of menstrual difficulties for female flight attendants. This seems to be the price one must pay for making several phase shifts in a short period. These studies have shown that adaptation differs with each body rhythm. For example, it takes five days for urinary electrolytes to adjust to a new schedule, eight days for heart rate, ten days for urinary steroids, and six days for temperature. Concerned and forward-looking companies have increased layover time for airline crews and business travelers, correctly reasoning that the extra cost of room and board is a good investment when weighed against the potential costliness of accidents, poor business decisions, or illness.

Stop here and complete Self-Assessment Exercise 10 before reading the next section.

With jet lag, it is estimated that it takes about twenty-four hours to adjust to each one-hour time difference. Jet travel alters more than sleep-wake cycles; it also affects heart rate, blood pressure, respiration, body temperature, urinary output, hormone secretion, and mental functioning because these are all regulated on a twenty-four-hour cycle. To beat jet lag, it helps to manipulate your blood chemistry by providing proteins that affect the brain's biochemistry in the direction of wakefulness and alertness and by providing carbohydrates that tend to calm the mind and damp out distractions (Anderson and Vail 1998, Inlander and Moran 1997). The following routine is suggested for the day of departure:

> Flying west to east:
>   Exercise in the morning
>   Breakfast and lunch high in protein
>   Dinner and evening snacks high in carbohydrates
> Flying east to west:
>   Carbohydrate breakfast
>   Protein lunch and dinner
>   Exercise in the afternoon

Plan your arrival for the morning so that you have all day to acclimatize by eating and exercising in the manner just given. Exercise raises the body's temperature, so when you arrive in the east in the morning, vigorous exercise helps you wake up. Vigorous exercise in the afternoon when you arrive in the west helps you stay awake past what would be your bedtime at home. Eating fatty foods within the first day or two after your arrival

SELF-ASSESSMENT EXERCISE 10

Choose the most appropriate answer for each of the following ten statements, and place the letter of your response in the space to the left of the question.

_____ 1. How many cups of caffeinated coffee do you drink in an average day?
  a. 0 or 1   c. 4 or 5
  b. 2 or 3   d. more than 5

_____ 2. How many cigarettes do you smoke in an average day?
  a. 0 to 10   c. 21 to 40
  b. 11 to 20   d. more than 40

_____ 3. Do you add salt to your food?
  a. yes   b. no

_____ 4. How many cups of caffeinated tea do you drink in an average day?
  a. 0 or 1   c. 3 or 4
  b. 1 or 2   d. more than 4

_____ 5. How many soft drinks do you consume in an average day?
  a. 0 or 1   c. 3 or 4
  b. 1 or 2   d. more than 4

_____ 6. How much alcohol (liquor, wine, or beer) do you consume during an average week?
  a. 0 to 7 drinks   c. 15 to 21 drinks
  b. 8 to 15 drinks d. more than 21 drinks

_____ 7. Do you eat a nutritionally balanced diet?
  a. no   b. yes

_____ 8. All together, how many pastries, pieces of pie, pieces of cake, donuts, or candy bars do you eat in an average day?
  a. 0   c. 3 or 4
  b. 1 or 2   d. more than 4

_____ 9. Do you eat a well-balanced breakfast most mornings?
  a. no   b. yes

_____10. How many slices of white bread do you eat during an average day?
  a. 0   c. 3 or 4
  b. 1 or 2   d. more than 4

_____ Total Score

Calculate your total score as follows:
For questions 7 and 9
a. = 4 points   b. = 0 points

For all other questions:
a. = 1 point   c. = 3 points
b. = 2 points   d. = 4 points

Place your total score in the space provided and then read the sections "Eating and Drinking Habits" and "Drugs."

counters the effects of a dietary regimen of protein and carbohydrates; alcohol exacerbates the fatigue of jet lag, so it is best to drink alcohol only in the evening, if at all.

Another way to alleviate the stress caused by jet lag is to schedule a buffer day after you arrive at your destination. Use that day to relax and adjust your internal clock.

Eating and Drinking Habits

Everyone knows that good nutrition contributes to healthful living, but few realize the extent to which our eating and drinking habits contribute to our daily stress levels. The consumption or lack of consumption of certain foods and the consumption of some kinds of beverages can add to the stress of everyday life by stimulating the sympathetic stress response directly or by contributing to its stimulation through creating a state of fatigue and increased nervous irritability (Althoff, Svoboda, and Girdano 1996). Either condition lowers your tolerance to the common stresses of day-to-day living. There are several eating and drinking habits that may be involved in stress. Some of the more common ones are examined in this section.

Sympathomimetic Agents

Sympathomimetic agents are chemical substances that mimic the sympathetic stress response. Many foods naturally contain these substances. When consumed, they trigger a stress response in the body, the severity of which will depend on how much of the chemical was consumed. The most common of these sympathomimetic stressors in the modern diet is caffeine, a chemical that belongs to the xanthine group of drugs. Xanthines are powerful amphetamine-like stimulants that increase metabolism and create a highly awake and active state. They also trigger release of the stress hormones that, among other actions, are capable of increasing heart rate, blood pressure, and oxygen demands on the heart. Extreme, prolonged stress-hormone secretion can even initiate myocardial necrosis—that is, destruction of the heart tissue.

Coffee (Coffea arabica) is the most frequently consumed source of caffeine (Dusek and Girdano 1993). Americans over the age of fourteen consume an average of three cups of coffee a day! The average brewed six-ounce cup of coffee contains about 108 milligrams of caffeine. Caffeine consumption of more than 250 milligrams per day is considered excessive and will have an adverse effect on the human body. A lethal dose of caffeine could be consumed in the form of twenty cups of coffee if drunk all at once! Frequent side effects of excessive coffee drinking are anxiety, irritability, diarrhea, arrhythmia (irregular heartbeat), and inability to concentrate, in addition to a host of symptoms characteristic of the stress response. Coffee may also stimulate the secretion of the digestive enzyme and other biochemical substances necessary for arousal and adaptation responses.

During stressful times, high levels of certain vitamins (such as vitamin C and B vitamins) are needed to maintain proper function of the nervous and endocrine systems. They are also called on to help carry out carbohydrate metabolism and gluconeogenesis (the process whereby the body forms glucose for more energy). Vitamin C and choline

TABLE 8.1 Sugar in Common Foods

Food	Portion	Tsp. Sugar*
Chocolate bar	1 average size	7
Chocolate fudge	1½ square	4
Marshmallow	1 average size	1½
Chocolate cake	1⁄12 cake (2-layer, icing)	15
Angelfood cake	1⁄12 cake	6
Doughnut, plain	3″ diameter	4
Brownie	2″ × 2″ × 3/4″	3
Ice cream	½ cup	5–6
Sherbet	½ cup	6–8
Apple pie	⅙ medium pie	12
Cherry pie	⅙ medium pie	14
Pumpkin pie	⅙ medium pie	10
Sweet carbonated beverage	12 oz.	9
Ginger ale	12 oz.	7

*100 grams sugar = 20 teaspoons = 1/2 cup = 3 1/2 ounces = 400 calories

are necessary elements in the production of adrenal hormones, which are secreted during the stress response. Deficiencies of these vitamins lower tolerance to and ability to cope with stressors. In turn, excessive stress over prolonged periods may deplete the body of these vitamins, making an individual more prone to vitamin deficiency.

One common dietary component implicated in depletion of the B-complex vitamins is refined white sugar. Another is refined white flour. Sugar—and therefore sugar products such as cakes, pies, cookies, and candy (see Table 8.1)—is a good source of energy but has no other redeeming feature. For sugar to be utilized for energy, however, the body must have B-complex vitamins. Natural foods that need these vitamins for their metabolism contain the necessary vitamins, but because sugar contains none of them, it must borrow them from other food sources. This may create a B-complex debt in the body. If this borrowing occurs frequently or if the body does not have sufficient sources of B vitamins from nutritious foods or supplements, the result may be a B-vitamin deficiency and symptoms such as anxiety, irritability, and general nervousness. This vitamin depletion may be exacerbated by stress because of the increased utilization of these vitamins in the stress response.

Hypoglycemic Stress

The third way in which diet may predispose an individual to distress is through *hypoglycemia*, or low blood sugar. Symptoms may include anxiety, headache, dizziness, trembling, and increased cardiac activity. These symptoms may cause normal stimuli to become severely acute stressors by making the individual highly irritable and impatient. In effect, they lower the individual's stress tolerance. This is routinely seen in people who get "crabby" when they are hungry. Although there are numerous causes for hypoglycemia, we are most interested in the two directly related to dietary behaviors. Reactive hypoglycemia is caused by high intake of sugars within a limited amount of time. Eating a meal high in sugars or even snacking on foods high in sugars may cause a hypoglycemic reaction in individuals prone to this disorder. Functional hypoglycemia occurs when meals are missed, and it may be exacerbated by sugar intake that results over time in a lower overnight (or fasting) blood-sugar level than would be considered normal.

The process by which such dietary behaviors lead to hypoglycemia is somewhat paradoxical because hypoglycemia is preceded by a state of high blood sugar (hyperglycemia). The high intake of sugar first raises the sugar level in the blood. This high blood-sugar level stimulates the release of insulin (almost instantly), which allows the excess sugar to enter all the body's tissues. Therefore, the blood sugar is not selectively saved for the central nervous system, whose function and vitality depend on it. Generally, if blood-sugar levels drop below 60 milligrams of glucose per 100 milliliters of blood, symptoms such as irritability, anxiety, and fatigue occur.

In extreme cases of high sugar intake, the symptoms of hypoglycemia may occur within a short period and may be so severe as to cause nausea, staggering, slurred and mixed speech, and fainting. Extreme hypoglycemic shock can result in coma and death, but in this situation there is generally some underlying cause, such as a pancreatic tumor or insulin shock, as seen in diabetics. Whether due to perpetual high sugar intake or other physiological conditions, a low blood-sugar level due to hypoglycemia may be responsible for "midmorning slump" and continual hunger that seems to be sated only with sugar products such as cookies, sweet rolls, candy bars, or soft drinks. Because many people eat only a jelly roll, doughnut, or bowl of highly sweetened cereal for breakfast, it is to be expected that low midmorning blood sugar will bring about increased response to stress situations and diminished ability to perform. The same situation may occur in midafternoon or at any other time of day after high sugar intake—or merely from not eating. The best way to avoid the stresses of hypoglycemia and its glucocorticoid stress response is to eat well-balanced meals (the size of which should be determined by the energy demands for the next few hours) containing a minimum of sugar and processed foods.

Sodium Intake and Fluid Retention

Salt (sodium chloride) is the mineral most responsible for regulating the body's water balance. The sodium ion in salt causes retention of water within the body; therefore, high levels of table salt or of foods naturally high in sodium may result in excessive fluid retention. Excessive fluid retention has the effect of increasing nervous tension (through edema, an abnormal accumulation of fluid) in the general nervous tissue and cerebral tissue.

Excess fluid retention can also lead to high blood pressure (Haythornthwaite 1993). In many people, increased blood pressure is the most common manifestation of the stress reaction. However, if a person's blood pressure is already high due to excessive fluid retention, the pressure elevation during distress may reach a danger point. It may become high enough to increase the risk of stroke or heart attack or perhaps become chronically elevated.

The body has the ability to store salt, so daily survival needs are relatively low (less than 1 gram). However, the average person consumes 4 to 8 grams per day (an average shake of salt from the salt shaker is 100 milligrams). A good, nutritious diet provides the necessary daily intake of sodium.

Table 8.2 lists foods high in sodium, and Table 8.3 lists seasonings low in sodium that may be used as substitutes for table salt. Also, many salt substitutes are becoming popular, the most frequently used one being potassium chloride. You can switch to one of the commercial substitutes and derive some of the same taste benefit without risking stress.

TABLE 8.2   Foods High in Sodium

Most Canned Foods	**Cheeses**	**Baking Soda**
meats	processed cheese	(sodium bicarbonate
soups	cheese dips	contains about 1000 mg
stews	snack cheese spreads	of sodium
sauerkraut		per level teaspoon)
Pork Products	**Seasonings**	**Most Fast Food**
ham	prepared mustard	
bacon	catsup	
sausage	Worcestershire sauce	
hot dogs	soy sauce	
	pickles	
Snack Foods	relishes	
pretzels	meat tenderizers	
popcorn	peanut butter (most brands are	
potato chips	heavy in sodium additives)	

As a rule, processed foods contain more sodium than fresh foods.

TABLE 8.3   Seasonings That May Be Used in Low-Sodium Diets

almond extract	ginger	paprika
bay leaf	lemon	parsley
caraway seed	lime	pepper
chili powder	maple extract	pimiento
chives	mint	sage
cinnamon	mustard (dry)	sesame seeds
cloves	nutmeg	thyme
coconut	orange extract	vanilla extract
curry	oregano	vinegar

The conscious manipulation of eating behavior to provide the nutrients essential for fighting stress is called *nutritional restructuring*, and it can be a powerful addition to the holistic pattern for stress control.

Eating Guidelines

To combat everyday stressors and prevent further stress from the foods you have chosen to include in your diet, it is important to develop healthful eating habits. In 1990 a major study in *epidemiology* (the branch of science that studies the causes and control of diseases) disclosed some important nutrition research facts to the public, all of which relate to the effect diet has on stress levels. This study, called the China Health Project (CHP), began in 1983 and tracked the daily living habits of 6500 Chinese in 65 counties across rural China. The study has been called "The Grand Prix of Epidemiology" because of its longitudinal nature (the same people are studied over a period of years), its breadth (it studied a wide range of dietary, environmental, and health factors), and its validity (a very stable population in each of the 65 counties). The people were genetically quite similar within each province, and there was a great deal of ethnic variation from region to region.

The researchers of this study, who were from Cornell University in the United States, Oxford University in England, and two Chinese academies, have confirmed some nutrition-disease relationships that American nutritionists have been hedging on for years. Some of the general results and recommendations of particular importance to stress and disease are the following:

- A high cholesterol level is a major predictor of disease, especially cardiovascular disease.
- Diets high in protein, fat, calories, and calcium are good for early childhood growth but are related to higher breast cancer rates among women later in life.
- A diet high in fiber can protect against colon cancer (a major killer in more affluent societies).
- A vegetable-based diet is completely safe and much healthier than an animal-based diet.

The following recommendations should help make your diet more healthful and less stressful (Harris 1996):

1. Replace animal-based protein with plant-based protein and carbohydrates such as whole grains, beans, and tofu or other look-alike foods such as vegetable- or soy-based burgers and hot dogs.
2. Cut down on dairy consumption by substituting soy beverage for milk, tofu for cheese, soy- or fruit-based desserts for ice cream, and fruit preserves for butter.
3. Shop more frequently, and buy fresh foods. Buy locally grown foods when possible.
4. If you have to eat in a fast-food restaurant, choose salads, vegetables, pasta, and potatoes rather than the high-fat foods.

5. Eat smaller meals evenly spaced rather than loading up on dinner (or any one other meal).
6. Plan your daily menu each morning, and save time by preparing ahead for dinner, including such tasks as soaking beans.
7. Change your eating habits slowly, incorporating one thing at a time. Note how your health changes with your dietary changes.
8. Buy a good vegetarian cookbook and/or take a cooking class featuring vegetable-based foods.

The USDA Food Guide Pyramid (1992) also provides a general guide to healthful eating (see Figure 8.1). At the base of the pyramid are the foods that should be consumed in the greatest amounts: 6–11 servings per day of breads, cereal, rice, and pasta. The next layer on the pyramid is vegetables (3–5 servings) and fruits (2–4 servings). The pyramid gets smaller as the next layer of milk, yogurt, and cheese (2–3 servings), and red meat, poultry, fish, dried beans, eggs, and nuts (2–3 servings) is added. At the small peak of the pyramid are fats, oils, and sweets, to be eaten sparingly.

The food pyramid gives only general guidelines and must be modified to fit the caloric needs of each individual. Within each category, there are additional health rules (Moog 1993; Harris 1996).

Bread, cereal, rice, and pasta group: Use a variety of whole-grain products and prepare them with little or no fat or sugars.

Vegetable group: Eat at least one cruciferous vegetable per day (broccoli, cauliflower, cabbage, etc.) and at least one vegetable that is high in beta-carotene (broccoli, tomato, carrots, etc.).

Fruit group: Eat fresh fruits in season, preferably raw rather than canned in syrup or cooked as a sauce. Red and orange fruits are high in beta-carotene.

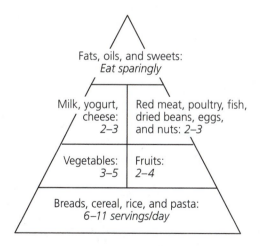

FIGURE 8.1 USDA Food Guide Pyramid

Milk, yogurt, and cheese group: Choose low- or no-fat dairy products.

Red meat, poultry, fish, dried beans, eggs, and nuts group: Avoid fatty red meat and poultry; prepare meats by broiling or grilling rather than frying.

Fats, oils, and sweets group: Use vegetable oils in moderation, remove animal fats from the diet as much as possible, and don't load up on sweets at any one time.

Drugs, Alcohol, and Tobacco

Drugs. Although people take drugs (including alcohol) for various reasons, a common motive is to get "high" or experience an altered state of consciousness, often in an attempt to reduce stress. An altered state can be defined as a deviation from the "normal" state of consciousness, in which most of us communicate, are goal-directed, and use rational, cause-and-effect thinking. Figure 8.2 shows some ways states of consciousness may be altered.

The sense of unreality and lack of self-awareness that result from some forms of drug use may be calming in the sense that the drug temporarily blocks one from actively thinking about a problem. Unfortunately, the problem still exists. It is stored in parts of the brain and is producing feelings and other body alterations even though the drug-taker is not actively aware of them. The psychoactive drugs, both legal and illegal, typically consumed to promote relaxation, do not change body physiology. Problems are still present and continue to stress the system. The only difference is that the flow of active, here-and-now thoughts has been temporarily blocked. The feelings of self-transcendence vanish once the drugs wear off and can be regained only by repeated use of the drug. There is little positive carryover, little is learned in the drug state, and few people experience long-term positive change from the drug experience. Their world, their problems, and their coping mechanisms are the same as

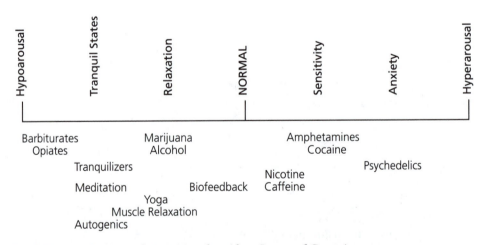

FIGURE 8.2   Drugs and Activities that Alter States of Consciousness

before. Drugs have fulfilled a limited goal, an altered state of consciousness, but they have not fulfilled the dream—that the experience would somehow grant the user greater insights and the ability to naturally transcend the ego and live a calmer, more relaxed and enlightened life.

The passivity of the drug experience is in itself a drawback. Experiences in which the individual just rides along, seeing, feeling, and experiencing are somehow not as satisfying as those in which the individual is the active, creative center of the experience. Creative activities increase one's self-esteem and in a circular pattern increase motivation and readiness for future unknown ventures.

An altered state can also be induced through such activities as meditation and daydreaming or by hypoarousal or hyperarousal of the central nervous system. It is healthier to induce these states by mind direction than by using drugs. There are many popular techniques for inducing a self-transcendent, altered state of consciousness through mind direction or control. Yoga, meditation, muscle relaxation, autogenic training, and biofeedback are but a few examples. These constitute a more positive approach than drugs, not only because they are less dangerous, more socially acceptable, and more controllable but also because they are active and creative, requiring and promoting self-control and self-discipline. They are learning exercises that result in temporary feelings of self-transcendence, thus providing the foundation and motivation to reeducate one's thoughts and coping processes. If mastered, they lead to an even higher state—that of conscious self-transcendence, a less conscious, or self-expanded state in which boundaries are infinitely extended. This is a health-promoting state because it is integrated with ongoing life and provides benefits to the individual, society, and humankind in general.

Research in the 1990s has offered strong evidence that two common "oral" habits, cigarette smoking and caffeine consumption, may be highly deleterious to health, either singly or when combined and that much of this effect is attributable to excessive stress.

Go back to Self-Assessment Exercise 10 and examine items 1, 2, 4, and 5 (if the soft drinks contain caffeine). If you responded with c's or d's for those items, your diet could be hurting your health, regardless of your total score on the exercise.

Throughout history, people have used drugs and become dependent on them. During the twentieth century, however, drug use and abuse reached epidemic proportions. No one reason can be offered as an explanation. However, the most often mentioned reason was a way to cope with stress.

Whatever the reason, researchers have found that each type of drug produces a specific psychological state, or an altered reality, and that chronic users choose a specific drug because of the state it induces. From the first experience of an altered state, the person may or may not seek that experience again. If the reason is "just to see what it's like," the person's motivation is experimental or curiosity. If the altered state is sought repeatedly, the motivation changes. It may be for perceived pleasure, escape from a world that seems stressful, or to satisfy physical and psychological addictions. Compulsive users find that virtually every aspect of their lives revolves around obtaining, maintaining, and using the drug. These individuals, described as being drug dependent, are controlled physically, psychologically, and socially by their drug habit.

Although that does not seem like competent coping to most of us, it actually is a coping mechanism to those in the cycle because it is predictable and makes many stressful decisions for the individual.

Drug rehabilitation research has documented lack of self-identity as a deep-seated cause of drug abuse. This is a common theme for individuals who also experience excess stress as well. In contrast, people who are comfortable with who they are are less inclined to try to alter their self-perception through drugs. Many drug and alcohol rehabilitation programs are aimed specifically at the formation of a positive identity (Gerstein and Lewin 1990; Sales 1999).

Alcohol.   The human organism does not require alcohol, yet throughout history alcohol has been an integral part of life in most parts of the world. Alcohol has gained the reputation as the ultimate stress-relieving drug, and relaxation and recreation are the most often cited reason for consuming it. Political leaders celebrate important agreements with a toast. Glasses are raised to toast the bride and groom and the New Year. Elaborate establishments are built to provide places to gather and consume alcohol. The average household contains some form of alcoholic beverage. In the United States a temporary prohibition of alcohol from 1920 to 1933 produced the largest episode of civil disobedience in the U. S. history. Alcohol is not consumed only when one feels deviant or defiant. It is not used only to mask stress, insecurity, or depression or to give a person courage. It is a cultural adjunct. To some extent and for some people, alcohol consumption is pleasant and pleasurable. For many others, however, especially people with emotional problems and those who overindulge, alcohol presents a problem—a self-inflicted, individual problem for which society as a whole pays a great price (Sales 1999).

You can protect yourself from alcohol abuse in several ways. Best advice: Don't drink at all if you have any reason to suspect that you are prone to alcohol abuse. Second best: Drink in moderation. Don't glorify alcohol or your ability to consume it. Learn to recognize the signs of overdrinking and use these as a signal to slow down. Common signs are loud talking, slurred speech, walking unsteadily, dropping things or spilling drinks, perspiring, turning red or pale in the face.

Don't drink and drive. Car pool, select a designated driver who will not drink, call a friend, take a taxi, hitch a ride, or stay the night. Don't let your friends drive if they've been drinking. Stay in control. Learn how to keep track of your blood alcohol level by knowing your weight, the amount of alcohol you've consumed, and your drinking time. Keep yourself busy with interesting and active pursuits. Avoid friends who do little else besides drink for their recreation.

If you find that you are:

- drinking, even in moderation, every day
- in a habit of constantly talking about your drunken exploits
- arriving late at work or missing early classes because of hangovers
- getting drunk regularly
- drinking to dull the hurt of loneliness and to counteract frequent depression
- driving after drinking
- needing to brag constantly about your ability to drink,

you should seriously consider cutting down on how much and how often you drink, for you are developing an addictive behavior pattern. If cutting down is difficult for you to do alone, seek help. NOW. Talk to your doctor or a counselor about the possibility that you are drinking too much. Be honest. If you aren't comfortable in doing this, look up the telephone number for Alcoholics Anonymous (AA) and call. Ask how you can tell whether you are drinking too much and whether AA can assist you in finding help (Brown and Lewis 1999, Dusek and Girdano 1993, Meyers and Smith 1999).

To avoid slipping past a pleasurable social interaction into intoxication for you and your guests at parties and other recreational functions, try some of these suggestions:

- The party atmosphere should be relaxing, and whatever can be done to make everyone mix should be done. One reason people drink too much at social gatherings is that they cannot seem to get conversations going.

- The volume of music should be low enough to allow people to socialize. Again, when you cannot talk, you drink more.

- Food should be served. It not only slows down the absorption of alcohol but also satisfies some oral needs to supplant the continual sipping of drinks. Good food also takes some of the spotlight off alcohol. Foods that have some protein content are best: for example, cheese and crackers, Swedish meatballs, hard-boiled eggs, cheese fondue, pizza, and bite-sized cold cuts.

- Activities should be going on, with some effort to get everyone involved. Dancing, games, sports, and good conversation quickly become the focus, and drinks become supplementary only.

Tobacco.   The final consideration in this section is the use of tobacco products. The harmful effects of smoking and chewing tobacco are well known. Less known is how the drug nicotine contributes to distress. Nicotine stimulates the adrenals, which release hormones that elicit the stress response—increased heart rate, force of cardiac contraction, blood pressure, respiration rate, and release of fatty acids and glucose into the blood, among other body reactions (Lee and Lee 1997).

Tobacco contains nicotine. Like caffeine, nicotine is a sympathomimetic chemical, and as such it is capable of stimulating all the adverse effects of the arousal response noted earlier. It causes a stress response each time it is taken into the body, whether by smoking a cigarette, inhaling the smoke of others, or chewing tobacco. The smoker and the person facing almost any everyday stressors exhibit the same physiological state. One difference is that the chronic smoker's physiological functioning is continually elevated to the point where this arousal state becomes the "normal" state. Being without the stimulating effect of nicotine creates a mild depression and a generally uneasy feeling that lead to the desire for additional nicotine for a pickup. As the chronic smoking habit develops, the stress tolerance to nicotine is increased, and the adverse stress-related effects become somewhat reduced, but the constituents of the smoke continue to affect the smoker's respiratory system. They also affect the nonsmoker. Because the nonsmoker has developed little if any tolerance to nicotine, the smoke can cause decreases in work performance. A smoky working area can irritate the nonsmoker's eyes and nose, impeding detail work, concentration, and tolerance for more difficult work tasks.

Following alcohol, the nicotine present in tobacco is the second most widely used drug in the world. Nicotine meets the established scientific criteria for classification as a dependency-producing drug. Tobacco use, like use of other abused drugs, often is peer initiated, and the primary reason given for its use is again pleasure and relief from stress. Social support for tobacco use allows for tolerance and habitual patterns to develop with repeated use. Tobacco use may produce both psychological and physical dependence. Quitting smoking is one of the more difficult dependencies to end, perhaps because smoking was acceptable for so long, and smokers developed the dependency early and continued it for decades. Smoking cessation treatment results in short-term success rates as high as 70 percent, but these rates decrease significantly to an average of between 6 percent and 15 percent one year later. The reasons some people succeed and others fail are not well understood, but many researchers believe that success is a result of a combination of personal motivation, an effective plan of action, and not trying to quit during periods of high stress.

Successful smoking cessation programs tend to include the following core elements (Girdano and Dusek 1988):

1. Healthful lifestyle. An essential component of an effective program often is not included in smoking cessation programs, and this oversight undoubtedly contributes to the high failure rates. This phase focuses on psychological needs that smoking traditionally has satisfied. The goal is to extinguish these needs and develop lifestyle skills that will help the nonsmoker remain a nonsmoker. The basic components are as follows:
2. Relaxation and stress management skills. Part of almost every smoker's habit is the use of cigarettes to control one or more of the following factors: excess anxiety, low self-esteem, excess anger, depression, a stressful lifestyle, and the inability to relax.
3. Diet. Many smokers are nervous eaters who have substituted smoking for eating; often, when smoking stops, eating and weight gain problems emerge. This creates fear in weight-conscious smokers. Close attention to diet and weight-management counseling are essential to the success of most smoking cessation programs.
4. Exercise. Exercise not only is integral to a healthful lifestyle but also may be essential to smoking cessation programs because it builds confidence and self-esteem, reduces anxiety and excess stress, burns calories, and is antithetical to the physical deterioration caused by smoking.

Noise Pollution

The study of noise as a stressor is somewhat complex because noise, more than the other environmental stressors examined in this chapter, has a strong social component (Blair 1998). Noise can produce a stress response by doing one or more of the following:

1. stimulating the sympathetic nervous system
2. being annoying and subjectively displeasing
3. disrupting activities

Noise also has a psychological aspect: It may be perceived as unwanted or somehow inappropriate. This reaction—and the accompanying stress response—can occur at any frequency level. For example, a conversation at a distance of three feet generates only about sixty decibels, far below the pain threshold; yet if you are trying to figure out your income tax or study for a final exam, this conversation could be highly stressful because it disrupts your activity. Similarly, what may be music to you may be noise to someone else. Thus, the music you play every day and find relaxing might be very annoying, and thus stressful, to another.

Whether noise has a predominantly physical or psychological effect, it is clearly capable of producing the stress response. Research has demonstrated that noise can produce cardiovascular changes. Studies of the effects of noise on blood circulation found that acute exposure to moderately high noise frequencies was capable of decreasing circulation to the arms, legs, hands, and feet. A more recent study discovered that repeated exposure to noise may result in a permanent rise in blood pressure due to structural adaptation of the heart and blood vessels. Finally, studies in an industrial environment demonstrated that workers exposed to moderate and high levels of noise had higher blood levels of the stress hormones. Such findings prompted the National Institute for Occupational Safety and Health (NIOSH) to go on record stating that noise is capable of stimulating changes in essential physiological functioning suggestive of a general stress reaction (1977). Workers under noisy conditions tend to suffer from shorter concentration spans and a lower frustration threshold. The U.S. Department of Labor has stated that government employees should not be exposed to steady noise levels in excess of ninety decibels per eight-hour day. Table 8.4 gives the noise level of various activities.

Finally, we should consider adaptation to noise. Adaptation requires energy and therefore can deplete the body of biological and psychological stamina. Selye (1976) notes that, although humans can adapt to stressors, they ultimately pay the price in biological depletion and, should the exposure become chronic, in eventual breakdown. It appears that prolonged exposure to noise can have physiologically and psychologically damaging effects on the human organism. Prolonged loud noise results in the diminished capability to hear.

Learning to avoid loud, obnoxious sounds is an effective stress management tool. There are several ways to remove yourself from the harm of noise: (1) remove yourself from the noisy environment; (2) protect yourself with earplugs while staying in the noisy environment; (3) avoid noisy environments whenever you have a choice; and (4) assert your right to have a quiet environment when others are encroaching on your boundaries.

TABLE 8.4   Noise Levels (in Decibels) of Various Activities

Sound	Decibel Level
Jet takeoff from 200 feet	140 dB
	120 (painful to humans)
Rock music	110
Automobile horn from 3 feet	110 (extremely loud)
Motorcycle	100
Garbage truck	100
Pneumatic drill	90
Lawn mower	90
Heavy traffic	80
Alarm clock	80
Shouting, arguing	80 (very loud)
Vacuum cleaner	75 (loud)
Freight train from 50 feet	70
Freeway traffic	65
Normal conversation	60
Light automobile traffic	50 (moderate)
Library	40
Soft whisper	30 (faint)

Music Therapy

Sound has a major impact on all of us. Soft ballads soothe us, anthems stir us, heavy metal sends some into a frenzy. It is natural that therapists have adopted sound and music for a variety of therapeutic uses.

Music therapy can reduce heart rate, blood pressure, pain, and anxiety. In hospitals, music is used to help alleviate pain, improve patients' moods and counteract depression, promote movement during physical rehabilitation, calm or sedate, induce sleep, counteract fear, and reduce muscle tension. In nursing homes, it is used to boost the residents' level of physical, mental, and social functioning.

There has been little if any scientific testing of music therapy, and the few available reviews are quite mixed. The treatments are unlikely to cause harm unless they are used as substitutes for proven therapies. However, they may not be extremely helpful, either.

Music therapy ranges from listening to music to improvising tunes, writing songs, discussing lyrics, performing compositions, using music and imagery, and learning through music. Because music therapy is used in so many different ways, there is no one typical approach. Music intended for relaxation should have about 70 to 80 beats per minute, similar to the heart rate. A faster beat may create tension. It should be low in pitch because a high pitch also fosters tension. Volume should be kept low because high volume can cause pain. When used to reduce anxiety, music should have a slow, steady rhythm, a low pitch, liberal orchestration, and relaxing melodies. Instrumental selections are considered more effective than vocal music because patients may focus on words and their meaning rather than relaxing with the music (Cassileth, 1999).

Climate and Altitude

When the body is exposed to changes in temperature, humidity, and altitude, it responds with stress arousal and then goes into the resistance phase, which readies it for prolonged exposure to the stressor. Carrying the concept of the general adaptation syndrome to completion, if the exposure to the stressor is too extreme or continues too long, the body can no longer protect itself, and the individual perishes. Every winter in the mountains, hunters, snowmobilers, skiers, and others become lost, disabled, or caught in an avalanche and suffer from frostbite or hypothermia as a result of the low temperatures, the altitude, or both. Likewise, fall football practice may take its toll in heat prostration or heat stroke.

Many skiers or summer vacationers from the "flatlands" arrive at high altitudes and want to perform the same as they do at home. Oxygen is not as available to the cardiovascular and muscular systems at these higher altitudes, so demands on these systems must be reduced. Preparing both of these systems before vacation time helps alleviate some of the altitude stress.

The sun is also a factor, especially when rays are reflected off snow or water. A total sun block or high-sun-protection-factor lotion is a must, especially for winter vacationers who have not exposed their skin to the sun since the previous summer.

Altitude sickness also hampers many mountain visitors. It is especially exacerbated by sudden changes to a higher altitude and by drinking alcohol.

Ask an athlete from the Colorado mountains what it is like to compete in the summer heat and humidity of Florida. Just as change in altitude causes stress, so does change in climate (to a hotter, colder, drier, wetter, more humid, or less humid place).

Cold climates demand special clothing. Down-filled or other insulating outerwear, polypropylene or wool underwear, and wool outerwear are especially suited to cold weather. Dress in layers with wool or some other "wicking" material next to the skin to take the perspiration away from the skin and the material next to the skin. (Winter sports enthusiasts know that cotton kills through hypothermia.) A warm hat, a good pair of gloves or mittens with glove liners, and insulated boots are also necessary for comfort in cold climates. If the weather is bitterly cold (either ambient temperature or because of added wind-chill factor), a scarf and/or face mask may also be helpful in staying safe and comfortable while outside.

Hot and humid climates are especially stressful to those who are not acclimated to them. When traveling in these conditions, slow down activity until some acclimation occurs. Because of fluid loss, drink ample liquids, especially good, clear water. Some water-soluble vitamins are lost through sweating, so it is best to maintain adequate intake of the B vitamins and vitamin C. Because potassium and sodium are necessary for water balance in the body, intake of these minerals should also be monitored. A good, balanced diet of fresh fruits and vegetables, calcium-rich foods, whole-grain products, and fish or lean meats normally provides the vitamins and minerals needed for maintaining water balance in the body.

Dry climates also demand that one focus on water balance and care of the skin. However, dry skin does not necessarily mean that low humidity is the culprit. Healthy skin protects itself with natural oils, the production of which is at least in part dependent on the presence of the water-soluble vitamins A, D, E, and K. When the skin cannot lubricate itself, a good natural moisturizer is called for.

SOURCES CITED

Althoff, S., Svoboda, M., and Girdano, D. (1996). *Choices in health and fitness.* Scottsdale, AZ: Gorsuch and Scarisbrick.

Anderson, N., and Vail, R. (1998). *The backseat flyer.* New York: Safe Goods.

Blair, C., ed. (1998). *Garbage and other pollutions.* New York: Information Plus.

Brown, S., and Lewis, V. (1999). *The alcoholic family in recovery.* New York: Guilford Press.

Cassileth, B. R. (1999) *The alternative medicine handbook.* New York: W. W. Norton.

Chen, J., Campbell, T. C., Li, J., and Peto, R., (1990). *Diet, lifestyle and mortality in China: A study of the characteristics of 65 counties.* Ithaca, NY: Cornell University Press.

Costs of Illegal Drug Use, The (1992). In *Drugs, crime and the justice system: A national report from the Bureau of Justice Statistics.* Washington, D.C.: U.S. Government Printing Office.

Dusek, D., and Girdano, D. (1993). *Drugs: A factual account,* 5th ed. New York: McGraw-Hill.

Gerstein, D. R., and Lewin, L. S. (1990). *Special report: Treating drug problems.* New England Journal of Medicine, 323, 14–18.

Girdano, D., and Dusek, D. (1988). Smoking cessation. In *Changing health behavior.* Scottsdale, AZ: Gorsuch and Scarisbrick, 215–38.

Harris, D. (1996). *Diet and nutrition sourcebook.* Ft. Lauderdale, FL: Omnigraphics.

Haythornthwaite, J. A. (1993). *Behavioral stress, sodium intake and blood pressure.* Homeostasis in Heath and Disease, 34, 302–12.

Inlander, C. and Moran, C. (1997). *Sixty-two natural ways to beat jet lag.* New York: St. Martins Mass Market.

Lee, R. S. and Lee, M. P. (1997). *Caffeine and nicotine.* Center City, MN: Hazelden Information Education.

Mead, N. (1990). *The champion diet.* East/West Journal (September), 45–50, 98–104.

Meyers, R. J., and Smith, J. E. (1999). *Clinical guide to alcohol treatment.* New York: Guilford Press.

Moog, S. (1993). *A guide to the food pyramid.* Freedom, CA: Crossing Press.

NIOSH. (1977). *Occupational diseases: A guide to their recognition.* U.S. Printing Office, Washington, D.C.

Sales, P. (1999). *Alcohol abuse: Straight talk, straight answers.* Calabasas, CA: IXIA Publications.

Selye, H. (1976). *The stress of life.* New York: McGraw-Hill.

Shiftwork Alert Editors (1998). *The practical guide to managing 24-hour operations.* Cambridge: Circadian Information.

Toates, F. (1998). *Control of behavior (biology, brain, and behavior).* New York: Springer Verlag.

U.S. Department of Agriculture (1992). *The food guide pyramid.* Washington, D.C.: USDA.

CHAPTER

9

Stress in Relationships

We initiated the discussion on relationships in the very first chapter of this book because we believe that relationships are the proving grounds upon which we show how well we have learned to manage stress. The greatest challenge to your serenity is human relationships: intimate partners, friends, children, parents, employers, co-workers, teachers, siblings, even campus cops and store clerks. However, nowhere are emotions so raw and vulnerable as in love relationships.

All of the issues discussed in the last few chapters such as self-esteem, anxiety, decision-making, patterns of behavior, and so on will definitely influence how well you handle that stress. Stress in human relationships comes from a combination of failure to meet the expectations of others and failure to get your needs met. Intimate relationships test us on such issues as loyalty, values, morals, defending lifestyle choices, competition, rivalry, compatibility, jealousy, and control.

Love

Violins and valentines, roses and romance—this is the stuff relationships are made of. Or is it? It is difficult to pin down because love, romance, and relationships are some of the most intangible phenomena known to humanity. Love itself completely defies definition, for it is not a product of a logical, analytical, left side of the brain. Love emanates from the right side of brain, which feels rather than thinks. Although the two sides of the brain do communicate well with each other, feelings cannot be described adequately; only the expression or outward behavior caused by the feeling can be explained. One of humanity's greatest frustrations throughout history has been the inability to define and explained feelings, especially love. That, of course has been a boon to poets, Valentine's Day card manufactures, florists, and others who make a living from our inability to express the feelings we have for that special person in our life.

Love is like a stimulant drug. It lifts our spirits and makes us giddy, and the crash from a lost love is comparable to the depression that follows the withdrawal from a powerful drug. In between are the highs and lows, trials and tribulations of stress and serenity that make our emotions feel like the amusement park roller coaster ride. Actually, there are degrees and stages of love. Being in love occurs at the beginning of a relationship. This stage is an exhilarating druglike high. After a period of time, the "in love" stage fades, and a couple either breaks up or develops what is referred to as second-stage or mature love. This kind of love is what sustains a relationship or marriage. Although everyone is capable of this type of love, some people never do accomplish it, for they seem so disappointed that the "in love" period is over that they work to destroy the relationship in order to find another person to fall in love with. These people must have the druglike high to be happy; thus they continuously seek new partners and experience merry-go-round romances. Obviously, for these people relationships are constant sources of stress in their lives. (See table 9.1.)

You probably know some people who are continually jumping in and out of relationships. They are the ones who just seem to love falling in love and do not seem able to develop mature love. Usually those who need to be always "in love" cannot stay with any one relationship for long. They ride the adrenaline-filled, breathless high of being in love until it wanes and wears out; then they seek a new source for another high. Their egos are tremendously inflated with the bombardment of positive strokes, only to be deflated again during the inevitable burnout and separation phase. They're not able to make the transition to a mature love and thus are robbed of the happiness that comes from building a strong foundation of mutual support. Their love life goes around and around but stays in the same place. They slow down periodically to pick up a new partner. It is interesting to contemplate how such a positive emotion can result in such confusion and pain when it is lost.

Freud described human psychosocial development in terms of six stages of love: narcissistic love in infancy, imitated love in the first few years, Oedipal love between the ages of four and seven, homosexual love in later childhood, idealistic love at puberty, and heterosexual love in early adultdhood. Children first learn how and whom to love from those who provide pleasure, security, or relief from pain; later they learn how to voluntarily control and inhibit expressions of love according to personal feelings and social dictates. In essence, this process is one of learning the voluntary control over a basic emotion: love. If you inhibit the expression of love, you may eventually lose the ability to feel the emotion. If you overcontrol it, you may begin to manipulate it. The result is that an involuntary, natural phenomenon becomes a servant of the logical, analytical self; love becomes a servant of the social psychological self: I will love you if . . . I will love you when . . . In this way love becomes conditional: I will love you if you are pretty, . . . thin . . . smart . . . kind . . . obedient . . . I will love you if you love me, or when I need you, or when I am not busy, or when I am not angry with you (Bailey 1995).

As we learn what and whom to love and when to love, love may become a consciously and subconsciously manipulated commodity—because it has so many conditions attached to it—a scarce commodity. And we may learn to save it for a certain person to show that person and us that this relationship is indeed special.

So we learn voluntary control over the outward expression of love, and to a large degree, the inner feelings of love as well. We maintain that control most of the time. At other times our natural physical emotions break through. We may fall in love with the "wrong person" at the "wrong time." Wrong person means someone who does not fit our "I will love you if . . ." criteria or someone other than our established partner; and "wrong time," a time in which we cannot afford to make lifestyle decisions or changes based on love. After reading the chapter on emotions and stress, we can understand how this roller coaster of emotions—the frustration and the anger of not getting expectations met and the fear of not being loved—can create intense stress in our lives (Fisher 1994).

TABLE 9.1   People in Love

People in Love

According to Nathaniel Branden (1981), people who are in love exhibit the following traits:

- They express love verbally.
- They are physically affectionate with each other.
- They express their love sexually, making love frequently.
- They express their appreciation and admiration for one another.
- They participate in mutual self-disclosure, sharing more of themselves and their inner lives with each other than with any other person.

- They offer each other an emotional support system, being there for each other in illness, difficulty, hardship, and crisis.
- They express love materially, with big or small gifts, but on more than the routine occasions, or with tasks performed to lighten the other's burden.
- They accept demands or put up with short-comings that would be less acceptable in another person.
- They create time to be alone together.

Relationships

It has been said that staying together is a matter of chemistry, the mixing together of true personalities in a social and cultural milieu. It is very difficult to predict which two people will be able to maintain a relationship. Some people tire of sameness (same partner, same job, same city), whereas others thrive on it. Some people do not seek change or excitement and avoid harmony and turmoil like the plague. They are stable people who find pleasure in security and predictability. It may be that they are terrifically adaptable and can roll with whatever adversity befalls them, or they may be so terribly dependent that they find it impossible to separate themselves from their crutches. In a society such as ours, which externally glorifies the ability to keep a relationship together, many people stay together out of fear of social recrimination. Breaking up is considered to be an admission of failure; and even though times are changing, staying together is still seen as a sign of stability and a mark of success. Staying together without love or in the face of great adversity is extremely stressful.

Relationships are said to have three phases: (1) physical; (2) psychological; and (3) philosophical, or spiritual. The physical is the most obvious. The physical attraction meets our biological needs and our emotional needs for closeness. It provides us with the feelings of being touched and cared for. The physical relationship provides the motivation and energy to stay in contact long enough to get to know one another. Physical closeness also provides a demonstrative way to heal hurts. In the most basic form, it is necessary for the reproduction of the species. This is the "in love" stage that we spoke of earlier.

Physical intimacy has its dark side. Sometimes we become too attached to a person and stay with the relationship longer than otherwise might be beneficial to both. That is assuming you accept the concept that hurt feelings are negative and not a growing experience. Also a negative aspect to the physical is that when we becomes less attractive and attached to the other person or bored with the same person, physical intimacy suffers. Absence of that is a source for anger and its companions: withholding, passive aggressiveness, and guilt (Harley, 1997). By now you recognize these behaviors as sources of emotional paths of stress and unhappiness.

The psychological phase of relationships, likewise, has its positive and negative sides. Relationships are the best proving ground for achievement of the mastery of life skills. If you are loved, you are important, touched, listened to, and taken care of, all of which boost self-esteem. Plus, you are not alone, not bored, and have a partner with whom to share your mutual dreams, if such exist.

We are attracted to another person and desire them in our lives because they fill a perceived need. Introverts often are attracted to extroverts. They recognize that they need some extroversion in their lives, so they are attracted to that person. On a subconscious level they find it easier to couple with the desired trait than develop it themselves. Often a relationship becomes a substitution for self-development, and because self-development is life's path, you have an eventual confrontation with your self. Some philosophers call this an existential crisis. Letting the other person really know you and still love what they come to know is the ultimate gamble. We are looking for unconditional love, rather like the way your mother loved you, or loves you—only better, but that is a nearly impossible situation in relationships.

What stops love and kills relationships? One love-stopper is when love is offered only to get love in return: "I'll love you if you love me," in which love is offered as a barter and not as a gift. I will love you if you are good to me, or I will love you as long as you fit my expectations of the perfect partner. What consumes most of the time and energy in relationships is trying to shape other people to fit our idea of a perfect partner. Another killer is guilt: the chief tool to keep one's partner in line. The message usually given to the partner is, "If you do this behavior, I will feel bad, and you will hurt me." The other person internalizes the message, "If I hurt you, I feel bad" (and subsequently guilty). Guilt is a suppressed form of anger, so when we succumb to the guilt game, we are really feeling angry with the one who created the situation. We have learned that anger is not acceptable, but guilt somehow is. You get to feel bad about yourself, and if you know how to also play the game, your guilt behavior will be so bad that your partner will feel guilty!

Equally devastating to a relationship is trying to make ourselves fit our own image of what we think we should be to our partner or how we should conduct ourselves in the relationship. This is not to say we should not try to please our partner. However, if we are trying too hard to be the perfect partner, and it goes against our natural tendencies and creates a strain. It is as if we are saying to ourselves we are not good enough the way that we are.

The third aspect of relationships, the philosophical or spiritual aspect, is the hope that the heart's eye can see the soul of the other person and understand their dream. You need to know your dreams and theirs and respect each other's dreams and understand each other's path and lovingly help them get where they want to go. Sometimes we cannot directly help with the other person's dream. Sometimes we can. However, we must determine whether our gifts are the ones we are most authentically able to give. If we try to give gifts we cannot easily give, we end up "sacrificing" ourselves for their dream, which will only make us more miserable.

It is interesting to note that the word "sacrifice" actually means "to make sacred." It has been changed into a term that means to give up what you care for so someone or something else can get what they want. The highest form of love is sacred. And it never dies. It is called unconditional love because it does indeed come without condition. What most people commonly call a love relationship is not unconditional at all. It is filled with the expectation that the other person will fulfill their needs.

Dreams are real life, the part of life that really sustains us. One needs the energy to want a fulfilling relationship. Many people do not have even this. They are willing to live quiet lives of discontent. Additionally, one needs the energy to do what needs to be done to make it work. There are seldom quick fixes and miracles to change our lives and make all that is wrong right and change effortlessly to a new course. Like anything else, it is step-by-step work that needs to be done. However, if it is a path with heart, it flows effortlessly.

Happiness comes from looking at what you want to be and moving toward that dream. Perhaps the real essence of life is not logical or even observable. Science cannot predict or explain dreams; perhaps they are the soul's calling. To reach for a dream, you must have the energy for the extra effort needed to excel, to work harder to really understand and to apply it to your lives, to recognize that your dream can coexist with a special someone and their dream. And that life can be lived with passion, excitement, and wonder.

The trials and tribulations, the joys and anguish of relationships, or the absence thereof are but other forms of the wake-up call we have been referring to in this book as stress. The ultimate question to ask regarding a relationship is, "What do I want to become in this relationship?" You are the only one who knows that (for help, see Table 9.2).

TABLE 9.2   Finding Mr./Ms. Right: Being Mr./Ms. Right

Finding Mr./Ms. Right: Being Mr./Ms. Right

The work of finding the right partner starts with some realistic and honest soul searching. When a few great dates turn into an almost constant togetherness, you should come up for air long enough to assess the situation. Logically, how does this relationship stack up?

- How do you feel about yourself when you are with this person?
- Does he/she bring out the best in you, or do you feel inhibited, put down, confined? Does this person energize you or drain your energy when you are with them and after you have been with them?
- How does your partner feel about himself/herself?
- How do you feel about yourself?
- How well does your partner express feelings and emotions?
- How well does this person let his or her needs and wants be known?
- Does this person give you positive feedback frequently?

- Is he/she able to express appreciation, affection, and caring by word, deed, and touch?
- How does this person handle anger, conflict, and differences? Is he/she placating, explosive, and sulking?
- Are this person's goals, values, and viewpoints on life generally similar to yours? More specifically, what are their attitudes toward money, sex, fidelity, roles, children? Have you ever discussed these topics?
- What changes would you like to see this person make?
- What changes would this person like to see you make?

Making a Relationship Work

No one really knows the exact ingredients for a successful relationship between any two people, but one thing is known: Whether as a result of a conscious effort by the couple or a natural way of relating, most successful relationships seemed to possess the following qualities: love, independence, self-authenticity, openness and honesty, room for personal growth, and personal freedom.

First, there must be love. Obviously you cannot have a love relationship without love. After a relationship stales due to "incompatibility," there is a tendency to try to save it by appealing to logic, to stay with a person with whom we should be able to make a go of it. No matter how intelligent, handsome, or beautiful the other person is, no matter how mutual the interests, without love there can be no real love relationship. Although you can have a relationship without love, you cannot have a love relationship without love, and there is no way to fool your emotions. Stress is the inevitable consequence of living with this deception (D'Angelis 1996).

Every relationship must have some independence. To reduce the chance of relationship failure, couples often seek "togetherness insurance" by trying to be everything to each other. Most couples are convinced that relationships fail because of a lack of togetherness, when just the opposite, too much togetherness, may be at the root of the problem. Nothing is as stressful as being smothered and forced to buy your partner's expectations. Both partners must be able to keep their own friends, male and female, and must be free to interact with them on a regular basis. Each partner must feel free to participate in the activities they enjoy, regardless of whether the other person is involved.

Both partners must remain authentic, true to their own selfhood, and true to their values. They each should live a lifestyle based on their own values and not sacrifice their own needs for their partner's needs. They should always move toward being their own person. Stress has often been defined as the distance between who you really think you are and how you act. Stress will tell you through physical symptoms or behavioral manifestations exactly how big the difference is.

Each partner should strive to remain open, honest, and assertive and not be held back by fear of hurting, fear of being rejected, or guilt. Both need to feel free to verbalize their wants and not expect their partner to somehow "know" what they want. Each needs to be able to talk about everything openly and honestly, and most of all to express hurts, anger, and disappointments as they occur and not allow resentments to build up.

There should be room for personal growth (that is, room to change and room to be independent). Expectations should be kept to a minimum, or resentments will follow. A healthier love relationship is just that, the love relationship. Each should realize that the other is not a business partner, playmate, housekeeper, or errand runner.

Each partner needs to be allowed to do those things they enjoy and not be expected to give them up just because the other person may be able to do them more efficiently. Interest should be more important than expertise or cultural bias (usually sexist) in the choice of activities.

Obligation—out of guilt, prior commitment, or security needs—should not rule the relationship. Binding commitments and lifetime security are a myth and usually work to increase complacency.

Partners, to the best of their ability, should strive to keep themselves healthy, physically active, fresh, interesting, playful, and growing. Neither partner should change or postpone change in order to stay in place with their partner. Mutual support is essential, but becoming a crutch or excessively leaning on a partner usually spells disaster for a relationship. And as the relationship goes, so go your health and happiness.

There's nothing new or profound in any of these statements, but by recognizing them and reminding yourself of them, you might keep a relationship with real promise from dying of neglect. If you are a free, loving, honest, and interesting person who is working to become the best possible you and acting to foster your partner's growth, and if you love each other and have a fair number of mutual interests, then the relationship will be fulfilling. If not, it will become old, boring, dependent, and stifling, and you'll be better off finding someone else and starting over.

It seems as though the philosophers, marriage counselors, and other professionals in this field are saying that success for a relationship adds up to experiencing mature love, maintaining independence, self-sufficiency, and being in touch with personal need fulfillment. When two people can respect where they are and work to develop their own identities, it is impossible for them to become clinging, jealous, and dependent—the three factors that most often undermine a relationship. The experts also seem to agree that although love may just seem to happen, good relationships do not. A strong, lasting relationship is not a matter of luck; it is a matter of two healthy personalities being realistic in working to make it work (Blanche 1998, Harley 1997, Gottman and Silver 1999).

Living Together

If you are lucky enough to have a good loving relationship going for you, then life together should be a stress-free walk in the park. Well, perhaps not. No matter how healthy and happy you are, trying to fit two lives together is a recipe for excess stress. The next step, living together or marriage, puts all of your positive psychological traits to the test. If the relationship continues beyond dating, the next step for many couples is marriage or living together, and once that blissful train starts to rumble, it is much more difficult to stop. Little things tend to be overlooked until one day, after the other person hangs their toothbrush next to yours, you may find that the candlelight and wine dinners with soft music have turned into pizza and beer in front of a TV and that leisurely discussions of love and life become play-by-play accounts of the NCAA basketball finals.

Dating, no matter how frequent or fantastic, does not prepare a couple for living together. After months of dinners out, breakfast in, studying together, vacationing together, and so on, you may feel you know everything there is to know about this person. But life is made of many more routine things than dating is. Meals need to be fixed, floors and furniture dusted, dishes and laundry done, and bills paid. People also need time to be alone. Everyone has his or her own living habits. Men sometimes leave the bathroom sink full of whiskers, guzzle orange juice from the bottle, and expect to have their dinners cooked, not to mention leaving the lid up! Women often leave their makeup all over the bathroom sink, want the garbage to be taken out, and expect their cars to be in running order and filled with gas. Little annoyances, perhaps, but they often precipitate arguments and make you wonder why you ever gave up the romance for the routine. There are more serious difficulties when the "strong silent type" is in reality sulking, withdrawn, and continually depressed; when the forceful, take-charge type turns out to be extremely pushy; when knowing just what is wanted turns into unforgiving perfectionism with high expectations of the right way to do everything; when the seemingly insatiable appetite for sex starts to take a backseat to other needs, pressures, and activities; when the cozy little apartment that made a great little love nest affords little space for privacy and time alone.

While you were dating you had time to spend alone, wind down from the day's work or school, and rejuvenate yourself before going out. Now you both come home needing that time, but there you are together with new, constant demands. You expect to see the same warm, witty, wonderful person alive with enthusiasm—the one you used to date. Unfulfilled expectations can engender excess stress that can eat away at a relationship, so the time to learn exactly what to expect is before you make the big move.

Although toleration of those little idiosyncrasies does grow, some major problems must be worked out if the relationship is to survive. Some problem areas in a relationship are handling money, basic communication, and jealousy. Of these, basic communication compatibility is probably the most important factor in keeping you and the relationship healthy.

Communication

Good communication is mandatory. It means being open and honest with your feelings; it means being assertive enough to get your needs met; it means not being so afraid of losing your partner that you always give in; and it means knowing how to fight fairly and constructively. As we discussed in Chapter 6, one essential to honest communication is learning assertiveness.

Assertiveness promotes the best communication in a relationship; people who are assertive are able to state their likes and dislikes without demeaning the other person. Aggressive people, on the other hand, make demands and state their likes and dislikes in a way that damages the other person's self-esteem. Passive placaters do not have the skill to ask for what they want; instead, they manipulate others by means of guilt and blame into getting what they want. Being assertive makes for happier communication in all facets of life, including sexuality. You can determine your verbal impact on others by watching the effect your words have. If you think that the words you use will intimidate or give the other person a feeling of low self-worth, you're probably being aggressive. However, if you tell the other person what you like or dislike without degrading them, then you're probably being assertive. Being assertive does not always guarantee that the other person will not choose to be hurt. For example, you may have had an instance in which a very good friend of yours wanted your friendship to become sexually intimate, but you did not want that kind of relationship. If you were assertive, you told the person that you regarded their friendship very highly and that you really liked having them as a friend but preferred to keep your relationship on a best-friend basis rather that let sex enter into it. At that point the friend could choose to be hurt or to continue to be one of your best friends. You asserted your rights in a caring way, and the response is up to the other person. If they choose to be hurt, it was not because you said something degrading.

Feeling assertive is incompatible with stressful feelings and anxiety. The more you feel one, the less you feel the other. Assertiveness is sometimes called "feel-good communication." If you feel good after a conversation or confrontation, you have communicated effectively and positively. When people choose to respond in nonassertive, passive ways, they do so for some payoff. Some reasons for not being assertive are fear of retaliation, fear of losing affection or esteem, being rewarded for not rocking the boat, and being unaware that it is all right to be assertive. Recall a situation in which you did not say how you felt, did not stand up for your rights, or did not express your opinion. What kept you from being assertive?

Aggression also carries payoffs. Among them may be the feeling of power, of being right, or of getting others' attention. When was the last time you were aggressive? What was the payoff? There may indeed be a short-term period of feeling good or righteous or smug after having been nonassertive or aggressive, but there's a long-term effect of feeling good that goes with assertiveness. We always have these three elements: the monster, the mouse, and the assertive me. The goal of assertiveness is responding less and less as a monster or a mouse and more and more as the assertive me.

Suggestions for assertive communication were given in Chapter 6. With regard to relationships, a good way to start being assertive is to tell others when they're doing something right—it will make both of you feel good. The next step might be to work on saying out loud what you like and what you dislike without expressing a judgment of the other person's personality. A good follow-up to this step is to also suggest out loud a positive alternative for the thing you dislike. Remember that the most powerful block to communication in a relationship is being negative. Use positive words and give positive suggestions instead of filling your sentences with "don't," "shouldn't," or "can't."

Many people have the most trouble being assertive in sexual situations. This is probably due to society's lingering attitude that sex is something that we should not discuss. Being able to talk about sex with a sex partner in an assertive way greatly enhances the sexual relationship and makes for a more mature relationship. In the sexual silence of the bedroom, neither partner knows what the other one wants or enjoys, but knowing how to ask and then asking for what you want enhances your chance of getting that need met.

Perhaps the most important sexual assertive communication is letting your partner know whether you wish to engage in sexual activity. It is important to say what you feel instead of giving vague signals. No matter how you ask for your needs to be met, you always risk being rejected, but having been asked to join a partner in sex, there are assertive ways of making rejection less painful. It is well to remember that, although you are not being assertive or not being entirely truthful verbally, your body/subconscious will communicate your true feelings somehow. This stressful behavioral communication will in the long run be much more damaging to the relationship and your health than just saying honestly how you feel. If you're feeling anxiety or resentment about saying "yes," you may carry that bad feeling about the same experience to the future. A caring, assertive "no" frees you from that anxiety.

Fighting Fair

Quarrels between daters are usually less frequent and less intense than those between couples who are living together. Couples who are just dating spend much of their time pleasing each other; they do not like to waste time arguing. When a couple is living together, there is no escape; the disagreement usually concerns the entire lifestyle, and each partner is more apt to want his or her own way. Also, the preliminary period of trying to continually please each other and impress each other ended when they began to live together.

No two people want to live exactly the same way, so disagreements are bound to arise. The "we never fight" couple usually spends a lot of energy burying the problem, and resentment builds up over time. If these resentments are triggered, a major battle that can undermine the relationship is apt to occur. The "we always fight" couple is usually a pair of unhappy individuals who are dissatisfied with themselves and the relationship and are venting a lot of emotion without really discussing the issues. Fighting too much is a sign of real problems in a relationship, problems that are never really resolved. Fights that resolve problems can strengthen a relationship, whereas those that do not are merely emotional outbursts that destroy the relationship. Most couples, furthermore, do not know how to fight fairly. The major obstacles to fighting fairly are the following:

1. The concept that there must be a winner and a loser. Actually, no one ever wins a fight. Each time one wins a point, the other feels resentment. The point is to resolve your differences and continue living with and loving each other. The basis for diplomatic negotiations applies—that is, give a little, receive a little. The outcome should be a win/win situation rather than a lose/lose or a win/lose one.
2. Charged emotions and hurt feelings. Attacking with the use of statements such as "I don't like the way you. . ." elicit defensiveness, and the real issues become sidetracked as the attacked tries to protect his or her feelings.
3. Trying to change the behavior of a partner by nagging, sulking, or withholding. This is manipulation, and true feelings never get expressed.
4. Killing effective communication with verbal and nonverbal turnoffs. These techniques signal that you do not wish to discuss the issue. Another technique is punishment—making your partner pay for weeks for bringing up the issue. This usually takes the form of recurrent sarcastic remarks, sulking, and withholding.

Effective, productive fighting consists of the following:

1. Stating in a matter-of-fact manner what is bothering you and how the situation makes you feel.
2. Opening up communication by listening to your partner's point of view. The tendency is to want to talk and to get your point across, but you must be a good listener, also. Be thankful that your partner wants to strengthen your relationship. Once you have both made some initial statements and have a discussion going, you're halfway there.

Once communication is underway, you may experience an emotional overload before the issue is resolved, so feel free to say that you need a break or time to think things over. Stress builds up over time. Too much stress in a short time and too much emotion inhibit communication. You are wise to know your limits and realize that more will be accomplished by coming back to this at a later time when you are less stressed and tired. The key is to make it known that the issue is not resolved and that you would like to resume the discussion later. In the meantime, try not to withhold affection. Do something fun together—it signifies that things are basically all right and that you just have to work out a few details. Many couples live by the rule that they will never go to bed angry. Fatigue may cause you to bury the problem for a while, but unresolved problems do not go away; they will reemerge later, usually dragging along a train of resentment. Try to maintain a normal existence while resolving the problem. Do not allow problems to get buried under a "return to normal." Renew the discussion the next day simply by saying that you do not feel the issue has been resolved. By then there is usually less emotion, and elapsed time has helped each to absorb the other's position. Always resist the temptation to play "shrink," which gives the impression that anyone holding those views has serious psychological problems. Use the model of labor and management, and enter into good-faith negotiations. With labor and management, both parties come in wanting everything and settling for less. Changes can be made only if parties consent, and that occurs only if both parties give some.

Areas of Stressful Conflict

It is no secret that unhappy couples fight more than happy couples. Many times the problems are due more to style than to the issues, and those unhappy couples have problems with their quality of interaction. Unhappy couples often use aversive problem-solving styles, show less appreciation for the other person, and have more difficulty initiating interesting conversation and expressing emotions clearly. The actual issues and fights do not really differ that much between happy and unhappy couples. The major issues most couples fight over involve sexual relations, money, personal habits, jealousy, and in-laws. When these problems become overwhelming or go on for a long time, the couple may have reached the "burned-out" stage.

Sexual Relations

One standard problem area is sexual relations. An inability to be close and get sexual needs met eventually leads to frustration. Partners become irritable over this issue, and they begin to haggle over other areas. Sexual problems are related more to intensity of feelings than to skill deficiencies. Frequency of sex is usually a matter of need and satisfaction. Even though many couples complain about infrequent sex, the fact is they're not enjoying sex and therefore do not engage in it as often. Time limitations are often mentioned as one of the major limiting factors in decreased frequency of sex; however, studies show that a large proportion of young adults who work sixty hours a week have sex more than eighty times a year, far out distancing fifty-eight times per year average for most couples (Welch 1995).

As it is difficult to have sex with someone you're not happy with, sexual problems usually grow out of other hostilities, and mutual resentments are often carried over into the sexual arena. Sexual problems are also bound up with communication problems. The inability to solve long-standing problems invariably has repercussions in the bedroom. Likewise the fatigue of stressful lifestyle usually catches up with a person by making them self-absorbed and a less considerate romantic partner.

Sex is sex—not a manipulation. You can't trade sex for getting the trash taken out. Even if sexual ploys garner the desired attention or win some other battle for its perpetrator, the real problems go unsolved. Feelings of disappointment, anger, and frustration begin to take over. Sex, which should be enjoyable on a physical, emotional, and spiritual level, is degraded. When you use sex as a tool of power, it interferes with the pleasure and togetherness it could bring to the relationship, and the beauty of the sexual experience is impeded.

In some cases, couples have a healthy relationship, but only outside the bedroom. This can be a problem in the long-term monogamous relationship, especially for couples busy with careers. Fatigue and pressure can leave them vulnerable. They may see their declining sex life as a symbol of a decline in their relationship. Sex sometimes becomes just something you do because you're supposed to—a habit. The greatest challenge confronting monogamous relationships today is maintaining the sexual passion. A couple needs to set aside time to make their partner and sex life a priority (Barbach 1997, Barbach and Geisinger 1993).

No one can instinctively know what his or her partner enjoys. A frequent obstacle to complete sexual fulfillment is a lack of communication on the part of one or both partners. Whether due to fear, embarrassment, or a general reluctance to discuss sex, an honest and open dialogue will help you to have sex the way you want it—in the manner that will bring you the most enjoyment possible.

Recall Exercise

Recall a time in your life when you felt you had a very special sexual or romantic experience. Who was your partner? Where were you? What was the setting? What made that particular experience so enjoyable? It may help to close your eyes, relax, and let the images come to you.
Describe the experience in the following terms.

1. When was it? _____
2. Who were you with? _____
3. Look around; describe what you see; describe your feelings and sensations:
   _____
   _____

Next recall a time in your life when you felt you had a not-so-pleasurable sexual or romantic experience. Who was your partner? Where were you? What was the setting? What made that particular experience less enjoyable?

Describe the experience in the following terms.

1. When was it? _____
2. Who were you with? _____
3. Look around; describe what you see; describe your feelings and sensations:

   _____

   _____

Now compare your favorite experiences with your not-so-good ones. Make a list of the significant factors that made the sexual experience good for you. Was it the location, the person, or other circumstances?

_____	_____
_____	_____
_____	_____
_____	_____

Now rewrite the list, placing the most meaningful items at the top and the least important on the bottom. This revised list will identify the conditions you associate with more enjoyable experiences, as well as those that are less satisfying.

_____	_____
_____	_____
_____	_____
_____	_____

Finally, analyze the items that appear high on your list. Are they reasonable? Which apply to your current partner? Can you work with your current partner to achieve more of the "optimal" conditions and to eliminate the ones that are less fulfilling?

Take this a step farther into the realm of fantasy. See yourself in the best possible sexual or romantic experience. Make a list of the significant factors that made this fantasy special. How does this list compare with the other two? This is what you really want. What keeps you from getting it? What can you do to make it happen for you? Can you communicate this to your current partner?

It is impossible to have a good sexual relationship without clear communication. But an amazing number of people find it difficult to talk honestly and openly about their sexual desires. The best time to broach the subject with your partner is when you are both feeling warm and intimate. The worst time to try to communicate your needs is when you or your partner feels angry, frustrated, or resentful. If you choose the time and the words carefully, you run little risk of offending or intimidating your partner. If you speak out of anger, you risk offending your partner. Remember that sexual criticism cuts deep and is not easily forgotten, and your attempts at reducing stress will only cause more stress instead.

Money

Money, how is it made and the style of spending, is another major area of conflict in most households. More than married couples, cohabiting couples often feel that "what is mine is mine," not "ours." How the money is spent is often a bone of contention. If spending and savings styles and values are incompatible, major negotiations are usually necessary to save the relationship. If couples cannot agree on this issue, then separating money is essential. Passivity in this area always results in resentment, long-term low-level stress, and an attitude of "getting even."

Personal Habits

Poor personal habits, or perhaps better stated, incompatible personal habits, are often the source of conflict in a relationship. The list here is endless, and often the items seem trivial. Things such as bad temper, jealousy, discourtesy, poor driving habits, moodiness, chronic lateness, household neglect, unhelpfulness, drinking too much, over emphasizing cleanliness, nagging, and infidelity may signal that a couple is mismatched or cannot communicate well enough to resolve these issues. Either way, if differences exist, they must be resolved or overlooked or the stress will eventually trigger conflict.

Jealousy

Still another area of frequent conflict is jealousy and the way it limits the freedom and independence of partners in a relationship. What makes the problem of jealousy so difficult to solve is that jealousy entails a threat to self-esteem as well as to a valued relationship. It does not really matter if that threat is real, potential, or just a figment of the imagination. In other words, jealous individuals will be jealous even if there is no actual, physical reason for that jealousy. Jealousy, then, is more a personal behavioral trait of persons who may themselves be faithless and have a tendency to stray. Jealous persons often have poor self-images and constantly feel that because they're basically not good enough for their partners, their partners will eventually stray. Interestingly enough, even persons who are not particularly happy with their partners or the quality of their relationship are nevertheless very often jealous. Thus, it is more the loss of self-esteem than the loss of the relationship that threatens them. Naturally, individuals whose self-esteem is heavily dependent upon their partner or emotionally overdependent upon their partner or the relationship are more often jealous than individuals who are healthily independent (Friday 1997, Pines 1998). As was outlined in Chapter 6, this is a good example of how poor self-perception can be at the root of stress problems.

It is also interesting that the sexes customarily react to jealousy in different ways. Jealous women tend to concentrate on enhancing their attractiveness and strengthening the relationship, whereas men tend to concentrate on saving face by becoming more sexually aggressive with other women and seeking new relationships. In addition, men are more likely than women to end a relationship because of their partner's

infidelity. Jealousy always limits freedom in a relationship; it leads to suspicion, insecurity, and resentment, and if not resolved, usually spells the end of the relationship
in one form or another.

In-laws

Even though you may not be married, if your partner has parents, you have "in-laws,"
and in-laws are often a source of conflict in a relationship. Young adults have usually
not been out of their parents' control and influence for very long—not long enough
to establish themselves as adults in their parents' eyes. Thus, parents still try to influence their children's decisions and the young adult children are trying to live up to
their parents' expectations. There is a big difference between "you and I" and "we."
If a couple is really getting close and starting to think of themselves as " we," then each
needs to be more important to the other than to either set of parents. This is a giant
step in the development of a relationship. Often young couples get caught between
pleasing their partners and pleasing their parents—a good definition of stress if ever
there was one. Parents often create difficulties by not accepting partners, thus making
it uncomfortable, to say the least, for partners to interact with them. Parents often
have a difficult time accepting the living-together arrangement, and consciously do
whatever they can to break it up. They make no attempt to get to know their child's
live-in partner. The presence of the parent or even a telephone call can be the source
of stress or conflict. If the couple cannot stand together as one in the face of such
opposition, their relationship will be short lived.

Although there are many more areas of potential conflict in a relationship, the
ones just described are most often mentioned. As discussed earlier, a couple's communication style is usually more important than the substance of their differences. If
there are too many differences or if there are too many communication problems,
then chances are the relationship is not worth saving. After a prolonged period of
damaging interaction, a couple can become "burned out," and the individuals will
exhibit the same burned-out symptoms as mentioned in Chapter 7, a state usually
associated with work-related overloads.

Separation

Is separation a personal tragedy, a family embarrassment, or a social problem? Or is it
a new lease on life, a chance to start over, and a chance to make something positive
out of something that has turned negative? It is a matter of perspective, but either way
it is the most stressful aspect of relationships. The end of a relationship may be
accompanied by an introspective period often filled with self-doubt.

Did I give up too soon, did I not try hard enough, or was it obvious that it was
a failure and I was not seeing it for what it was? Did I bail too soon or too late? After
a separation friends will tell you they never thought the two of you were right for each
other. Do they say that to make you feel better, or did they see something you were
unwilling or unable to see?

What happens when two people do not see the incongruities in their paths? They are unhappy for a long period of time and resent the partner, which allows the low-level stress to fester for long periods of time. When loves dies, it is difficult to overlook the partner's faults. It is as though there is a hole opened in the dike. Without love the wear and tear from the stress and strain of everyday life come rushing in that hole, making it bigger and bigger. Gradually you start to dislike yourself for putting up with things that you feel diminish you. On the surface, at least, you deny your anger, keep it bottled, and don't talk to anyone about it, especially your partner. People often say, "Hindsight is perfect. Looking back now, I realize that I didn't know what was going on. I let our love erode to the point that we were fighting over whose turn it was to take out the trash. I couldn't seem to stop it, or I didn't want to stop it."

However, we are not victims of life circumstances. The stress of overwhelming financial, social, and professional responsibilities are challenges presenting opportunities for us to join together and find ways to be happy with what we have. Relationships are supposed to add to our feelings of joy and abundance. When they don't, it may be time to move on.

For any one of a thousand reasons, a couple may suddenly see each other as being worlds apart. Usually it is not because the personality for which each was chosen is not there, but because the unrealized, unallowed-for differences are deeper than either bargained for. After months or even years, living with these differences and experiencing the frustration, fights, hurts, and angers, a couple may see that going their separate ways is the only viable alternative. Everyone should be allowed to change their minds, to change jobs, move to a new place, or choose a new partner. People move into relationships to prove their sense of commitment and to find security. However, many find that commitment is situational and security is a figment of their imagination. With all couples there is a real possibility that the day may come, no matter how strong the prior commitment, no matter how much love was shared and shown, that the relationship may end. One may find oneself companionless, jobless, childless: and in a matter of a few months, one's entire life can change. Although separation cannot help but be stressful, the length of time one remains in this stressful state is an indicator of how well they manage stress and will be the determining factor in how quickly they return to positive health and happiness.

When children are involved, separation and divorce take on a whole new aspect. No longer can each partner think of himself or herself first (unless violence and abuse are involved in the issue).

Loneliness

One of the more stressful aspects of relationships is the absence of relationships. In a society in which the culture gives a high rating to togetherness, it is often very stressful to find yourself alone without a partner. Here again the relationship arena provides the proving grounds for how well you deal with the stress of boredom and loneliness. There is a difference between being alone and being lonely, and that is most often determined by the spiritual health of the individual. Very often being single does not mean being alone at all. The singles who seem to enjoy being single tend to be young; most are in college or just out of college. They like themselves and are content with what they are; they have many friends and many interests, are physically active, have fulfilling jobs, are emotionally fit, have a sense of humor, and generally are content with their lives and not overzealous in their search for a mate. A sharply increasing number of young people are choosing to remain single for reasons such as freedom and privacy (Sanders 1998). Table 9.3 shows pros and cons of being single.

In our society being alone is seen as a symptom of social pathology, being less worthy, less lovable, something to be pitied. If being coupled is the norm, then everyone who is not part of a couple is abnormal. Few people consider that being alone is an integral part of everyone's journey. It may be even more noticeable in the lives of those people who are working on self-reliance issues. What do you learn from being alone? Many things, especially, how to be alone. Only in your aloneness will you find out who you really are. If you are concerned about aloneness, reframe the reason you are alone. There is a large difference between being lonely and unlovable or undesirable and experiencing aloneness as a precondition to philosophical integration. If you need to be alone to gain that experience, you'll find some reason to be alone. And if you need to be alone, you're going to have to practice being alone, or you're not going to be able to pull it off. Even if it's sometimes painful, you're learning how to do it. If you cannot be alone, or "pull it off," then you will not be able to be alone, and you will constantly seek the comfort of relationships. As a rule we fixate our loneliness on other people and thus try to rid ourselves of loneliness by being with other people or being entertained. People are more afraid of what being alone means to them and society than the actual state of being alone (Middleton 1999). Even battered women are reluctant to get out of their relationships not because they love the creeps but because they are terrified to be alone.

How does one go about being comfortable with being alone? By trying it in varying degrees. One might start out with short sessions of solitary meditation. That is quality alone time. When rewards and insights come from being alone, the time will increase. One may learn that relationships, especially dependency relationships, hinder. And if you are at a point in your path where you need to integrate what you have learned about who you really are, then you will seek aloneness.

When being alone hurts, that is, causes us to feel lonely or incomplete, it is a purely physical or material state. Our physical body is alone, but our spiritual bodies are still joined. When we access our spiritual bodies, we are able to know the soul's will. We are able to be alone in our physical bodies and at the same time be in constant oneness with our divine part, or God part, if you prefer. What we find in our quality alone time is that we are never alone. Each of us is a part of the whole.

There is a difference between "alone" and "lonely." Both are free-will choices, but being lonely carries with it the negative baggage of the ego, that of self-doubt, and lack of self-respect, self-regard, and self-love. We have an agenda for the time we spend alone—it's part of our experience. How can we resent being alone when we have chosen it as our tool? Resentment of being alone is the feeling we are trying to overcome. Lonely is on a physical level, an emotional choice we can make to know our aloneness. When we integrate that emotion with the sense of free will, we can choose to experience joy in our aloneness.

Experiencing your aloneness as being lonely with its accompanied socially- and psychologically-promoted pathology is an indication that you have not understood the purpose of the aloneness and that you are not ready to give up either the loneliness or the debilitating fear of it. Fear, as we know, has as its companion, anger, and the antisocial behavior that goes with it.

If you do not know what you need, look at what you have. If you do not know what you want, look at what you have. You create what you need and what you want. What have you created? You could also be ready to create relationships if that's what you think you want. Or you could create a whole new attitude about aloneness.

Relationships! Both the advantages and disadvantages inherent in them have their accompanying stressors. Relationships can, and will, be as stressful as your perception allows them to be. Perhaps more than any other arena, the stress of relationships is largely dependent upon one's perception. One's self-perception, patterns of behavior, communications skills, ability to deal with change, frustration, and overload, and one's ability to manage stress before it gets out of control will greatly affect the stress engendered by relationships or the joy they can bring.

TABLE 9.3   Being Single

Being Single	
Advantages:	*Disadvantages:*
■ privacy ■ no one to clean up after ■ money goes a lot farther; you can spend your money on whatever you want without answering to anyone or feeling guilty ■ not being tied to a schedule; working when you feel like it, not having to prepare meals on time or when someone else is hungry ■ generally not being responsible to or for anyone else ■ enjoying the feeling of being in control of your own life	■ loneliness; not having anyone to talk with, to share with, to support you when you are down ■ lack of emotional intimacy, no one to touch, hug, share thoughts and moods with ■ lack of steady sex ■ having to find a date, and being stuck with someone undesirable ■ lack of opportunity to meet companions; most singles do not like the "meat market" atmosphere of single bars ■ fear that being single will become permanent ■ an overemphasis on looks and outward appearance in the singles scene; there is little opportunity to really get to know someone ■ not being able to have children

SOURCES CITED

Adams, V. (1980). *Jealous love.* Psychology Today. May, 38–47.

Bailey, L. (1995) *The original lovers questionnaire.* Raleigh, NC: Lormax Communications.

Barbach, L. (1997). *Fifty ways to please your lover.* New York: E. P. Dutton.

Barbach, L. and Geisinger, D. (1993). *Going the distance: Finding and keeping life-long love.* New York: Plume Books.

Blanche, C. (1998). *The book of love.* New York: Time Life.

Branden, N. and Branden, E. D. (1981) *The romantic love: Question and answer book.* Los Angeles: Torcher Publishing Co.

D'Angelis, B. (1996). *One hundred and one ways to transform your love life.* Springfield, VA: Nataraj.

Fisher, H. (1994) *Anatomy of love.* New York: Ballantine Books.

Friday, N. (1997). *Jealousy.* New York: M. Evans.

Gottman, J. and Silver N. (1999). *The seven principles for making marriage work.* New York: Crown Publishers.

Harley, W. F. Jr. (1997). *Five steps to romantic love.* Grand Rapids, MI: Fleming H. Revell. Co.

Middleton, D. (1999). *Dealing with feeling left out.* Center City, MN: Hazelden Information Education.

Pines, A. M. (1998). *Romantic jealousy.* New York: Routledge.

Sanders, J. (1998). *Facing loneliness.* New York: Discovery House.

Welch, L. (1995). *Sex facts.* New York: Citadel.

10 Crisis, Violence, and Posttraumatic Stress

For years it was said that we were living in an "age of anxiety." As the new millennium is born, we find ourselves in an age of crisis and violence. Stressful events are commonplace as we live our lives in modern society. Indeed, this book discusses many varieties of stressor events that you, the reader, may likely encounter. In this chapter, however, we move beyond the discussion of more commonplace stressors to the discussion of a form of stressor that is uniquely acute and may yield the most severe form of human stress response known.

Historical Background

Have you ever experienced a crisis? Just what constitutes a crisis, from a psychological perspective?

A crisis is a response to some threatening or adverse event wherein three conditions are evident:

1. your normal state of psychological balance (homeostasis) is disrupted, leading to a state of distress;
2. your normal coping strategies are not successful, and;
3. you are unable to perform at your normal level of effectiveness, that is, some level of impaired functioning is evident (Everly 1999).

As a physical crisis threatens your physical health, a psychological crisis threatens your psychological health. The most severe form of crisis is the psychological trauma, and a traumatic event is the most severe form of stressor. Psychological trauma has existed as long as humanity. The earliest accounts of posttraumatic stress reactions come to us from the battlefield. Terms such as *battle fatigue, soldier's heart, war neurosis,* and *shell shock* were often used as labels for posttraumatic stress reactions (Chalsma 1998, Parrish 1999). But such reactions are not limited to warfare.

In 1865 Charles Dickens wrote of a railway accident in which he was involved (Trimble 1981). Dickens's diary contained numerous accounts of the accident, and he subsequently described his reactions to the disaster in the following way: "I am curiously weak—weak as if I were recovering from a long illness." The description is intriguing in that Dickens himself was not physically injured but rather was an observer of several hours of "horrifying" sights and sounds during which many people did indeed die.

The year 1666 was the year of the Great Fire of London. Trimble (ibid.) in his historical account of posttraumatic stress notes that the fire not only destroyed lives and property but also engendered numerous accounts of posttraumatic stress reactions including phobic reactions, nightmares, flashbacks, and many stress-related physical complaints.

In 1980 the American Psychiatric Association officially described a mental disorder that may develop in response to psychological or physical trauma. That disorder is now referred to as posttraumatic stress disorder (PTSD). Thus, with PTSD's recognition as an official "legitimate" affliction in 1980, further inquiry and preventive programs became possible. Recent events in the world have further underscored the need to recognize and investigate posttraumatic stress reactions. In 1992 the American Red Cross and the American Psychological Association cooperated to create a national disaster mental health network. The purpose of this network was not only to provide disaster mental health services to Red Cross personnel working in disaster venues but more important, to provide acute mental health support for primary disaster victims throughout the United States. Shortly after this network was created, the United States saw a virtual plague of disasters including Hurricane Andrew, Hurricane Iniki, the Los Angeles earthquake, the floods in the Midwest, the California firestorms and floods, the World Trade Center and Oklahoma City bombings, numerous airline disasters such as TWA 800 and Swiss Air 111, and internationally, the earthquakes in Turkey.

Recognizing the fact that emergency response professionals such as law enforcement, fire suppression, emergency medical personnel, and rescue workers were at high risk for PTSD, another organization was formed, which actually predates the network just mentioned. In 1989 the international Critical Incident Stress Foundation was formed to provide support for all emergency services professionals because they are at greatest risk for developing PTSD. While this foundation predated the national disaster mental health network of the American Red Cross and the American Psychological Association, it has a far more selective constituency.

Just how widespread is crisis? Consider the following:

- Recent evidence suggests that 90 percent of adults in the United States will be exposed to a traumatic event during their lifetime;
- The rate of trauma exposure for children and adolescents has been estimated at about 40 percent;
- Suicide rates have been seen to increase after natural disasters;
- The lifetime prevalence of criminal victimization was assessed among female HMO patients and was found to be about 57 percent;
- Violence at work costs over 1.75 million lost workdays;
- Homicide is the third leading cause of death from injury at the worksite (NIOSH) in the United States, but in California and the District of Columbia it is the leading cause of workplace death;
- Each year, approximately one million persons become victims of violent crime at work;

- The prevalence of PTSD was found to be 13 percent in a sample of suburban law enforcement officers;
- Law enforcement officers are 8.6 times more likely to die from suicide than from homicide and are 3.1 times more likely to die from suicide than from accidental circumstances;
- Clinical healthcare staff sampled reported that 62 percent of their employees were exposed to a traumatic stressor at work;
- The prevalence of posttraumatic stress disorder ranged from 15 to 31 percent for samples of urban firefighters based on a traumatic exposure prevalence ranging from 85 to 91 percent.
- Symptoms of distress and PTSD are correlated with exposure to traumatic stressors, such that there exists a virtual dose-response relationship, that is, the more crises you are exposed to, the greater your risk of developing PTSD (adapted from Everly and Mitchell 1999).

Posttraumatic Stress Disorder

Widespread research and prevention programs did not develop until PTSD became an official psychiatric phenomenon in 1980. The American Psychiatric Association's diagnostic nosology, *Diagnostic and Statistical Manual of Mental Disorders* (APA 1994), retains the PTSD diagnosis under the heading "Anxiety Disorders." The official diagnostic criteria are as follows:

1. The person has been exposed to a traumatic event in which both of the following were present:
   - The person experienced, witnessed, or was confronted with an event or events that involved actual or threatened death or serious injury or a threat to the physical integrity of self or others.
   - The person's response involved intense fear, helplessness, or horror.
2. The traumatic event is persistently reexperienced in one (or more) of the following ways:
   - recurrent and intrusive distressing recollections of the event
   - recurrent distressing dreams of the event
   - acting or feeling as if the traumatic event were recurring
   - intense psychological distress at exposure to internal or external cues that symbolize or resemble an aspect of the traumatic event
   - physiological reactivity on exposure to internal or external cues that symbolize or resemble an aspect of the event
3. The person persistently avoids stimuli associated with the trauma and numbing of general responsiveness as indicated by three or more of the following:
   - efforts to avoid thoughts, feelings, or conversations associated with the trauma
   - efforts to avoid activities, places, or people that arouse recollections of the trauma
   - inability to recall an important aspect of the trauma
   - markedly diminished interest or participation in significant activities

- feeling of detachment or estrangement from others
- restricted range of affect
- sense of a foreshortened future

4. The person presents persistent symptoms of increased arousal (not present before the trauma), as indicated by two (or more) of the following:
   - difficulty falling or staying asleep
   - irritability or outbursts of anger
   - difficulty concentrating
   - hypervigilance
   - exaggerated startle response
5. Symptom duration is greater than one month.

The disturbance causes clinically significant distress or impairment.

Consequences

The consequences of prolonged PTSD are nothing less than profound. There exists evidence that prolonged PTSD represents chronic neurotransmitter and neurohumoral cascades that may result in a wide variety of behavioral and health-related consequences that extend far beyond the diagnostic criteria themselves, for example:

1. irritability and aggressiveness;
2. difficulty concentrating;
3. difficulty in assimilating new information;
4. reclusive, avoidant behavior;
5. self-medication;
6. symptoms consistent with attention deficit hyperactivity disorder (ADHD) formulations;
7. narcoleptic symptoms;
8. symptoms consistent with those of complex partial seizures;
9. existential crises;
10. compulsive eating, buying, and/or sexual behavior;
11. an acceleration of physical diseases of degeneration;
12. presenile dementia-like symptoms.

The Nature of Posttraumatic Stress

The symptoms just listed provide a working definition of a complex psychological condition. As we can see in Criteria 2, 3, and 4 of the preceding list, PTSD exhibits three specific symptom clusters that reveal the pathological nature of the disorder:

1. Reexperiencing the traumatic event;
2. Numbing and withdrawal symptoms: persistent avoidance of people, places, and things associated with the trauma, and/or a psychological numbing in which the victim seems to withdraw into a shell;
3. Persistent increased stress arousal.

PTSD may also be seen as a combination of recalled images and excessive arousal, especially of the sympathetic nervous system (Everly and Lating 1995). The numbing and withdrawal is then understood as a secondary reaction to the intrusive recollections and increased arousal. Figure 10.1 depicts the postulated relationships.

This latter formulation may help us to better understand PTSD and other traumatic stress syndromes. For example, PTSD may represent an extreme variation of survival mechanisms. Remember that PTSD arises from exposure to some event that is life threatening or otherwise capable of overwhelming normal coping mechanisms. The mind's survival response may be to deeply ingrain that event in the memory so that similar situations may be avoided in the future (or so that the person will be better prepared to cope with them). The body's survival response may be to create a chronic state of arousal that keeps one prepared for fight or flight at the slightest provocation or threat. Finally, the numbing, and especially the withdrawal symptoms, may represent an energy-conservation mechanism designed to allow recovery of strength after a traumatic event (Everly 1991).

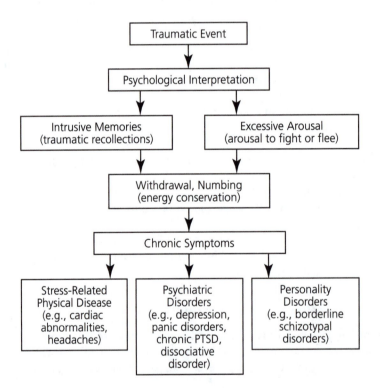

FIGURE 10.1   A Process Model of PTSD

Source: Adapted from Everly and Lating 1995.

Figure 10.1 indicates that chronic acute traumatic syndrome has three potential outcomes:

1. Stress-related physical disease
2. Psychiatric syndromes such as depression or chronic PTSD itself
3. Posttraumatic personality disorders such as borderline personality disorder

An analysis of PTSD reveals two underlying factors: a neurological hypersensitivity and a psychological hypersensitivity (Everly 1991). In neurological terms, exposure to a traumatizing event may result in a hypersensitivity within the neural networks of the subcortical limbic system (described earlier in Chapter 2). Functionally, such a hypersensitivity represents a lowering of the threshold for excessive arousal or excitation. Thus, the slightest irritation or provocation could result in rage, impaired general memory, panic, withdrawal, impulsive reactions, or other forms of extreme stress reactions. The biological foundations for such neurological hypersensitivities and abnormalities may include massive catecholamine release, abnormal cortisol secretions, and endogenous opioid release (Everly and Lating 1995). Mukerjee (1995) has even reviewed evidence that suggests that nerve centers in the hippocampal area of the limbic system of PTSD victims may be so adversely affected by trauma that a 13 to 26 percent reduction in cellular mass may result. Semple and colleagues (1993) found that persons diagnosed both with PTSD and as substance abusers show abnormal blood flow patterns in the frontal cortex as well as the subcortical hippocampus.

Psychologically, exposure to a traumatizing event may create a hypersensitivity within important mechanisms used by all individuals to maintain psychological homeostasis. More specifically, trauma shatters some important assumptions about the nature of our world. It was Abraham Maslow (1968) who noted that a basic human need, second only to the need for food and shelter, is the need for safety.

To make the unknown aspects of the world somewhat safe, we all create assumptions about life in general. For example, one assumption many people hold is that life is "fair." Another is that you get what you deserve and you deserve what you get—it is a "just" world. Another assumption might be that "good" always conquers "evil." Traumatic events by their very nature violate, challenge, and sometimes destroy these presuppositions about life and the world around us. In so doing, they create a psychological void. This void represents a "psychic puzzle" that yields a hypersensitivity to perceptions of threat, demoralization, and panic.

PTSD is not the only form that posttraumatic stress can take, however; it is the most severe. In addition to physical illnesses and personality dysfunctions, a posttraumatic reaction may manifest itself in the following ways (Horowitz 1997):

- fear of a recurrence of the trauma
- shame over being a victim
- rage over being a victim

- rage toward the person or thing that caused the trauma
- phobic reactions
- fear of a loss of control
- depression
- mourning
- guilt

Traumatic Events

What sort of events can cause traumatic stress reactions? Initially, psychologists defined a *traumatic event* as any event outside the usual realm of human experience that would be markedly distressing to virtually anyone who encountered it. That definition has been drastically narrowed to not only embrace particular events but to also include one's appraisal of the event, for example, appraisals of helplessness, fear, or horror. Table 10.1 contains a list of potentially traumatic events.

Even though all of the factors listed in Table 10.1 can clearly lead to traumatic stress reactions, one's psychological appraisal of the adverse experience can serve to mitigate or augment one's personal traumatic response. This phenomenon not only helps us explain why not every person exposed to a traumatic stressor develops the same level of posttraumatic reaction, but it also gives us clues into how we might more effectively treat and even prevent PTSD in high-risk individuals.

TABLE 10.1   Traumatic Events

Personal Traumas	Community Traumas
robbery	flood
physical assault	earthquake
rape	fire
automobile accident	building collapse
a "life-or-death" struggle	airplane crash
physical abuse	multiple-injury accident
psychological abuse	terrorism
sexual abuse	injury or death of a child
a perceived serious threat to one's well-being	
a perceived serious threat to a family member or close friend	
observing any of the personal or community traumas listed here	

Coping with Traumatic Stress

A number of strategies that consider both neurological and psychological hypersensitivity have been used to cope with traumatic events. Neurological hypersensitivity manifests itself in the form of excessive arousal. This arousal is based upon either a biological propensity for arousal or a failure of the brain to dampen arousal.

Relaxation training is usually the best generic approach to lower the level of arousal. No one technique appears to be superior to others. One should practice the relaxation technique that seems easiest and most convenient to utilize. However, some individuals will find that during relaxation they tend to recall the traumatic experience. Such recollection can be stressful and therefore counterproductive. It is sometimes recommended that a more active relaxation technique be employed to reduce the intrusive ideation. Biofeedback is one such technology. In some instances, psychotropic medications are used to dampen the excessive arousal that is a natural constituent of PTSD.

Psychological hypersensitivity arises from a violated world view, or assumption about the world. The strategies often employed to reduce the disequilibrium associated with a violated world view include (1) reinterpreting the traumatic event, (2) reinterpreting the role that one played in the event, (3) active behavior oriented toward increasing one's sense of control over similar events, (4) behaviors designed to increase one's general sense of control, (5) utilization of social support, and (6) changing one's world view so as to assimilate the trauma and thus reduce the anxiety associated with disconfirmation. Let us take a closer look at each of these.

One of the most common coping mechanisms for reducing stress and a sense of chaos is to reinterpret the traumatic event, perhaps by trying to find some positive aspect to it. For example, one might say that the trauma allowed one to finally "grow up" and face problems like an adult. Or one might say that the trauma revealed a previously unknown inner strength. In general these strategies allow the person to find "meaning" in an otherwise meaningless catastrophe. Although it may seem like a pedestrian effort to find the "silver lining" in a cloud of trauma, reinterpretation can prove quite useful as long as it doesn't stifle further growth and development or create new problems of its own.

Another strategy is to reinterpret the role one played in the trauma itself. Survivors of disasters sometimes cope by considering themselves fortunate even to have survived. A similar strategy might be to compare oneself to victims who were more adversely affected. Often, victims of physical harm cope by focusing not on the event but upon recovering from it beyond anyone's expectations. If one tends to blame oneself for the traumatic event, it is sometimes helpful to search for other reasonable explanations for the event. If one is truly responsible, however, one should try to accept responsibility and then consider how to assist the recovery process and/or reduce the chances of similar events occurring. Also, viewing oneself as partially responsible for the traumatic event, one quickly discovers a reason for it. This coping strategy of self-blame is commonly used by victims, even when their role in the trauma was minimal, as a means of restoring order and predictability to the world.

The third common coping mechanism is engaging in some action that reduces the likelihood of a similar event, actively pursuing rehabilitation, or even pursuing punitive action through proper authorities. For example, a burglary victim may place locks on windows and dead-bolt doors or even install an electronic alarm system. These strategies are likely to reduce the probability of a repeat trauma. The victim of an automobile accident may install an air bag in the car. Often, traumatized persons who are physically injured will not only pursue rehabilitation but will use the opportunity to become more health conscious. Finally, the victim of a crime or of human negligence may pursue punitive action through the court system. Such action may not only reduce the likelihood of further crimes or negligence, but it often results in a feeling of empowerment for the victim.

A fourth strategy to reduce psychological hypersensitivity after trauma is to engage in any activity that creates a sense of empowerment and control. It is well known that victims of trauma commonly suffer feelings of self-doubt, helplessness, and a general lack of control. Any activity that helps develop a sense of self-control tends to restore order to a world view whose assumptions have been violated. The activities do not have to be related to the trauma; rather, any activity that increases self-esteem will prove valuable.

Trauma often leaves the victim believing that the world may be a malevolent place. This is in direct contradiction to the more deeply ingrained assumptions that the world is safe and secure. A strategy that helps refute the malevolent-world perspective is social support. We all need some form of social support; humans are social animals. Trauma increases our inherent need for social support. Yet trauma victims often hesitate to seek social support out of a dislike for showing "weakness," a concern over being taken advantage of, and even a reluctance to have others feel sorry for them. Nevertheless, trauma actually increases the need for social support, and thus appropriate social support can have powerful healing effects. Sometimes that support must be obtained from a trained mental health professional such as a psychologist. Failure to obtain social support can needlessly protract psychological suffering. Pennebaker (1995, 1997) argues that translating emotional events into language increases both physical and emotional health. On the other hand, "holding it all inside" can be destructive to both in the long run.

In some cases the trauma may be so overwhelming, the victim's ability to cope may be so meager, or one's previously held assumptions about the world may have been so ineffective (or blatantly inappropriate) that the only reasonable coping strategy is to change one's world view rather than try to salvage it.

A brief summary of the various coping strategies follows:

1. Dampen the tendency for overexcitation, overreaction, and excessive arousal.
2. Reinterpret the traumatic event.
3. Reinterpret your role in the trauma.
4. Increase your control over the traumatic situation.
5. Increase your personal sense of control.
6. Obtain social support (perhaps professional support).

7. Verbalize or journal your feelings.
8. Change your assumptions about the world.

The earlier one recognizes the symptoms of psychological trauma and seeks help, the more rapid the recovery is likely to be. The victim of psychological trauma usually requires assistance to recover. Professional help should always be sought in fully developed cases of PTSD. This information is offered not as a way of treating trauma but rather as a way of familiarizing you with this extreme stress response so that formal treatment can be sought more readily when and if trauma strikes.

Violence: A Special Form of Crisis

In his book *Violence in America*, Dr. Raymond B. Flannery Jr., a leading expert on violence, points out a disturbing trend from 1960 through 1992:

	Homicide	Robbery	Aggravated Assault
1960:	5.2/100,000	49.6/100,000	72.6/100,000
1992:	10.2/100,000	263.6/100,000	441.8/100,000

Regarding youth violence, a 1998 Department of Education report covering a sample of 1,200 schools indicated that there were 11,000 fights using weapons, 4,000 rapes and other sexual assaults, and 7,000 robberies (Flannery 1999). In April 1999, a mass murder and subsequent suicides of the perpetrators took place in a Colorado high school. This tragic event has led to a closer scrutiny of violence in the United States, especially youth violence. Dr. Flannery concludes that there is an *epidemic* of violence in the United States. He notes that Americans do not feel safe because *we are not safe!*

In the search for the causes of our violent society, Flannery lists the following contributing factors:

- Disrupted familial relationships and domestic violence
- Poverty
- Discrimination
- Inadequate schooling
- Media portrayal of violence as acceptable/desirable
- Disruption of prosocial values
- Drug abuse
- Disruption of caring attachments with others

As a solution, Flannery (1998) notes the remedy to the epidemic of violence resides in the restoration of a sense of community, restoration of the family and caring attachments to others, improvement of the educational system, and restoration of religious values. It is likely that the pursuit of such outcomes will result not only in a less violence society but a less stressful one as well.

SOURCES CITED

American Psychiatric Association (1994). *Diagnostic and statistical manual of mental disorders*, 4th ed. Washington, D.C.: APA.

Chalsma, H. W. (1998). *The chambers of memory: PTSD in the life stories of U.S. Vietnam* vets. London: Jason Aronson.

Everly, G. S. (1991). Neurophysiological considerations in the treatment of PTSD: A neurocognitive perspective. In *International handbook for traumatic stress syndrome*, ed. J. Wilson and B. Raphael. New York: Plenum, 356.

Everly, G. S. (1999). *A primer on critical incident stress management: What's really in a name?* International Journal of Emergency Mental Health, 1, 77–79.

Everly, G. S., and Lating, J., eds. (1995). *Psychotraumatology: Key papers and concepts in posttraumatic stress*. New York: Plenum.

Everly, G. S., and Mitchell, J. T. (1999). *Critical incident stress management*, 2d ed. Ellicott City, MD: Chevron.

Flannery, R. B. Jr. (1998). *Violence in America*. New York: Continuum.

Flannery, R. B. Jr. (1999). *Preventing youth violence*. New York: Continuum.

Horowitz, M. J. (1997). *Stress response syndromes: PTSD, grief, and adjustment disorders*. London: Jason Aronson.

Maslow, A. (1968). *Toward a psychology of being*. New York: Van Nostrand Reinhold.

Mukerjee, M. (1995). *Hidden scars: Sexual and other abuse may alter a brain region*. Scientific American, 273, 14, 20.

Parrish, I. S. (1999). *Military veterans' PTSD reference manual*. Buy Books on the web.com.

Pennebaker, J. W. (1997). *Opening up: The healing power of expressing emotions*. New York: Guilford Press.

Pennebaker, J. W., ed. (1995). *Emotion, disclosure, and health*. Washington, D.C.: American Psychological Association.

Semple, W., Goyer P., McCormick, R., Morris, E., Comptom, B., Muswick, G., and Nelson, D. (1993). *Preliminary report: Brain blood flow using PET in patients with posttraumatic stress disorder and substance-abuse histories*. Biological Psychiatry, 34, 115–18.

Trimble, M. R. (1981). *Post-traumatic neurosis*. Chichester, England: Wiley.

CHAPTER

11 Stress in the Workplace

According to the popular press, the jobs of an inner-city high-school teacher, a police officer, and an air-traffic controller rank among the most stressful careers you can pursue. On the other hand, a forester, bookbinder, and civil engineer rank among the least stressful jobs. Most young men and women, by the time they reach college, have worked at some kind of job—perhaps for spending money, to save for college, or to help with the family finances. If you are not working at outside employment now, consider that your job is being a student, housewife, or other pursuit even though you do not receive a paycheck for it. This chapter will have more meaning for you if you can apply it to your current "occupation" or job. Have you ever considered that job stress could play a significant role in your life?

The workplace is the natural extension of our discussion of the causes of stress. Most individuals spend one-third of their adult lives at the workplace. Thus, not only is the workplace a natural venue within which to search for sources of stress, it is also a natural venue within which to apply stress management interventions. Worker's compensation costs have tripled in the last ten years and in the United States alone is in excess of 60 billion dollars annually (LaDou 1997). When decreased production costs, delays, training, and placement costs are added, the figure jumps to 350 billion dollars. Stress-related conditions increased 500 percent in the last decade and represent 15 percent of that 350 billion dollars. These are mainly mental conditions and do not reflect the stress contribution to physical diseases, which makes the stress-related figure even more staggering.

In general the work pace has increased over the last decade. Half of today's workers feel they work at an increasingly higher pace, three-fourths see poor possibilities for promotion, and one-third see no fit between their work and their education. Thus stress and anxiety on the job and at school contribute significantly to the total stress level of the average person in our fast-paced society (Keable 1999).

Job Stress

Swedish researchers have helped clarify some of the broadest conceptual aspects of work-related stress. Bertil Gardell (1976) was among the first to demonstrate that work environments that contribute to feelings of powerlessness and alienation are stressful for most workers. Marianne Frankenhaeuser (1986, Frankenhauser, Lundberg, and Chesney 1991) focused on the variables of effort and distress. She defined *effort* as active coping and a striving to gain and maintain control and distress as feelings of dissatisfaction, boredom, and unpredictability. In her model of job stress, she shows that high effort creates a condition of elevated catecholamines (epinephrine and norepinephrine) in the body, while high distress is related to elevated levels of cortisol. (Conversely, low effort and low distress are related to lower levels of catecholamines and cortisol.) High levels of both effort and distress represent the most stressful environment, one in which the worker attempts to overcome boring, routinized, repetitive, or unpredictable constraints. Such environments give rise to extraordinary catecholamine and cortisol secretion, which contributes to cardiovascular disease (Karasek and Theorell 1992). Environmental conditions that engender feelings of loss of control, helplessness, and hopelessness are associated primarily with elevated levels of cortisol, depressive syndromes, and perhaps even neoplastic formation (Diberardinis 1998, Fletcher 1991, Karasek and Theorell 1992). Workers who are motivated and who see productive results enjoy a strong sense of personal control, accompanied by a sense of accomplishment and job commitment. Catecholamines increase moderately under these conditions, and cortisol seems to be suppressed.

Whereas Frankenhaeuser's research focused largely upon psychophysiological dynamics of the workplace, Robert Karasek and his colleagues (Karasek 1981, Karasek and Theorell 1992) advanced the study of occupational stress by focusing upon the psychological dynamics of the workplace. Karasek's work yielded a model of occupational stress that analyzes job stress by two primary interacting variables: (1) the psychological demand of the job and (2) the degree of control (or decision latitude and flexibility) that the worker possesses with regard to the job function.

The combination of high job demands and low control over the job combine to create an unhealthy, pathogenic environment. Table 11.1 is an adaptation of Karasek's and Frankenhaueser's models.

For some, it may be surprising that the condition that yields high job satisfaction is the high demand-high control condition. Just remember, there are many workers who genuinely enjoy the challenge of their work; they simply wish to have some control over the working conditions. Since the advent of Karasek's model, repeated empirical investigations have not only demonstrated the validity of the model (Radmacher and Sheridan 1995) but have also consistently validated the pathogenic nature of a work environment characterized by high psychological demands and low decision latitude (see Karasek and Theorell 1992). Such work situations appear to put people at greater risk for heart disease, a risk similar to that of smokers or those with elevated serum cholesterol levels.

Examples of high-risk jobs according to this model are sales clerk, receptionist, secretary, nurse's aide, police personnel, fire-suppression personnel, construction laborer, computer operator, telephone operator, assembly-line worker, food server, and cashier. These jobs typify a condition in which demand upon the worker is high

TABLE 11.1 Job Stress, Psychological Demands, and Control

		Control	
		High	*Low*
Psychological Demands	*High*	High job satisfaction	Most pathogenic, high catecholamines, high cortisol
	Low	Least pathogenic	Second most pathogenic

and often unpredictable and the worker's control over the job function is generally minimal.

Karasek's research underscores two critical concepts in the study of occupational stress: (1) Beware of any job that gives you high levels of responsibility but provides you with low levels of authority, and (2) the essence of most jobs from a psychological health standpoint resides not in the actual job responsibilities, but in the worker's perceptions of the job.

Occupational Stressors

Smith and his colleagues (Smith, Everly, and Johns 1992; Smith, Davy, and Everly 1995) have attempted to answer the question of just how important one's psychological perception of the workplace is in the process of stress and disease. The results of their investigations demonstrate that the primary work-related stressor is not a direct one; rather, the primary influence of job stressors on stress-related illness is through the psychological discord allowed to be caused by the stressor. Such psychological discord has been previously shown to be highly correlated with biological mechanisms of disease. Thus, it may be that stressors, like beauty, lie in the eye of the beholder.

Having made the case that the worker's perception of the workplace is an essential element in workplace-related stress and disease, there is still great value in understanding what workplace factors seem to be almost universally stressful or at least highly likely to be perceived as stressful. In this section of the chapter we look at three main categories of job stressors:

1. Organizational stressors
2. Individual stressors
3. Work environment stressors

SELF-ASSESSMENT EXERCISE 11

Choose the response that best answers the question, and place the corresponding letter in the space provided.

Questions 1–7: During the typical course of your job, how often do you . . .

_____ **1.** face important time deadlines that you have difficulty meeting?
    a. once a day or more   c. once a week
    b. more than once a week   d. less than once a week
       but less than once a day

_____ **2.** feel less competent than you think you should?
    a. once a day or more   c. once a week
    b. more than once a week   d. less than once a week
       but less than once a day

_____ **3.** wish your work were less complex?
    a. once a day or more   c. once a week
    b. more than once a week   d. less than once a week
       but less than once a day

_____ **4.** feel overwhelmed by your job?
    a. once a day or more   c. once a week
    b. more than once a week   d. less than once a week
       but less than once a day

_____ **5.** feel that you're in the wrong job?
    a. once a day or more   c. once a week
    b. more than once a week   d. less than once a week
       but less than once a day

_____ **6.** feel frustrated by "red tape"?
    a. once a day or more   c. once a week
    b. more than once a week   d. less than once a week
       but less than once a day

_____ **7.** perceive yourself as lost in the bureaucracy?
    a. once a day or more   c. once a week
    b. more than once a week   d. less than once a week
       but less than once a day

Questions 8–10: During the typical course of my job, I . . .

_____ **8.** feel guilty for taking time off work?
    a. almost always true   c. seldom true
    b. usually true   d. never true

_____   9. have a tendency to rush into work that needs to be done before knowing
           the procedure you will use to complete the job?
    a. almost always true   c. seldom true
    b. usually true   d. never true

_____ 10. whenever possible, attempt to complete two or more tasks at once?
    a. almost always true   c. seldom true
    b. usually true   d. never true

_____   Total Score
Calculate your total score as follows:
a = 4 points   c = 2 points
b = 3 points   d = 1 point

Place your total score in the space provided.

Organizational Stressors

Organizational variables greatly influence employee job satisfaction. Very few
employees report high job satisfaction in high-stress situations. Organizational factors
tend to center on financial rewards and opportunities for individual growth.

Lack of Financial Rewards

It has often been said that pay is important only on payday, when employees are
reminded that they are more or less valued. Even so, substantial financial rewards are
a constant reminder that the work is valued and the employee is probably hard to
replace. On days when immediate rewards are absent, a high salary may help to bol-
ster self-esteem and reduce frustration. Low pay may increase stress in exactly the
opposite way, fueling the negative self-image and self-talk that destroy concentration
and deflate the energy often necessary to fight simple depression and anxiety. Employees who are highly satisfied with most other aspects of their work will often overlook
low pay, but low pay and lack of job satisfaction represent a deadly duo that greatly
contribute to stress.

Lack of Career Guidance

Another potential source of stress from occupational frustration exists in the area of
career development. Especially in this technological, computer-driven age, advanced
skill training is expected in many jobs. The following aspects of career development

are considered important components of the working environment and are useful in contributing to job satisfaction and preventing occupational frustration:

- the opportunity to fully use occupational skills
- the opportunity to develop new, expanded skills
- counseling to facilitate career decisions

Thus, it is important for managers to realize that workers on all levels are demanding intrinsic rewards from their jobs more than ever before. Many large corporations and even branches of the federal government (NASA, for example) have instituted formal career counseling and career-development programs.

Such programs have taken on increased importance as companies enter the age of down-sizing, sometimes called "right-sizing." Spawned by massive corporate mergers and efforts to decrease operating costs, many workers are being retired early or simply fired in order to achieve small corporate work forces.

Overspecialization

In this era of highly specialized work, another source of occupational frustration is overspecialization. It has been accepted wisdom in industry that a high specialization—that is, having workers become expert in highly specific job areas—is a way of increasing the efficiency and quality of work. Conceptually, this is a sound procedure. However, because workers are searching for greater intrinsic rewards from their jobs, having them work in an overly fragmented or specialized job area may frustrate them. In our own consulting work with industry and business, we are impressed with the number of employees on all levels and in all professions who express a desire to "see the completed fruits of their labor." Workers do not want to perceive themselves as an insignificant cog in an immense wheel of industry; they want to identify with their companies and products. Far too often overspecialization robs the worker of this reward. This problem is a serious one on the assembly line, and it may even reach into the professions. In a local hospital famous for its emergency shock-trauma department, we were surprised to find nurses expressing desires to follow patients through recovery rather than seeing them only in the emergency room and never knowing how their treatment progressed.

Work Overload

Job design and technology can contribute to occupational stress. Jobs without freedom produce more stress than autonomous and flexible ones. One of the most damaging situations involving a lack of freedom is excessive deadline pressure resulting in overload.

Sometimes there is simply too much work to do, or the work is too difficult. When these conditions result in mistakes on the job or contribute to ill health, work overload exists. Overload affects the individual by overstimulating psychological and physiological mechanisms. In effect, overload is a condition in which the individual is bombarded with excessive job demands—excessive in that they cause excessive stress when the worker attempts to meet all the demands.

There are three types of overload: (1) quantitative, (2) qualitative, and (3) a combination of both. Quantitative overload exists when too much work has to be done within a limited time. The individual is capable of completing all of the work, but the time restriction causes the reaction. This form of overload is most commonly found in the production industries and in clerical occupations. Qualitative overload exists when the work to be completed exceeds the individual's technical or intellectual capabilities at that time. This form of overload is encountered most often in research and development organizations as well as in many of the so-called professions—health care, law, and so on. Finally, the combination of quantitative and qualitative overload is commonly encountered in administrative-management positions in all industries, in all levels of the sales industry, and in entrepreneurial endeavors.

Three occupational conditions that seem to predispose one to overload are the following:

- time pressures, which may develop into quantitative overload
- job complexity, which may develop into qualitative overload
- decision making, which may evolve into a combination of both forms of overload

Time Urgency.   Our society's race against the clock has been proven to be a major source of stress. Virtually every organization exerts some form of time pressure over its employees. It may be in the form of deadlines for work projects, deadlines for reports, sales deadlines, seasonal working limitations, or even unit production quotas (as in assembly-line or other factory environments). Time urgency is the most obvious condition that fosters the development of quantitative overload because time limitations create restrictions on the quantity of work that can reasonably be completed. When the employee attempts to complete more work than is reasonable for the time restriction, a case of overarousal will arise—the heart will pump harder and faster as the individual attempts to work beyond his or her normal work rate. In addition, worry about what will happen if the work is not completed will cause the heart to work even harder. A vicious cycle is begun.

In some cases, deadlines will motivate a worker to achieve high levels of performance. However, when the time urgency causes mistakes or contributes to ill health, a condition of quantitative overload exists. At that point, time urgency becomes destructive. This condition has been referred to as the *hurry sickness.* You can perhaps recall instances when you were racing against the clock. How did you feel? Could you feel your temples pounding or your heart racing? Take a moment to remember the last time you were rushing against a deadline you couldn't meet. Medical research on the effects of time urgency on health is most revealing. Research by cardiologists Meyer Friedman and Ray Rosenman (1974) led them to conclude that chronic time-urgency appears to harm the cardiovascular system. Typically, the results are premature heart attacks and/or high blood pressure (Friedman 1996).

Even the threat of impending quantitative overload has an adverse effect on workers. Many employees tend to demonstrate contempt and suspicion for management—they resent management telling them how to do more work in less time. In some instances, the results are work slowdowns and sabotage if time/work output analyses are implemented from an authoritarian point of view.

Time urgency appears to be a way of organizational life. However, in Chapter 6 we discussed ways in which individuals may reduce the harmful effects of time urgency on their minds and bodies while still meeting most organizational demands.

Job Complexity.   Many people believe that life is growing more and more complex. The most common factor contributing to qualitative overload is *job complexity,* or the inherent difficulty of the work that must be done. The higher the complexity, the more stressful the job. The complexity of the work can easily evolve into qualitative overload if the complexity exceeds one's technical or intellectual capabilities at the time. Job complexity is usually increased by the following factors:

- increase in the amount of information to be used
- increase in the sophistication of the information or in skills needed for the job
- expansion or addition of job methods
- introduction of a contingency plan

Although these four strategies will increase the probability of a better product, when excessive they will also increase the individual's stress-arousal level to where it actually inhibits his or her performance. Therefore, there is a point at which increasing the complexity of the job no longer proves productive but instead becomes destructive. At this point the individual's abilities to reason and solve problems have been surpassed, and mental fatigue and emotional and physical reactions ensue—all forms of the stress response. Medical research suggests that emotional and mental fatigue, headaches, and gastrointestinal disorders are common outcomes of chronic qualitative overload.

Decision Making

Decision making pervades all aspects of life. Yet it has special applicability to the world of work (Smith 1998). Decision making represents a unique combination of factors that may eventually lead to the development of simultaneous quantitative and qualitative overload. Let us examine decision making as a potential source of occupational stress.

Decision making involves making a choice. Inherent in this process is evaluation—that is, determining the relative merits of one alternative versus another. The stressfulness of decision making is determined largely by the following factors.

- the importance of the decision's consequences
- the complexity of the decision

- the amount of available information
- the locus of responsibility for the decision
- the amount of time allotted for the decision-making process
- the expectation of success

The importance of the consequences of any decision greatly contributes to the stressfulness of decision making. You know, for example, that deciding what kind of car to buy is more stressful than deciding where to eat lunch. There is simply more at risk, more to be lost should your decision be a poor one. The key to successful handling of a complex decision is being able to ascertain what is meaningful and what is superfluous information and being able to organize and synthesize that information.

While too much information can make decision making stressful, insufficient information can lead to even greater stress. If you have ever lacked sufficient information to make a decision, you know how frustrating this can be. We have chosen to discuss this topic in terms of overload because of the way most people react to such a condition. If you are faced with insufficient information for making a decision, your first reaction is usually to guess or to extrapolate the needed information. In most cases this guessing game results in a significant psychological strain as you attempt to foresee all of the possibilities. This strain is nothing other than overload. Another factor that surely increases the stressfulness of decision making is the locus of responsibility—that is, who will be responsible for the decision? It is more stressful if one person alone has responsibility for a decision than if that responsibility can be shared. It is interesting to observe that many executives insist on single responsibility, for in many systems the individual will receive full recognition for a job well done. Such systems are also very quick to point out consistent incompetence. The fact remains, however, that single decision-making responsibility can be highly stressful and thus may stifle creativity in some individuals; upholding the status quo may be perceived as the safest decision.

Time is another factor in the stressfulness of decision making. With only a few exceptions, we can say that the shorter the amount of time allotted for decision making, the more stressful that decision process will be. One notable exception is the case in which far more time is allowed than is really required. Such conditions seem to breed worry and reconsideration; you might go back and change your mind, a habit that often leads to a less-effective decision.

Finally, the expectation of success figures into the stressfulness of decision making. Self-fulfilling prophecy suggests that if the decision maker fully expects to make a correct decision, his or her stress level will be lower than if there is doubt (Farmer 1999). Typically, the probability of making a correct decision will be enhanced as well. However, if the decision maker fully expects to fail, his or her stress level may be low also. Such a negative self-fulfilling prophecy may be used to cope with the stress involved in decision making because there will be no disappointment when the individual does indeed fail—after all, it was expected. The only problem with this stress-reduction strategy is that it greatly increases the probability of failure and loss of self-esteem. Therefore, it is a destructive coping mechanism.

The amount of stress involved in decision making may be expressed as follows:

Decision-Making Stress = Importance + Complexity + Lack of Information + Responsibility + Lack of Time + Lack of Confidence

The multifaceted nature of the decision-making process explains why decision making can result in quantitative and/or qualitative overload. How many of these factors adversely affect your day-to-day decision making?

Organizational policies—not to be confused with human interactions and politics, which will be covered later—contribute to the stressful climate of the workplace. Policies that are rigid and insensitive to employee needs increase employee stress levels and can create an atmosphere in which decision making, the job of most employees and all managers, is fraught with stress.

Individual Stressors

Individual stressors are perhaps the greatest contributors to occupational stress because they include human interaction, the greatest source of stress in general. Another stressor of special concern is occupational frustration, which in turn is influenced by such stressors as job ambiguity and role conflict, stifled communication, discrimination, bureaucracy, inactivity, and boredom.

Occupational Frustration

Have you ever thought that your job was holding you back? Have you ever considered yourself lost within the organization? Have you ever wished for more of a chance to use or develop your job skills? These are the types of thoughts that result from being frustrated on your job. Occupational stress from frustration exists when the job inhibits, stifles, or thwarts desired expectations and/or goals. The body reacts adversely to the frustration of psychological desires, resulting in what we know to be the stress response. If we understand occupational frustration as this sense of being inhibited, then several major sources of occupational frustration immediately come to mind.

Job Ambiguity and Role Conflict

Two of the major contributors to frustration on the job are job ambiguity and role conflict. Job ambiguity refers to the condition in which the job description or the level of job performance is confusing or virtually unknown to the employee. In a case like this, you might find yourself asking questions such as "What should I do now?" or wondering "How did I do on the last assignment?" Job ambiguity may be caused by the following:

- unclear work objectives (goals)
- confusion surrounding responsibility

- unclear working procedures
- confusion about what others expect of you
- lack of feedback or uncertainty surrounding your job performance

Consistently, such conditions result in job dissatisfaction and significant stress levels. Role conflict exists when a job function contains roles, duties, or responsibilities that may conflict with one another. This is most commonly found among middle managers who find themselves caught between top-level management and lower-level management. Research has clearly demonstrated the middle-management position to be the most stressful of the three management levels. Role conflict may also be caused by work roles that conflict with personal, familial, or immediate societal values. Individuals in the law-enforcement profession are those most frequently caught in this conflict. Once again, the result of such role conflict is job dissatisfaction and stress from frustration.

Stifled Communication

The term *organizational communication* refers to the patterns and networks along which communications flow through an organization. Stifled organizational communication has been found to be the single most prevalent source of frustration in organizations today. Do you find yourself feeling isolated in your job or relying on information that comes too late or not at all? Have you ever had a conversation with someone and walked away asking yourself what that person had really said? These are common communication problems. Proper planning and organizing depend on effective communication. Ideally, communications flow upward from subordinates to superiors and horizontally from department to department, as well as in the traditional downward direction from superiors to subordinates. In many cases, organizations frustrate employees by keeping open only the downward channels. Typically, the last channel to be maintained is the upward channel. This is not only frustrating but a gross waste of human resources. Efficient organizational communication is perceived as so important that organizational communication is becoming a field in itself. University graduate programs are offered in this area. Efficient communication can be a powerful source for stress reduction and increased performance on the job. Unfortunately, it is often overlooked or assumed to be working well.

Discrimination

Hiring, pay, and promotional policies are discriminatory if they are based on nonwork-related factors. Discrimination has long been known to be correlated with intense frustration and anger. Occupational discrimination has been found to be a major concern of the working middle class. This topic is of special interest in today's job market because the discrimination that plagued nonwhites and females in the work force is being replaced to some degree by so-called *reverse discrimination*, wherein nonwhites and females are being looked upon favorably for jobs and promotions (Burnbach 1998). Discrimination of any type is harmful to the organization and the individual worker because it leads to job dissatisfaction, anger, resentment, and a sense of hopelessness embodied in the "what's the use of trying to do a good job?" attitude.

Bureaucracy

Another source of occupational frustration, and perhaps the most insidious source of this form of stress, is bureaucracy. Bureaucracy is a form of organizational planning. The man most responsible in the twentieth century for formalizing and advocating bureaucracy was Max Weber (1864–1920). Weber was concerned with designing an "ideal" organizational structure based on logic and rational thought. According to Weber, there are four major characteristics of a bureaucracy:

1. Specialization and division of labor
2. A set of rules governing all aspects of organizational behavior to ensure uniformity and organizational stability
3. Emotionless management; relationships within the organization should be typified by objectivity and a lack of enthusiasm, hatred, and so forth.
4. A hierarchy of positions; the entire organizational structure must follow the principle of centralized hierarchy—that is, offices built upon offices—so that there exists absolute control over subordinate functions. (*Bureaucracy* literally means "rule by office.")

It must be understood that Weber's design was to be an ideal one. No bureaucracy yet created has lived up to his expectations. The major reason for this failure is probably that the complexity of the human personality is simply not applicable to the bureaucratic structure. In theory, bureaucracy is the most logical and efficient organizational structure possible; in practice, it may be the most counterproductive form of organized work effort.

The most common criticisms of this form of management are the following:

- frustration or thwarting of personal and professional development
- fostering mediocrity on the job
- the reinforcement of complex rules (red tape)
- stifled communication due in part to excessive paperwork (more red tape)
- impersonality of supervisors and supervisory practices
- arbitrary rules virtually written in stone
- stifled creativity

Especially in this age of participation, most new, eager, creative workers find bureaucracies stressful places to work (McLagan and Nel 1997, Pinchot and Pinchot 1994).

Inactivity and Boredom

Have you ever noticed that some people become nervous when they don't have enough to do? Have you ever gone looking for something to work on when you didn't really have to? Inactivity and boredom on the job can cause a stress response. They may manifest themselves as nervousness, an inability to sit still, or a noticeable tenseness. Hans Selye categorizes this form of stress as *deprivational stress.*

If you suffer from deprivational stress on the job, then your job is failing to provide you with meaningful psychological stimulation. Two occupational settings are noted for this form of stress: the assembly line and the large bureaucracy.

Perhaps the best place to begin to look at boredom is on the assembly line. Here the employee is asked to perform some highly repetitive task. After a relatively short orientation period, he or she will be able to perform the required task with minimal challenge. Before long the task will become boring, and stimulation of another kind will be sought—something to occupy the mind in a more meaningful manner. If such stimulation is found and does not distract from task performance, all will be fine. However, in some cases the thing that the employee chooses to occupy his or her mind with detracts from job performance; the worker makes more mistakes or works more slowly. In other cases the employee may be unable to keep his or her mind occupied; job satisfaction then begins to decline.

The industrial literature from the last half century is full of examples of worker reactions to job boredom. Cases of low production efficiency, alcohol and drug abuse, and even assembly-line sabotage have been recorded, not to mention employee turnover. The majority of cases seem to occur under the following conditions: (1) job boredom, (2) repetitive tasks on the job, (3) no opportunity for workers to communicate, and (4) low job satisfaction

Boredom and inactivity may affect white-collar workers as well. In our own consulting work with large bureaucracies, we have observed the results of the boredom that overspecialization and job redundancy create. A common complaint from white-collar workers in such organizations is that there is "not enough stimulating work to do." Many federal agencies appear to manifest this problem. To maintain sanity, people find ways of compensating for their low job satisfaction and stifled creativity. The most common compensation device we've seen is employees working at minimally acceptable levels of job performance during the week and then expressing themselves on the weekend through their avocational pursuits. This "living for the weekend" attitude is obviously debilitating to the organization.

Environmental Stressors

Environmental stressors range from the physical environment of the work station and the organization's location in the community to the location of the community itself (Sellers 1999). More often the stress in this category is that of adapting to the environment and living with the changes that accompany most work situations. As Dilbert working in his cubical has made famous, unfavorable environments and changes result in more severe stress; however, even positive changes require adaptation and can be stressful. As with most stressors, the severity level of environmental stressors forms a continuum. The competitive environment, for example, might range from boring and nonexistent to cutthroat.

Change and Adaptation

Change within an organization is a necessary and vital component of growth and continued productivity; yet it can also be a source of stress for many employees. Change is stressful because it disrupts the psychological and physiological rhythms that accompany all human behavior. Change requires the expansion of psychological and physiological energies, whether the change is good or bad. Hans Selye summarizes this point by stating that the expenditure of adaptive energy is what makes change stressful. Change becomes harmful at the point at which adaptive energy is depleted. The result is psychological or physiological breakdown or illness (Kompier and Cooper 1999).

There are numerous sources of *adaptive stress* (stress due to change) within the organizational world. Some of the more common ones are the following:

Technological Change.   Business and industry are ever more dependent on technology. Space-age technology has contributed to increased efficiency of all work functions from production to clerical processes to high-level managerial decisions. Computers, the Internet, and other modern forms of communication affect workers. Even though this technology is a very positive force in the working world, it still requires role changes for those whom it affects. Such changes require adaptation.

Relocation.   Another common source of adaptive stress is relocation, both vocational and residential. When you are forced to relocate, a great deal of stress generally follows. Even if the relocation is in conjunction with a raise and promotion, you will still have to cope with a new environment. The following factors intensify stress from relocation:

- the complexities of moving possessions from one location to another
- the severing of interpersonal relationships
- the formation of new interpersonal relationships
- the necessity of adjusting to new cultural and/or socioeconomic conditions

All of these factors are compounded if you must relocate residence and work setting simultaneously.

For many individuals change is exhilarating. Even so, change, whether good or bad, requires the expenditure of adaptive energy and is therefore stressful. So even positive changes should be carefully considered during periods of high stress unless of course the change removes you from the stressors.

Promotion.   The stressfulness of being promoted is considered by most to be a small price to pay for the rewards of the promotion. Take a moment to consider the impact of the following factors that generally accompany a promotion, in addition to the obvious rewards:

- significant changes in job function
- increased responsibility for people, production, and money

- changes in social role (Some promotions come with certain social obligations that cause intense social and even financial stress)

These factors involve considerable adaptation for most individuals. Even if they are all positive, they take some getting used to.

Reorganization and Down-sizing.   Departmental or organizational restructuring often happens when a new administration takes over. Such major reorganization happens rarely, but it can be a major source of adaptive stress. Feelings of insecurity, anticipation, and apprehension usually dominate the minds of those affected by reorganization. If you are ever in such a reorganization, the first thing on your mind will probably be job security. Your next question will typically be, "How do I fit into this new arrangement?" During such uncertain periods your work will probably fall off, or you may stress yourself through overload in an attempt to demonstrate your worth to the new management. In either case it behooves you as well as the new management to quickly resolve questions of job security following reorganization.

As the costs of doing business have increased, management has attempted to curtail cost increases by reducing the labor force—down-sizing. Massive corporate mergers, such as Walt Disney and Capital Cities/ABC television in July 1995 and Time Warner and Turner Broadcasting in August 1995, created huge corporate empires ($18.8 billion and $6.8 billion, respectively) but also resulted in significant changes in the labor force due to consolidation of corporate resources. In 1999 hardly a day went by that some megamerger did not make the business headlines. The trend definitely is moving toward larger and larger companies.

A generation ago, a worker would typically work for one or two employers throughout his or her career. It is estimated that the average worker starting in the 1990s will work for three or more employers throughout his or her working life. As workers progress through their working lives, change will likely be no longer an exception but the rule, the new way of the working world. The workers of this decade need to prepare themselves for the inevitability of occupational change and learn how to use it to their advantage. The first step in that process is learning to cope personally with adaptive stress.

Violence in the Workplace

While violence in the workplace seems to have become ubiquitous, the first landmark case of workplace violence occurred on August 20, 1986, in Edmond, Oklahoma (Kinney and Johnson 1993). On that day thirteen postal workers were shot to death. The Bureau of Labor Statistics counted 1,063 workplace homicides in 1993; 36 percent of all homicides occurred in retail sales, while 17 percent occurred in service industries (Thornburg 1993, 40). Beyond homicides, the United States experienced over 110,000 incidents of workplace violence in 1992 costing employers $4.2 billion (Kinney and Johnson 1993, 5). Other than motor vehicle accidents, it seems clear that violence in the workplace is the leading cause of worker death and injury on the job.

What is workplace violence? Workplace violence not only includes homicides of workers but encompasses injuries sustained from battery, assaults, sexual assaults, verbal abuse, threats, and mental anguish caused from actual or threatened violence.

According to Flannery (1995) preincident training and anger management and stress reduction programs can be useful deterrents to workplace violence. Also, employee counseling programs, especially in response to down-sizing, can be effective in reducing employee anger, frustration, and violence (Engel 1998; Kinney and Johnson 1993).

Retirement

Retirement is stressful for many people who have spent most of their adult life working. The association between self-esteem and job is a significant one. People who say "I am an engineer," rather than "I am employed as an engineer," reflect the tendency of employees to identify themselves in terms not so much of broad personal characteristics as of job-related characteristics and roles. Thus, when workers retire, and particularly if they are forced to retire from a very rewarding job, they typically suffer some of the following symptoms:

- depression
- a sense of worthlessness and a loss of self-esteem
- decreased appetite
- lack of motivation in general
- increased cardiovascular complaints
- decreased sexual drive

More important, the U.S. Bureau of Labor Statistics (1995) reports data that suggest that workers who are forcibly retired will survive, on the average, only thirty to forty months after their retirement. It will be interesting to see whether the first decade of the new century will reverse this trend as the older population works to fit the new active, involved image being portrayed in the media. In addition, the better health of older people in general, greater affluence, and the extended retirement age brought on by the pressure on the social security system should make life after work healthier.

Other factors that increase the stressfulness of retirement are as follows:

- a great number of years at the same job
- lack of interests outside the job, such as family, hobbies, and social involvement
- a high affiliation with the job
- lack of preparation for retirement—for example, retirement counseling or even informal mental preparation
- lack of alternative sources of income
- lack of alternative sources of ego gratification (self-esteem)
- knowing others who have retired and encountered difficulties adjusting

Biological Factors in the Workplace

Time Change

If you must rotate work shifts, you don't need this book to tell you that this is stressful and requires significant adaptation. Even changes in time zones during travel are stressful. Two common occupational examples of how stress affects the body when the natural biological rhythms have been disturbed are *jet lag* and *shiftwork fatigue*.

Jet Lag. Jet lag commonly affects transcontinental and transoceanic travelers (Inlander and Moran 1997). This problem can prove costly for business executives who must conduct high-level business affairs. Jet lag has also been found to be a major problem for pilots and airline crews who frequently make long flights.

Shiftwork Fatigue. Workers who must alternate shifts report many of the same symptoms found in jet lag. The most severe symptoms occur when changing to or from the 11 P.M.–7 A.M. shift. Some workers can adapt to the time change in about a week, others require three weeks, and some never properly adjust. It is important to note that the increased stress associated with shiftwork is not directly related to the shiftwork per se but is associated with one's efforts to adjust to an unnatural pattern of sleeping (Moore-Ede 1999, Shiftwork Alert 1998, Westfall-Lake and McBride 1997).

Workers who are subjected to shiftwork over long periods of time appear to have a higher risk for cardiovascular disease, neurotic disorders, dysfunctional alterations in appetite, diarrhea, constipation, and possibly depression (Monk and Folkard 1992).

Noise

Noise can affect the body in three ways: hearing loss, sleep deprivation, and stress. Noise as a source of stress is a rather unique variable. It can prove stressful because of its psychological characteristics—that is, by being unwanted or distracting. It can also prove stressful simply because of its physical characteristics—volume and/or frequency. According to the U.S. Census noise ranks higher than crime, traffic, and public services as a cause of dissatisfaction with urban environments. When New York City opened a hotline for complaints, 70 percent of all calls dealt with noise. Whatever its effect on health as a psychological irritant, noise is moving to the top position (Schafer 1998).

The physical characteristics of noise (intensity and frequency) are the points most often mentioned in discussions of noise as a stressor. Sound levels above 35 to 40 decibels will typically awaken a sleeping person, and sound levels in excess of 55 decibels are sufficient to make normal conversation difficult. Of greater biological significance are noise levels in excess of 65 to 70 decibels. Evidence suggests that at this level there is increased sympathetic-nervous-system arousal characteristic of a stress response. The major component of this response is increased adrenal functions. As decibel levels increase, the body reacts with greater cardiovascular responses characteristic of stress (ibid.). Reactions such as increased heart rate or increased blood pressure become evident.

As chronic noise levels approach 85 decibels, the potential for permanent hearing loss increases significantly. Perhaps the most insidious aspect of this process is that chronic noise exposure is typically selective in its attack on auditory acuity. The usual case of hearing loss occurs only on specific frequency levels, depending on the amount of the exposure. Therefore, it may be very difficult for a worker to notice a hearing loss until it becomes severe.

The federal government has mandated that workers exposed to an average eight-hour total of 90 decibels must wear protective ear equipment. In addition to the harmful effects caused by the intensity of noise, frequency can also be a factor. Frequencies in excess of 20,000 cycles per second are most often implicated in the harmful effects of noise. However, it has been shown that frequencies in the 15-to-20-cycles-per-second range appear especially stressful because of their extremely low vibration levels. Such levels appear to harm the internal organs of many humans. In some cases, frequencies between these levels may actually reduce the stressful effects of noise.

Lighting

Too little light or too much light can create a stress response. The luminance of a light source may be measured in nits (candles per square meter). Tasks that involve fine detail in workmanship (such as watchmaking) require a great deal of light. The recommended luminance for such tasks is around 800 to 1000 nits. General office work and general factory work require around 100 nits. Most stores require around 60 to 100 nits. Hallways usually require around 30 nits. When lighting is below these recommended minimums, the eyes must strain to see the work. The most common form of stress eyestrain results in tension headaches caused by the muscular adjustments needed to maintain proper visual acuity.

The most common characteristic of too much light is glare. Glare results from having the light source so bright that it interferes with focusing on the object being viewed. Computer screens are especially vulnerable to glare if care is not given to their placement. Lighting should be arranged so reflections and glare are minimized. Sometimes standard office lighting is too bright for comfortable video display terminal (VDT) use. If it is not practical to modify office lighting, hoods and neutral density or micromesh filters for the VDT may help. With glare, the light source competes within the retina with the object you are interested in viewing. The result is excessive retinal stimulation. Glare appears also to cut down on the length of time that a worker can spend at a given task without developing headaches.

Computers and Eye Strain

There seems to be no convincing scientific evidence that computer VDTs are harmful to the eyes. VDTs emit little or no harmful radiation such as X-rays or nonionizing radiation (such as ultraviolet) under normal operating conditions. In fact, the amount of ultraviolet radiation produced by VDTs is a small fraction of that produced by fluorescent lighting. The levels of radiation from VDTs are well below those required to produce cataracts or other eye damage even after a lifetime of exposure (American Academy of Ophthalmology 1999).

VDTs are, however, associated with eyestrain, with symptoms such as eye irritation (red, watery, or dry eyes), fatigue (tired, aching heaviness of the eyelids or forehead), and difficulty focusing. Headaches, backaches, or muscle spasms can also occur. These complaints can often be relieved by either changing the arrangement of the workstation or providing proper glasses for the user.

Eyestrain can be prevented by placing the top of the VDT screen at or slightly below eye level, and reference material should be as close to the screen as practical to minimize head and eye movements and focusing changes. Periodic rest breaks are also important because use of a VDT requires a fairly unchanging body, head, and eye position, which can be fatiguing. Frequent blinking will lubricate the eyes and prevent them from drying out.

Carpal Tunnel Syndrome

Carpal Tunnel Syndrome (CTS) appears to be another computer-related condition, and it may occur in any occupation where forceful and repetitive hand and finger movements are necessary. Before the pneumatic nail gun revolutionized the building industry, many "nail-pounders" nursed this condition. CTS occurs when the median nerve is compressed in the carpal tunnel between the transverse carpal ligament and the bones of the wrist and hand. In addition to nerve compression, many people with CTS also have associated problems such as tendonitis, arthralgia (joint pain), and muscle strain (Cherniack 1992).

Carpal Tunnel Syndrome (CTS) is a common cause of numbness or tingling over the thumb side of the hand; pain in the hand, wrist, and arm; or in severe cases, weakness or atrophy in those muscles in the hand that are supplied by the median nerve. The sensory symptoms are often more pronounced after forceful or repetitive use of the hand and are often present at night. Common clinical signs of CTS include decreased sensation in the thumb, index, middle, and half of the ring finger; a tingling, electric sensation in the hand when the base of the palm is firmly tapped; and onset of symptoms when the wrist is held in sustained flexion (the fingers pointed in toward the body) (Neurology Staff 1993).

OSHA's guidelines on CTS state that unless the illness was caused solely by a nonwork-related event or exposure off-premises, the case is presumed to be work-related. OSHA also points out that it is appropriate to make all reasonable efforts to apply the principles of ergonomics to the workplace to reduce the physical and psychological factors that may contribute to Carpal Tunnel Syndrome (1998).

When there is a strong suspicion that activity at work is a contributing factor to CTS, a worksite analysis may be done. Its purpose is to identify and minimize contributing risk factors such as positioning and repetitive activity.

Temperature

As most readers will confirm, working conditions that are too hot or too cold can be stressful. The ideal average temperature (at 50 percent relative humidity) for sedentary work ranges from 70 to 75 degrees Fahrenheit for someone wearing a suit and long-sleeved shirt. Light standing work is done best at about 66 to 72 degrees. Manual labor appears to be done best at a few degrees lower (McIntyre 1973).

Ambient temperature in excess of 81 degrees Fahrenheit appears to erode productivity on tasks that consist of complex reasoning or minute detail and require intense concentration. This is especially true in temperatures in excess of 86 degrees Fahrenheit. This decline in productivity appears to be due to the psychophysiological arousal characteristic of the stress response. However, temperatures in the low 80s have little effect on light mental tasks such as basic arithmetic or typing or on light manual tasks such as most production-line work.

High humidity can significantly increase the stress from heat. The body cools itself by evaporation of perspiration, but evaporation is retarded by high humidity; the result is greater retained heat in the body. Fresh circulating air tends to assist in the cooling process. Although most stress caused by temperature is heat related, cold can also affect industrial performance. As the work environment gets colder, blood flows out of the hands and feet to curb heat loss through radiation. When this happens, fine motor control is gradually lost, and manual performance is hindered. Such performance declines significantly when hand temperatures drop below 55 degrees Fahrenheit. In general, however, excessive heat appears to be a larger contributor to stress and decreased occupational performance (ibid.).

Physical Posture

Cramped muscles and inactivity plague anyone who is deskbound for a period of time, especially at the computer. Muscle tension in the head, neck, and shoulders is the most prevalent example of what can happen from laboring over the computer or piles of paper every day. Leg cramps and even some lower-back problems can result from chronic sitting. Computer workers know all too well the aching forearms, wrists, and fingers that can result from hours of typing at a keyboard. Neck problems, carpal tunnel syndrome, and eye strain are now the leading occupational conditions caused, of course, by logging excessive time on the computer. In addition to these specific problems are the effects of sedentary work on the cardiovascular system. Exercise is a necessity for a healthy mind and body; thus many office workers participate in some kind of exercise regimen.

Compassion Fatigue: The Stress of Caring Too Much

We are told that it is important to care about our jobs, to care about our "customers." But can we care too much? Earlier in this volume, we discussed the notion of "burnout" and described its three stages. Burnout is sometimes seen as a result of stress on the job. Charles Figley (1995) has described a special form of burnout that he refers to as "compassion fatigue." Compassion fatigue may be thought of as the stress of helping individuals during or after traumatic, or otherwise serious, life events. Examples could be working with persons who experience a terminal diagnosis, a disfiguring injury, sexual assault, a near-death traumatic accident, a mass disaster, or other traumatic incidents.

Compassion fatigue may be thought of as a beleaguering degree of sympathy for others who have experienced extreme suffering. Therapists, nurses, physicians, emergency response workers, and hospice workers are prime candidates for compassion fatigue. Symptoms may arise in two seemingly opposite forms: (1) symptoms of overidentification and enmeshment with the primary "victim," or (2) symptoms of anger, resentment, and even disgust directed toward the primary victims. An example of the first type would be the paramedic who felt so sorry for the victims of an automobile accident (an eighteen-year-old unmarried mother and her nine-month-old boy) that she took them both home with her and allowed them to live with her for three years. An example of the second type of compassion fatigue would be the emergency room physician who became extremely angry at the suicide victim who died while the physician was trying to save his life.

It is clear that compassion fatigue is a very real occupational hazard for some unique professions, namely the helping professions. Although contrary to the professional images conveyed by firefighters and law enforcement officers, they too may be victims of compassion fatigue.

Recent advances in occupational psychology have led to the development of training programs designed to "immunize" professionals who may be prone to compassion fatigue (Flannery 1999, Sheehan 1999).

Occupational Stress Management

In this chapter we have reviewed core concepts related to the understanding of occupational stress and occupational stressors. The integrative work of a number of researchers points us to an important conclusion: The worker's perception of the work environment and job itself plays a critical deterministic role in the creation of excessive occupational stress. Smith and his colleagues (Smith, Everly, and Johns 1992) have shown, as noted earlier, that the majority of occupational stressors reviewed in this chapter do not exert a direct stress-to-disease link. Rather, these stressors create a condition of psychological discord, which then leads to stress-related illness. This concept is captured in Figure 11.1. This model points out that adverse health consequences in the workplace may be mitigated by two intervention strategies: (1) creating a healthier workplace, and (2) reducing psychological discord by implementing personal stress-management programs. The latter has been the focus of several of the preceding chapters. By practicing personal stress management techniques, the worker not only mitigates the adverse effects of a stressful workplace but increases stress resistance.

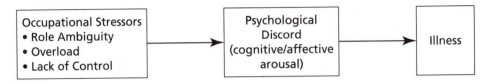

FIGURE 11.1   Stressors, Psychological Discord, and Illness

As for creating a healthier workplace, the following guidelines have been suggested (Cartwright, Cooper, and Murphy 1995, Everly and Mitchell 1995, Gauster 1995):

1. Job functions should be designed to provide the worker with sufficient control to mitigate overload and frustration. Responsibility must be followed by authority.
2. The work environment should provide sufficient social support for workers, including adequate leadership. Cohesive work teams and participative management should be encouraged to further involve workers' participation.
3. Workers should receive adequate clarification of work-related roles and policies.
4. Schedules should be flexible.

Provisions should be made to respond to work-related trauma, disasters, and crises. Despite the difficulty of objectively measuring the costs of stress to business and industry, the occupational stress epidemic is perceived to be severe enough to have prompted the mobilization of a stress-management industry to combat the problem. It is important to recognize that not all stress can be eliminated from work. Work is a place where people interact, and some stress is inherent in human interactions. Work is also very often done in an impersonal and hurried environment with little social support because the purpose of work is productivity.

Reduction of debilitating stress is the primary objective of occupational stress management. A secondary focus is aligning personality, skill level, and task to decrease stress and increase productivity. Turnover or functional transfers can reduce organizational strain caused by mismatches of skill and task. A more efficient approach is to find and reduce the stress situations before inefficiency, decreased productivity, and ill health occur. If stress-management programs are effective, we may soon see corporate savings sufficient enough to be passed on to consumers, thereby creating a lever that competition-minded corporations can use in the marketplace.

SOURCES CITED

American Academy of Ophthalmology. (1999). *Computers and eyestrain.* http://www.eyenet.org/public/faqs/computers_faq.html

Burnbach, J. (1998). Job discrimination: *How to fight and win.* Ojai, CA: Voir Dire Press.

Cartwright, S., Cooper, C. L., and Murphy, L. R. (1995). Diagnosing a healthy organization. In *Job stress interventions,* eds. L. Murphy, J. Hurrell, S. Sauter, and G. Keita. Washington, D.C.: American Psychological Association, 217–34.

Cherniack, M. (1992). *Disease of unusual occupations: An historical perspective.* Occupational Medicine, 7, 369–384.

Diberardinis, Louis, ed. (1998). *Handbook of occupational safety and health.* New York: John Wiley and Sons.

Engel, P. (1998). *The exceptional individual: Achieving business success one person at a time.* New York: St. Martins Press.

Engel, F. (1998). *Taming the beast: Getting violence out of the workplace.* New York: Ashwell.

Everly, G. S., and Mitchell, J. T. (1995). Prevention of work-related post-traumatic stress: The critical incident stress debriefing process. In *Job stress interventions,* eds. L. Murphy, J. Hurrell, S. Sauter, and G. Keita. Washington, D.C.: American Psychological Association, 173–84.

Farmer, R. E. A. (1999). *Macroeconomics of self-fulfilling prophecies.* Cambridge: MIT Press.

Figley, C. R. (1995). Compassion fatigue. In *Secondary Traumatic Stress,* ed. B. Hudnall Stamm. Lutherville, MD: Sidran, 3–28.

Flannery, R. B. (1995). *Violence in the workplace.* New York: Crossroad.

Flannery, R. B. (1999). *Critical incident stress management and the assaulted staff action program.* International Journal of Emergency Mental Health, 1, 103–8.

Fletcher, B. (1991). *Work, stress, and disease.* New York: John Wiley & Sons.

Frankenhaeuser, M. (1986). A psychobiological framework for research on human stress and coping. In *Dynamics of stress,* eds. M. Appley and R. Trumbell. New York: Plenum, 101–16.

Frankenhaeuser, M., Lundberg, U., and Chesney, M., eds. (1991). *Women, work, and health.* New York: Plenum.

Friedman, M. (1996). *Type A behavior: Its diagnosis and treatment.* New York: Plenum.

Friedman, M., and Rosenman, R. (1974). *Type A behavior and your heart.* New York: Knopf.

Gardell, B. (1976). *Reactions at work and their influence on nonwork activities.* Human Relations, 29, 885–904.

Gauster, D. (1995). Interventions for building healthy organizations. In *Job stress interventions,* eds. L. Murphy, J. Hurrell, S. Sauter, and G. Keita. Washington, D.C.: American Psychological Association, 323–36.

Gouldner, A. W. (1954). *Patterns of industrial bureaucracy.* Glencoe, IL: Free Press.

Inlander, C., and Moran, C. (1997). *Sixty-two natural ways to beat jet lag.* New York: St. Martins Mass Market.

Karasek, R., Baker, D., Marxer, F., Ahlbom, A., and Theorell, T. (1981). *Job decision, job demands, and cardiovascular disease.* American Journal of Public Health, 71, 694–705.

Karasek, R., and Theorell, T. (1992). *Healthy work.* New York: Basic Books.

Keable, D. (1999). *The management of anxiety.* New York: Church Livingston.

Kinney, J. A., and Johnson, D. L. (1993). *Breaking point.* Chicago: National Safe Workplace Institute.

Kompier, M., and Cooper, C. (1999). *Preventing stress, improving productivity.* New York: Routledge.

LaDou, J. (1997). *Occupational and environmental medicine.* Stamford, CT: Appleton and Lange.

McCarthy, M. (1988). *Stressed employees look for relief in worker's compensation claims.* Wall Street Journal (April 7), 34.

McIntyre, D. (1973). *A guide to thermal comfort.* Applied Ergonomics, 4, 66–72.

McLagan, P. and Nel, C. (1997). *The age of participation: New governance for the workplace and the world.* San Francisco: Berrett-Koehler.

Monk, T. H., and Folkard, S. (1992). *Making shiftwork tolerable.* London: Taylor and Francis.

Moore-Ede, M. (1999). *The twenty-four hour society: Understanding human limits in a world that never stops.* Cambridge: Circadian Technologies.

Neurology Staff. (1993). *Practice parameters for electrodiagnostic study in CTS.* Neurology, 43, 2404–5.

Occupational Safety and Health Administration. (1998). *Carpal tunnel syndrome.* Washington, D.C.: OSHA.

Pinchot, G., and Pinchot, E. (1994). *The end of bureaucracy and the rise of the intelligent organization.* San Francisco: Berrett-Koehler.

Radmacher, S. A., and Sheridan, C. L. (1995). An investigation of the demand-control model of job strain. In *Organizational risk factors for job stress,* eds. S. Sauter and L. Murphy. Washington, D.C: American Psychological Association, 127–38.

Schafer, R. Murray (1998). *The book of noise*. New York: Arcana Editions.

Sellers, C. C. (1999). *Hazards on the job: From industrial disease to environmental health science*. Chapel Hill: University of North Carolina Press.

Sheehan, D. C. (1999). *Stress management in the FBI*. International Journal of Emergency Mental Health, 1, 39–42.

Shiftwork Alert Editors. (1998) *The practical guide to managing 24-hour operations*. Cambridge: Circadian Information.

Smith, C. L. (1998) *Computer-supported decision making: Meeting the decision demands of modern organizations*. Norwood, NJ: Ablex.

Smith, K. J., Davy, J. and Everly, G. S. (1995). *An examination of the antecedents of job dissatisfaction and turnover intentions among CPAs in public accounting*. Accounting Inquiries, 5, 99–142.

Smith, K. J., Everly, G. S. and Johns, T. (1992). A structural modeling analysis of the mediating role of cognitive-affective arousal in the relationship between stressors and illness among accountants. Paper presented to the 2nd APA/NIOSH Conference on Occupational Stress, December, Washington, D.C.

Thornburg, L. (1993). *When violence hits business*. HR Magazine, 7, 40–45. U.S. Department of Labor (1995). Labor Statistics Report. Washington, D.C.: Government Printing Office.

Westfall-Lake, M., and McBride, G. (1997). *Shiftwork safety and performance*. New York: Lewis Publishers.

CHAPTER

12 Breathing and Relaxation

Breathing Correctly

Wouldn't you know it! The first thing in life we learned to do, and we learned it wrong. We are referring here to the act of breathing. But, you say, breathing is a natural, automatic body function. How can breathing be right or wrong? You should realize by now that any body process can be altered and, if the practice is prolonged, conditioned. For reasons too numerous and involved to discuss here, most of us have developed and conditioned inefficient and improper breathing techniques. And what could be more important than bringing in fresh air and revitalizing the body tissues? Ancient yoga philosophy states that mind is the master of the senses, breath is the master of the mind, and breathing is the elixir of life.

Actually, the exchange of air is only one aspect of breathing that is important to the relaxation process. Breathing is an involuntary, automatic function that reflects our general state of stress arousal. But breathing is also voluntary and can be manipulated. If we so desire, we can breathe fast or slow; our inhalations can be deep or shallow; our expirations can be partial or complete; and in some cases, we even "choose" difficult or pathological breathing patterns. By learning to breathe correctly, air is taken in more efficiently, the pulmonary system is strengthened and conditioned, the function of the cardiovascular system is enhanced, greater oxygenation is promoted, the nerves are calmed, and restfulness occurs. The breathing centers in the brain have a facilitating relationship with the arousal centers; therefore, constant, steady, restful breathing promotes relaxation. It is almost impossible to be tense and have slow, relaxed, deep breaths. Thus, control breathing and you control tension. Condition breathing, and you condition your system to be more tranquil. The power of deep, steady breathing is instinctual. When you want to control your energy—when lifting a heavy object, for example—you instinctively hold your breath. When you want to center yourself—when pulling the string of a bow or the trigger of a gun, for instance—you instinctively breathe deeply and hold. It is your most natural way of centering yourself or concentrating. Breath control is essential for control of the mind (Iyengar 1995).

Breathing is used in almost every relaxation technique that has stood the test of time and been evaluated as effective. Scientists have mapped the location of the neuropeptides associated with the relaxation response, and they can be found in the floor of the fourth ventricle, which is where breathing is controlled. Peptides are released into the ventricular fluid and affect how fast the breaths are, how shallow, and how deep. Breathing goes on automatically, but you can instantly take control of it without any training. You can make your will change your breathing, your peptides, and your emotional state (Pert 1995).

Most of our shifts in attention at the body level are subconscious. Although neuropeptides are actually directing our attention by their activities, we are not consciously involved in deciding what gets processed, remembered, and learned. But we do have the possibility of bringing some of these decisions into consciousness, particularly with the help of various types of intentional training techniques such as insight meditation (described in Chapter 16). In some instances the unconscious can be harnessed for healing or change without the conscious mind being involved. Hypnosis, breathing, and many of the energy-based therapies utilizing body work, massage, and therapeutic touch are all examples of techniques that you can use to effect change at a level beneath consciousness (Pert 1999).

Practicing breathing techniques not only facilitates relaxation; it also plays a vital role in the prevention of respiratory ailments. Individuals with respiratory disorders such as asthma and emphysema can benefit not only from increased oxygenation but also from learning correct, efficient, and less-stressful breathing patterns. But even for those individuals without respiratory-system pathology, breathing is often labored and inefficient. At rest we normally use only one-third of our lung capacity. Through breathing exercises, you will be able to vitalize these functions, regulate breathing patterns, build up respiratory reserve, and increase oxygenation capacity.

The biggest breathing muscle in the human body is the diaphragm, the lowering of which can take place only when the jaw and the throat are relaxed, the belly is free, and the hip joints allow free leg movement and flexibility in the lower back. When these conditions are not met, the body compensates by lifting the shoulders, pulling up the chest bone, and contracting the sphincter muscles in the throat, movements that weaken the muscles that assist the breathing process (Buchholz 1994).

In correct breathing the floating ribs (lower five pairs) are moved by the intercostal muscles between the ribs and the diaphragm as it descends toward the abdomen. This movement allows for expansion of the lower lobes of the lungs, creating a vacuum, and the air rushes in. If you keep the abdominal muscles tight during the breathing movement, your diaphragm cannot descend and the lower lobes cannot fill, so a deep breath is possible only by a hyperexpansion of the top lobes, a method that expends much more energy. Many people have developed the habit of high breathing because it is thought to represent a more "masculine" posture—stomach in, chest out. This is not to say that one should not have strong, taut stomach muscles; on the contrary, contraction-relaxation movements will further strengthen stomach muscles without a chronic shortening developing. It is also important not to neglect exhalation. You must exhale deeply to get the stale, used air out or there is less room for fresh air to enter. Generally, exhalation lasts longer than inhalation. Correct breathing, once mastered, becomes a chronic exercise that expands and contracts the lung tissue, building strength and endurance.

Learning more efficient breathing patterns can be facilitated by the ability to perform and differentiate between the following exercises.

Upper Costal Breathing

Use your hands to sense the action of the respiratory movements. Place your hands on the upper third of the chest wall, preferably crossing the hands with the fingertips resting comfortably over the collarbones. You can easily sense the expansion of the upper lobes of the lungs with your fingertips in the open space between the collarbone and the trapezius muscle, which runs behind that bone. Keeping your abdominal wall relaxed, inhale through your nose, expanding the upper ends of your lungs as fully as possible. Hold your breath for three seconds, then let go, exhaling slowly, letting the air gently flow from the mouth. Repeat the exercise five times, resting for five normal breaths between each one. The pause in between is important because as you want to avoid hyperventilation and allow yourself time to center your thoughts on the activity and reflect on what you sensed or felt.

Middle Costal Breathing

Again let your fingers be your sensors. Place your fingers on the middle third of the chest wall below the nipples (sixth rib). Keeping your abdominal and upper costal area relaxed, inhale through your nose, expanding the midchest region as fully as possible. Hold for three seconds and gently exhale through the mouth. Repeat this five times and then relax quietly. Remember to pause between each repetition.

Diaphragmatic Breathing

Breathing with the diaphragm is performed by taking a deep inspiration while the belly is pushed down and out by the movement of the diaphragm, thus allowing the lower lobes of the lungs to inflate fully. Your hands are placed on the lower ribs, where they should easily sense the breathing motion. With the upper chest relaxed, inhale deeply. The abdominal wall is pushed up and out. Hold for three seconds and exhale, feeling the abdominal wall descend toward the spine. Repeat this exercise five times. Diaphragmatic breathing stretches the lower lobes of the lungs, thus allowing more fresh air to enter. It also acts to correct shallow breathing habits, allowing increasing depth of inspiration.

Very Deep Breathing

Start by exhaling every bit of air from your lungs. Force the air out and feel the space between your belly and spine shrink. When all the air is out, inhale slowly, using the diaphragmatic technique. Picture your lungs as a glass being filled with water—bottom, middle, then top. Hold your breath three seconds and then exhale gently through your nose or mouth. This may sound like an exaggerated, strenuous action, but it is not. Breathe from your diaphragm naturally and effortlessly. Concentrate on the air traveling through the air passageways. With each expiration feel yourself relaxing and letting go. Begin to feel the looseness in your body, an uncoiling feeling as you settle down and pull your mind and body together. Repeat this exercise five times, resting between each repetition.

Now that you know how to breathe correctly, go on to the following breathing exercises. You may want to periodically repeat these learning-to-breathe exercises until you feel that you have fully mastered them. Once you do, start with the following exercises on breathing.

Breathing Exercises

Breathing Down

During the course of an average day, many of us find ourselves in anxiety-producing situations. Our heart rates increase, our stomachs may become upset, and our thoughts may race uncontrollably. In such moments we tend to make poor decisions or overreact. During such episodes we require fast-acting relief from our stressful reactions so that we can attempt to calmly solve the crisis or problem at hand. The following exercise has been found effective for quickly calming one down in stressful situations.

The basic mechanism for stress reduction in this exercise involves deep breathing. The procedure is as follows:

Step 1. Assume a comfortable position. Rest your left hand (palm down) on top of your abdomen. More specifically, place your left hand over your navel. Now place your right hand so that it comfortably rests on your left. Your eyes should remain open (see Figure 12.1).

Step 2. Imagine a hollow bottle or pouch lying internally beneath the point at which your hands are resting. Begin to inhale. As you inhale, imagine that the air is entering through your nose and descending to fill that internal pouch. Your hands will rise as you fill the pouch with air. As you continue to inhale, imagine the pouch being filled to the top. Your rib cage and upper chest will continue the wavelike rise that began at your navel. The total length of your inhalation should be three seconds for the first week or so, then lengthening to four or five seconds as you progress in skill development. Remember to concentrate on "seeing" the air move as you inhale and exhale.

Step 3. Hold your breath. Keep the air inside the pouch. Repeat to yourself the phrase "My body is calm."

Step 4. Slowly begin to exhale—to empty the pouch. As you do, repeat the phrase, "My body is quiet." As you exhale you will feel your raised abdomen and chest recede. Repeat this exercise four or five times in succession. Should you begin to feel lightheaded, stop at that point. If lightheadedness remains a problem, consider shortening the length of the inhalation and/or decreasing the total number of repetitions of the four-step exercise.

Practice this exercise ten to fifteen times a day. Make it a ritual in the morning, afternoon, and evening as well as during stressful situations. After a week or two of

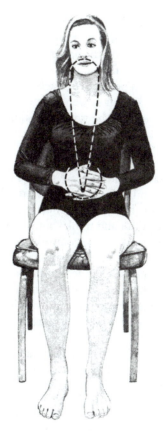

FIGURE 12.1   Breathing Down

practice, omit Step 1. This was only for teaching the technique. Because this form of relaxation is a skill, it is important to practice at least ten to fifteen times a day. At first you may not notice any immediate relaxation. However, after a week or two of regular practice, you will increase your ability to relax on the spot. Remember: You must practice regularly if you are to master this skill. Regular, consistent practice of these daily exercises will lead to a calmer and more relaxed attitude—a sort of antistress attitude—and when you do have stressful moments, they will be far less severe.

Controlled Tempo Breathing

This exercise develops powers of concentration, facilitates centering, and helps breath control. You may sit or lie down. Keep your eyes closed. The breathing will be diaphragmatic—quiet, natural, and effortless. Concentrate on your breathing. Become part of it. With one hand, find your pulse in the wrist of the other arm. Count your pulse for one minute. While still counting your pulse, bring part of your attention back to your breathing. Count the number of pulses during normal expiration. Do this several times until you have a rhythm. The average will be somewhere between five and ten. As an example, say the number is five. Still monitoring your pulse, breathe in with five beats of your pulse, hold for five, exhale for five, and remain quiet for five. Continue this for three minutes; then sit quietly and prepare for the Breath Counting Exercise. At first you may tend to lose count, but as your powers of concentration increase, you will make it all the way. You can then increase the time spent doing this exercise.

Breath Counting

This is another exercise to promote relaxation and increase powers of concentration. You may do this sitting or lying down. As in the Controlled Tempo Breathing Exercise, you will use quiet, normal diaphragmatic breathing. Concentrate on your breathing. As you breathe in, think "in." Let the air out and think "out." Think ". . . in . . . out . . . in . . . out." Now each time you breathe out, count the breaths. Count ten consecutive breaths without missing a count. If you happen to miss one, start over. When you get to ten, start at one again. Do this ten times, and then sit quietly. Concentrate, anticipate the breath, and block all other thoughts from your mind.

Controlling breathing is the simplest and most basic activity in the stress management arsenal because breathing is the simplest and most basic physiological, life-sustaining activity.

In the sense of brain development, breathing is ancient and basic, and so too is our sense of smell, the oldest, most primitive of the senses. Unlike vision, which must cross five synapses as it moves from the back of the brain to the frontal cortex, smell is only one synapse away from the nose to the amygdala, where it is directly routed to the higher centers of association in the cortex (Pert 1999). Because there is only one intervening synapse, there is little potential for erroneous associations to the smell that is entering the system. Therapists have revived the ancient art of using the sense of smell to alter emotional states and to affect a cure of dysfunctional systems. This stress management/alternative medicine therapy is called *aromatherapy*.

Aromatherapy

Aromatherapy is one of those rare forms of treatment that can improve your quality of life regardless of whether it has any other benefits. That's just as well because few medical doctors believe it has any significant effects on health. However, in the area of stress management there may be benefits from emotional response to aromatherapy's pleasing nature. Used as a comforting ritual to reduce stress, enhance relaxation, and relieve anxiety, aromatherapy may indeed relieve stress symptoms and alleviate some emotionally-related disorders (Holmes 1995). For some people, it has provided a respite from insomnia. Others have found it an effective remedy for impotence. A few people even report that it eases the pain of arthritis and relieves postpartum discomfort. However, medical science is still searching to document the physical reason for these effects.

Fragrant oils have been used for thousand of years to lubricate the skin, purify infectious air, and repel insects. However, aromatherapy as we know it today dates from the late 1930s. It increased in popularity in the 1980s, when there was an upsurge in the popularity of "natural," nontoxic healing methods that cost less than conventional medications and produce fewer side effects. Practitioners in California used essential oils to treat everything from viral and bacterial infections to depression, anxiety, and sexually transmitted diseases. They insisted aromas could heal wounds, stimulate the immune system, cure skin disorders, improve circulation, relieve pain, reduce swelling, and even improve memory. According to these enthusiastic therapists, fragrant oils had the power to heal malfunctioning ovaries, kidneys, veins, adrenal glands, and many other organs. However, none of these claims has ever been scientifically substantiated.

Indeed, relatively few attempts to verify aromatherapy's purported benefits have ever been made at all, and of those, only a few have delivered promising results. In one trial for arthritis pain, some of the participants were able to reduce the dosage of their potent antiinflammatory drugs. In another study, the scent of lavender successfully put insomniacs to sleep. Other research has documented improvement in cases of erectile dysfunction and a reduction in pain following childbirth. However, attempts to prove that aromatherapy can cure shingles have failed (although fragrant creams can reduce some of the pain). And a 1958 (Cassileth 1999) paper extolling the ability of essential oils to fight and conquer infections could cite no positive human or animal tests (Cassileth 1999).

Advocates of aromatherapy propose a variety of mechanisms for its reported effects. The most widely accepted theory suggests that fragrances do their work via the brain. When aromatic molecules enter the nasal cavity and stimulate the odor-sensing nerves, the resulting impulses are sent to the limbic system—the part of the brain that's believed to be the seat of memory and emotion (Cassileth 1999).

Depending on the scent, emotional responses then kick in to exert a calming or energizing effect on the body. Alternatively, some proponents suggest that certain aromas may work by stimulating the glands, prompting the adrenal glands, for example, to produce steroidlike hormones that fight pain and inflammation. Others believe that the essential oils, whether inhaled or rubbed into the skin, react with hormones and enzymes in the bloodstream to produce positive results (Holmes 1995).

Aromatherapists assign specific properties to each essence. According to Price (1991), here are typical claims for some of the more common essential oils:

Lavender: Heals burns and cuts; destroys bacteria; relieves depression, inflammation, spasms, headaches, respiratory allergies, muscle aches, nausea, and menstrual cramps; soothes bug bites; lowers blood pressure.

Peppermint: Alleviates digestive problems; cleans wounds; decongests the chest; relieves headache, neuralgia, and muscle pain; useful for motion sickness.

Eucalyptus: Lowers fever; clears sinuses; has antibacterial and antiviral properties; relieves coughs; useful for boils and pimples.

Tea tree: Fights fungal, yeast, and bacterial infections; useful for skin conditions such as acne, insect bites, and burns; helps clear vaginitis, bladder infections, and thrush.

Rosemary: Relieves pain; increases circulation; decongests the chest; relieves pain, indigestion, gas, and liver problems; lessens swelling; fights infection; helps alleviate depression.

Chamomile: Reduces swelling; treats allergic symptoms; relieves stress, insomnia, and depression; useful in treating digestive problems.

Thyme: Lessens laryngitis and coughs; fights bladder and skin infections; relieves digestive problems and pain in the joints.

Tarragon: Stimulates digestion; calms neural and digestive tracts; relieves menstrual symptoms and stress.

Everlasting: Heals scars; reduces swelling after injuries; relieves sunburn; fights infections such as bronchitis and flu; treats pain from arthritis, muscle injuries, sprains, strains, and tendonitis.

Although many gift boutiques have taken to marketing scented candles, pomanders, and potpourri as "aromatherapy," genuine treatments rely on the use of highly concentrated essential oils extracted from various healing herbs. In most cases, these oils are produced by steam distillation or cold pressing from a plant's flowers, leaves, branches, bark, rind, or roots. The volatile, flammable oils are then mixed with a "carrier"—usually a vegetable oil such as soy, evening primrose, or almond—or diluted in alcohol before being applied to the skin, sprayed in the air, or inhaled.

Rubbing aromatic oil into the skin may be either calming or stimulating, depending on the type of oil used. Some people use it as a remedy for muscles sprains and soreness. Most preparations contain five drops of essential oil blended with a light base oil. A higher concentration could irritate the skin. Bathing in aromatic oil is another popular practice for relaxation. No more than eight drops should be used in a tubful of water. Ten to fifteen drops might be added to a Jacuzzi or hot tub, four to five drops to a foot bath, or three to four drops to a hand bath (for chapped skin). During showering, a wet sponge or cloth may be dipped into an oil-water mixture and applied to the skin while the water sprays the body. This technique should not be used if a person has skin allergies.

Warning. Never take aromatherapy oils internally. They are extremely potent and many can be poisonous. Many essential oils can trigger bronchial spasms. Asthmatics should not use any form of aromatherapy without first consulting their doctor. Also, a person who has skin allergies should not use essential oils in their bath. To check for allergy to an oil, place one drop on the inside of the elbow and after 24 hours see whether it produces a reaction. As with any medication, it's best to avoid aromatherapy during pregnancy. Be especially wary of sage, rosemary, and juniper oils. These herbs have been known to cause uterine contractions when taken in excessive amounts. Infants and young children are especially sensitive to potent essential oils. Keep the oils away from their faces. Do not use peppermint oil on children under the age of thirty months. Because essential oils are highly concentrated, taking them internally can easily lead to a toxic overdose. Not even the tiniest amount should be ingested without a doctor's approval. Do not use highly concentrated, undiluted oils on the skin, and be careful to keep the oils away from the eyes. Many essential oils will cause skin irritation if used too frequently. They can also increase one's sensitivity to sunlight, making it easier to burn. Excessive inhalation of fragrant vapors can cause headache and fatigue. Remember, too, that certain oils, such as peppermint, can cause insomnia rather than relieving it. If a person develops an allergy to any of the products, stop the treatment immediately and seek another form of therapy (Fisher-Rizzi, 1991).

SOURCES CITED

Buchholz, I. (1994). *Breathing, voice, and movement therapy: Applications to breathing disorders.* Biofeedback and Self-Regulation, 19(2), 141.

Cassileth, B. R. (1999). *The alternative medicine handbook.* New York: W.W. Norton.

Fisher-Rizzi, S. (1991). *The complete aromatherapy handbook: Essential oils for radiant health.* New York: Sterling Press.

Holmes, P. (1995). *Aromatherapy: Applications for clinical practice.* Alternative and Complementary Therapies, 1(3), 117–82.

Iyengar, B. K. S. (1995). *Light on Pranayama.* New York: Crossroad.

Pert, C. (1995). *Neuropeptides, AIDS, and the science of healing.* Alternative Therapies, 1(3), 70–76.

Pert, C. (1999). *Molecules of emotion.* New York: Simon and Schuster.

Price, S. (1991). *Aromatherapy for common ailments.* New York: Simon and Schuster.

CHAPTER

13 Muscle Relaxation

Take a moment and shift your attention from this book to your body. First note your overall position. Are you sitting comfortably? Is your body supported by the chair, or are your back muscles being strained? Are your arms supported, or are you holding the book in the air? Are your fists clenched? Think back to times when you were writing something. Did you ever notice that you were holding the pencil or pen so tightly that it was leaving an indentation in your fingers? Think of another activity, such as driving a car. Have you ever found yourself with a death grip on the steering wheel, producing tension up your arms to your shoulders, neck, back, and even to your head and facial muscles?

These are examples of tension exhibited through the muscles. More specifically, it is excess and needless muscle tension because it is far more than what is needed to accomplish the task. This excess muscle tension is both a response to stress and a cause of stress. The often-mentioned fight-or-flight syndrome is muscular expression, as are speech, facial expression, and eye movements.

Most movements are readily observable; that is, you can see your fingers move a pencil as you write, but it takes a second look to notice whether there is excess pressure. Excess exertion has nothing to do with the writing movement. It is an outward expression of the anxiety or resentment over what you are writing and/or it represents the general state of tension constantly with you. It is no mystery that people experienced at observing stress can quickly pick out stressed people by analyzing certain characteristics of their penmanship.

Much of the harmful, stress-producing muscle tension is extremely subtle and almost impossible to detect. If you are thinking defensive thoughts, you start to assume a defensive posture. It is practically impossible to think of an action and not have your muscles prepare for that action. To illustrate this phenomenon, take a pendant on a chain, or tie a key to a string, and hold it out in front of you. Close your eyes and, without moving your hand, imagine the object swinging toward and away from you. After a minute, open your eyes, and chances are it will be moving. Move it side to side, or imagine it circling. Even though your hand did not actually move, the thought was translated to your fingers, and tension developed in a rhythmical pattern with enough force to cause the object to move. This shows that we have the ability to anticipate, and this ability is necessary for preparation. Unfortunately, we often spend so much time in unproductive imagined preparation that our bodies adapt by increasing general muscle tension. At several points in this book we mentioned Selye's concept of the disease of adaptation. Muscle tension represents a good example. The individual who is defensive and is constantly imagining actions creates a situation in which the body learns to adapt by maintaining a chronic state of muscle tension.

If such a condition is permitted to exist for an extended period, a wide variety of physical disorders may be produced or exaggerated.

The connection between inordinate muscle tension and disease was made hundreds of years ago, but it was not until the end of the 19th century that systematic relaxation programs were formulated. The names Schultz, Sweigard, Maja Schade, and Jacobsen became synonymous with relaxation training because their pioneering work formed the basis of most of the relaxation programs in existence today. There are literally hundreds of techniques now, but all have the same basic objective of teaching the individual to relax the muscles at will by first developing a cognitive awareness of what it feels like to be tense and then what it feels like to be relaxed. If one is able to distinguish between tension and relaxation, control over tension follows almost effortlessly (Jacobsen 1977).

Muscle relaxation techniques can also help the individual learn to remain calm throughout the day by differentially relaxing unneeded skeletal muscles during everyday activities. There are great variations in the actual techniques of muscle relaxation; some are true to the original Jacobsen Progressive Muscle Relaxation, and others are either a shorter version or are used in combination with hypnotic suggestion and emphasize the perception of relaxation rather than actual muscle relaxation (Bernstein and Carlson 1993).

The newer combination and shorter-version techniques have been widely used in recent years because they are thought to be more easily learned but produce good results nevertheless. Abbreviated progressive muscle relaxation training seems to be most effective when accompanied by training tapes and when offered to one individual at a time (rather than to groups). In addition, longer sessions offered more times have produced better results (Carlson and Hoyle 1993).

Neuromuscular Exercises

Neuromuscular relaxation trains not only the muscles but also the nervous system components that control muscle activity. The benefits are, of course, the reduction of tension in the muscles, and because the muscles make up such a large portion of the body's mass, this represents a significant reduction in total body tension.

The types of stress and medical problems that have been shown to be positively affected by muscle relaxation run the gamut from tension or muscle-contraction headaches, chronic neck and back pain, and essential hypertension to coping with general stress as an adjunct to cancer chemotherapy. It was also found very helpful in postsurgical recovery (Good 1995). In addition, this training helps develop a sense of tension awareness. If you use muscles as a biofeedback device, you can develop an inherent autosensory awareness to the point that a little internal alarm goes off when tension starts to rise.

Another benefit of this training is mental discipline, often mentioned throughout this book. To accomplish any of these techniques, one must learn to center on the task or problem and control the mind's tendency to wander aimlessly in daydreams. Neuromuscular relaxation requires concentration, specifically passive concentration. As you perfect your ability, you can practice relaxation anywhere, even in short spurts, for example, while stopped for a red light, waiting for an appointment, or watching television. Just think of how much time you spend each day just sitting around waiting for things to happen; you might view this "wasted time" as an opportunity to practice relaxation. Two things will happen: First, you will easily get in thirty to sixty minutes of practice a day, and second, you will lose the concept of wasted time—a very important philosophical development necessary for reducing stress.

The Learning Phase

What follows is a detailed set of instructions on how to practice muscular relaxation. The learning phase, of course, necessitates more structured time involvement, more concentration, and more commitment than will be necessary once you master the technique. Once you have perfected it, you will be able to choose the particular exercise sequence that is most beneficial to you and that meets your immediate needs. It is very important, however, that in the learning phase you follow the instructions to the letter. It is also important to note that individuals with heart conditions, high blood pressure, or any condition that results in sore, weak, or other compromised muscular systems should consult their physician for medical clearance before attempting muscle relaxation training.

The exercises presented in this chapter have been used for years in our clinical practice and have been proven to be quite effective and easily learned. Even though they are theoretically based on the concepts of the many relaxation techniques that have preceded them, significant differences exist. We follow a natural pattern to provide a constellation of exercises that we have found more effective and more easily learned than other current relaxation techniques. First you practice the gross muscle actions that you initially developed during the prenatal as well as the neonatal stage. These movements are innate to human locomotion and can be easily identified and controlled. Because these movements provide an excellent basis for cortical learning, you can gain awareness and conscious control over these motor actions. Then you can progress to higher levels of skilled muscle activity. Another important consideration taken into account when these exercises were developed was that they include group-muscle action rather than single-muscle activity. The brain knows nothing about muscles, only about movements involving many muscles working together. Trying to relax one muscle is difficult and retards learning. Finally, the exercises start from distal muscle groups (feet and legs) and proceed to proximal groups of muscles closer to the head and trunk.

Preparation

In order for the learning experience to be as effective as possible, you should do whatever you can to create an environment that enhances concentration. A few minutes spent preparing the environment and the body is a good investment.

First, concentrate on the environment. Do whatever you can to reduce external noise. Find a room away from traffic, with no telephone and with indirect or dim lighting. You may want to use earplugs or earphones or play soft instrumental music or environmental sounds. As you become more proficient at these exercises, you will not have to make such elaborate preparations, but anything that might enhance initial learning will reduce learning time.

Next, work on preparing your body. A reclined or semireclined position with proper support under the legs is best (see Figure 13.1). Lie down on a mat; place your arms at your sides, elbows flexed at about sixty degrees so that the hands and wrists rest on the abdomen. Your hips will naturally flex to about twenty-five degrees, so don't attempt to hold your legs together. Your legs will naturally rotate outward; don't force them straight. In other words, allow the body to assume a position that does not require muscle action to maintain it. If you wish, you may support your neck with a small, soft pillow. If it is difficult for you to maintain a lying position without pain in the lower back due to unusual pull on the lumbar spine, place a pillow under your knees. This helps flatten the back against its support and relieves strain on the lower back. Also, if you have a history of low-back pain, lumbar-disc disease, or any other musculoskeletal disorder or postural condition including round shoulders, overdeveloped muscle mass, or cervical lordosis, you should take individual precautions and adopt the most restful and comfortable position to promote maximum concentration and learning. Any tight clothing, jewelry, belts, and the like should be loosened or removed. In preparing for relaxation, if you experience tingling or numbness in a body area, change your posture to relieve the pressure on that area. Above all, if pain or cramps develop during relaxation, rest the muscle until they diminish, then proceed with less intensity.

Lower Extremities

The Ankle.   The first exercise involves the ankle joints (Figure 13.2). No other joints should be involved here. You should be lying in the preparatory position shown

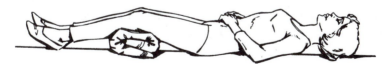

FIGURE 13.1   Preparatory Position for Relaxation Exercises

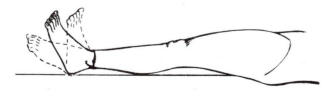

FIGURE 13.2   Ankle Exercises

in Figure 13.1 and should have proceeded through the breathing exercises. Now pull your feet toward the front of your legs (the movement involved in taking your foot off the gas pedal of a car). The contraction should be felt only in the muscles on the front and outside of the lower leg, not in the calf muscles, which will feel stretched.

Your toes should be pulled forward toward your legs as hard as possible until you feel uncomfortable (short of pain—if pain develops, rest for a moment and proceed less vigorously). Center your thoughts in the muscles experiencing the tension. Try to visualize the tension. Form an image in your mind about this tightness. Hold for a few seconds and let go. Repeat the exercise, this time being sure to synchronize your breathing. Breathe in, pulling the feet up, hold your breath, hold the contraction— then let the air out, relaxing the muscles. Lie quietly for one minute and then repeat.

After you have done this several times and feel comfortable with the activity and the breathing pattern, turn your awareness more toward the relaxation than to the contraction. As you breathe out and relax, allow the muscles to go limp. As you pass over the peak of the contraction, begin to unwind. Try to form a visual image of this relaxed state, and hold it in your mind. Repeat this exercise until you have gained confidence in your ability to relax those muscles.

Next, move on to another group of muscles called the plantar flexor group, or calf muscles. They are the exact opposite of the first group. Thus, tightness will be felt in the calf area, and the stretching sensation will be felt in the muscle group in the front of the lower leg. Start by taking a deep breath, then push your toes down (as in pushing down on the gas pedal) and away from the body as far as possible. Keep the heels down. When you reach the peak of your breath, hold the breath for five seconds, keeping your toes pointed. Now, slowly exhale while allowing the feet to come back to a resting position.

Repeat this exercise three to five times, attempting to synchronize your breathing with the contraction and relaxation phases. As you exhale and let go of the contraction, form a visual image of the tension in the calf muscle flowing out with the air from your lungs. Imagine an unwinding or letting go. Concentrate on the feelings of tension, the feelings of relaxation, and the difference between the two states.

Hips and Knees

The best exercise in this group is the extension of the knees and hips, the knees being pushed down into the mat while the legs are kept straight (Figure 13.3). For this exer-

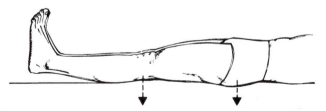

FIGURE 13.3 Hip and Knee Exercise

cise, remove the pillow from under your knees if you were using one. The tightness will be felt in front of the thighs and in the buttocks area. You will not be aware of any appreciable stretching force because these muscles are long and serve more than one joint. As always, begin with a deep breath, pushing your hips and knees down into the mat. Hold at the peak of your breath, then exhale and allow the muscles to rest. Again, form an image of the tension; feel the letting go.

Table 13.1 summarizes these lower-extremity exercises. Put these together in three successive movements. Allow about thirty seconds between each exercise.

Trunk

The first of these two exercises utilizes the extensor muscles of the lower back. This exercise is particularly good for you if you have lower-back discomfort not related to deformity or injury. Because a large proportion of our population suffers from tension-related low-back pain, remember the earlier warning: If this or any of these exercises produces pain or spasms, stop the exercise and rest. Then continue with only a moderate amount of contraction, gradually increasing the strength of contraction over several weeks. If pain persists, discontinue this type of relaxation training. In this exercise, you hollow or arch your back, as shown in Figure 13.4. Move your chest slightly toward your chin. The pelvis is fixed on the mat. You will feel the tension in the lower-back area. Synchronize the exercise with your breathing, concentrating on the feelings of tension and relaxation. Repeat five times.

The second exercise is pulling in the abdominal muscles. Keep the legs, pelvis, and shoulders in contact with the mat. Breathe in, contract the stomach muscles, and flatten the lower back against the mat. Hold for five seconds, exhale, and relax.

TABLE 13.1   Summary of Lower-Extremity Exercises

Dorsiflexion of Ankle Joints	Bend up the feet . . . Pull hard . . . Harder! And let go.
Plantar Flexion of Ankle Joints	Push the feet down as far as you can . . . Push harder! And slacken off the muscles completely . . .
Extension of Knee and Hip	Straighten the knees as much as possible . . . Now press the legs down into the mat . . . Hard . . . Harder! Now relax . . .

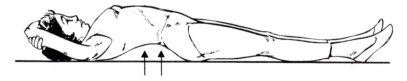

FIGURE 13.4   Trunk Extension

The trunk exercises are summarized in Table 13.2. Try them both, one after the other with three-second rest intervals between them. At this point, go back and repeat one time each of the exercises you have learned thus far. Concentrate on the feelings of tension and relaxation. The visual imagery is just as important as the performance of the muscular exercise.

Upper Extremities

This group of exercises is for the muscles in the upper limbs—around the shoulder, elbow, wrist, and fingers. Remember to start each exercise with deep breathing, and follow all the progressive steps (as discussed in Chapter 12).

The first exercise in this group is the extension of the wrist and fingers (Figure 13.5). Exercise both your left and right extremities at the same time. Pull your hands and fingers simultaneously back toward your forearms, keeping your fingers straight. You should feel the tension in the backs of your hands and the backs of your forearms below the elbows. A little pain might be felt near the wrist—this is ligament stretch; don't strain. Hold the tension for five seconds; then relax. Make sure you give yourself a proper rest period so you can focus on the relaxation. Repeat this exercise five times.

The next exercise (Figure 13.6) reverses the previous one. Turn your wrists in (stretching the back of your hand), and clench your fists very tightly. Hold the tension five seconds; then relax. Repeat five times.

TABLE 13.2 Summary of Trunk Exercises

Extensor Muscles of the Spine	Push the chest forward until you have hollowed the back strongly . . . Lift a little more! And let go . . .
Abdominal Muscles	Pull in the abdominal muscles until they are quite flat . . . Pull a bit more! And rest . . .

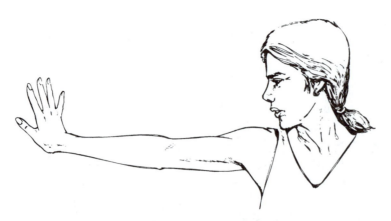

FIGURE 13.5 Wrist and Finger Extension

Next, straighten your arms against your sides, keeping your fingers straight (Figure 13.7). Press both arms tightly against your sides. Hold the tension for five seconds; then relax. Repeat this exercise five times.

Finally, do the following exercise for your shoulders. Shrug your shoulders up as high as you can—try to touch your shoulders to your ear lobes (Figure 13.8). Hold the

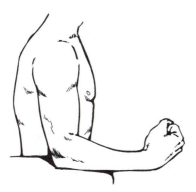

FIGURE 13.6   Wrist and Finger Contraction

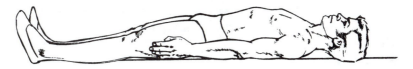

FIGURE 13.7   Arms Straight against Sides

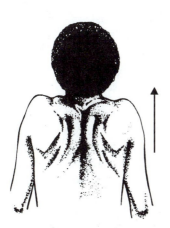

FIGURE 13.8   Shoulder Shrug

TABLE 13.3 Summary of Upper-Extremity Exercises

Finger and Wrist Extension	Straighten the fingers and pull back the wrists . . . Pull hard.
Flexion of the Fingers and Wrists	Clench your fists and curl your wrists inward.
Adduction of Shoulder Joints	Straighten the arms against your sides . . . Press tightly.
Shoulder Shrug	Shrug your shoulders high . . . Higher . . . Touch your ears.

tension for five seconds; then relax. Repeat five times. This exercise is excellent for stiff necks and shoulders caused by excessive desk work.

For a summary of upper-extremity exercises, see Table 13.3.

Head, Neck, and Face

The primary exercise in this group is rotation of the head. The muscles in this region become overworked because we tend to hold a steady partial tension for hours at a time, especially while doing desk work or driving. If you have chronic neck problems, use extreme care. To do this exercise (shown in Figure 13.9), first close your eyes. Touch your chin to your breastbone. Return, rest for a breath, and move the head backward toward the spine. Return, rest, and then rotate the head so as to look over the right shoulder. Return, rest for a breath, and then look over the left shoulder. Consider these four moves as one exercise, and complete them in succession, but do not hurry. Synchronize each movement with your breathing; contract, relax for a few breaths, and continue with the next movement.

Another group of overworked muscles is the facial muscles, especially those involved in talking and chewing. To exercise these, clench your teeth together and draw your facial muscles up tightly (Figure 13.10). Always remember the correct emphasis on breathing. Repeat five times and then relax.

Table 13.4 contains a summary of head, neck, and facial exercises.

The learning phase will take time and concentrated effort, but as learning progresses, it will take less time to complete the exercises. In the beginning, you may tend to fall asleep during practice or feel lethargic afterward. This reaction is due to your mindset. If the only time you relax is when you are too tired to do anything else, you may feel this way. However, these are precision exercises requiring concentration (albeit passive), and as you become more proficient you will feel rested, relaxed but alert, and full of vigor, strength, and enthusiasm for your daily activities. These exercises are more than relaxation promoting; they are a learning process that provides awareness of states of mind and body in relation to everyday

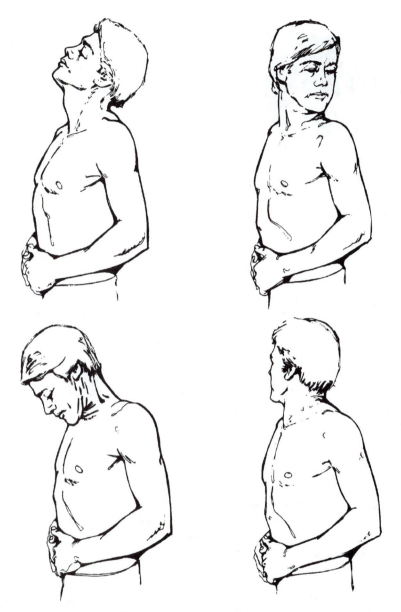

FIGURE 13.9   Head Rotation

life. Slowly you will begin to notice your posture, how your hand grips objects, your neck position, and your facial expression. Being aware of such neuromuscular states is the first step in the change process, and finally you will be well on your way to not only combating tension but preventing it.

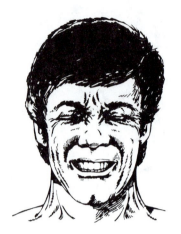

FIGURE 13.10   Facial Exercise

TABLE 13.4   Summary of Head, Neck, and Face Exercises

Rotation	Shut the eyes . . . Now roll the head slowly forward, then slowly back . . . Roll the head to the right, then slowly to the left . . . It's heavy . . . and it's rolling easily—front to back, side to side . . . Now stop, with the face turned forward, and rest . . .
Facial Exercise	Clench the teeth together. Now draw up the facial muscles very tightly . . . Tighter! And relax . . .

Biofeedback

When you become frightened, anxious, angry, or generally stressed, numerous changes occur in your body—most of them negative. If the stress is moderate to severe, you will have no trouble in recognizing the outward signs. For example, your heart rate speeds up, and often you can feel the palpitations in your chest. The palms of your hands become moist with increased sweating, your skin may flush or become excessively pale, the pupils of your eyes may change size, your mouth may become very dry, or in some instances salivation may become excessive, your muscles may tense to the point of pain or feel so limp that your legs threaten to give way, your stomach "turns over" and you may feel nauseated, your breathing rate may increase, and you may have a difficult time swallowing.

The body is constantly telling us about its activities. We have learned to key into some feelings, sounds, and outward signs of mind-body function. Stomach contractions are interpreted as hunger, diarrhea and constipation are indicators of gastrointestinal problems, and redness and swelling are indicators of possible infection. We have also learned to use physiological parameters such as heart rate and blood pressure to assess the body's functioning. When an increase in blood pressure is detected, the individual has some information about the cardiovascular system, and during treatment subsequent blood pressure readings are a constant measure of the success of treatment.

Biofeedback is to some extent a refinement of that feedback system. Instead of diarrhea, which is a rather gross measure of intestinal action, one could measure the minute muscle contraction of various intestinal segments. Thermal measurement of skin can indicate blood flow to a particular region of the body. Measuring contraction of skeletal muscles can detect muscle action before it reaches the stage of producing pain and discomfort.

Any system in the body that emits energy can be used in the biofeedback process. Because of anatomical and physiological considerations, some systems are more difficult to use than others, and the muscular system is by far the most accessible and useful especially to stress management.

There are two distinctly different applications of biofeedback to the muscular system:

1. Muscle tension and relaxation
2. Neuromuscular rehabilitation

Both of these utilize the electromyograph (EMG), an instrument that measures the activity of a muscle. More specifically, the EMG measures the electrical energy emitted by the flow of electrically charged particles in and out of a muscle cell just before contraction. The strength of the muscle contraction depends on the quantity of these particles; thus the EMG can give an instantaneous and continuous evaluation of muscle contraction.

A muscle is a mass of millions of cells with the ability to contract, or shorten, thus producing movement. As we learn how to perform activities, patterns of muscle movements are ingrained in our memory and become automatic functions. You do not have to think about how to pick up a pencil but rather just think of the act and the muscles respond. Other muscle-action patterns are learned as well, such as fighting back, running away, and bracing for anticipated harm, to mention a few. When a threatening situation occurs, each muscle does not have to be commanded to act; one just thinks of the action "run," and the legs move.

Sit back in your chair, close your eyes, and try to focus your thoughts on your muscles. Bend your arm up so that your hand touches your shoulder. The muscle tension is obvious as movement occurs. Next, just think of the same movement. You almost have to hold the arm back as it seems to want to move. Feel the muscles contract ever so slightly. Try the same activity with your forehead. Frown; feel the muscles contract. Then just think of an activity that is unpleasant to you, and try to feel the tension that may develop in that area. You are, of course, getting feedback of subtle muscle activity that does not produce movement only because you have not willed the movement.

But just as the gross movement can be controlled, so can the more subtle muscle tension if its existence is known. Unfortunately, most people possess limited ability to sense muscle tension. It is here that the EMG biofeedback instrument can be helpful. If sensing electrodes are placed on the skin over the muscle, subtle contractions can be measured. The signal is specially processed and converted to a light or sound signal and is fed back to the individual, who can use that information to direct the muscle to relax. In most tension-reduction or general-relaxation programs, muscles of the face and/or neck are used. Tension in these areas generally reflects moods and emotions.

As mentioned earlier in this chapter, Edmund Jacobsen, an expert on muscle tension and relaxation, popularized the concept of mind-muscle interrelationship. He indicated that anxiety and muscle relaxation are incompatible and formulated the idea that one effective way of reducing anxiety was to reduce muscle tension. This concept formed the basis for the most common biofeedback program, which uses EMG biofeedback as a technique to develop self-awareness and an awareness of the relationship between emotion and tension. EMG biofeedback has also been used to promote general relaxation, reduce anxiety, treat phobias, and relieve a myriad of other conditions such as tension headache, migraine headache, premenstrual distress, and insomnia commonly associated with muscle tension (Lehrer et al. 1994, Lehrer and Woolfolk 1999).

Massage and Bodywork

There is a substantial body of knowledge and research that indicates that we store emotional energy in all parts of the body, especially the muscles (Pert 1998). The Gestalt body work literature describes pain pockets as "depots" in which emotional energy is stored in the muscle and other organs. Manipulation of these pockets by a trained body work therapist can release this stored energy. Massaging pain pockets not only alleviates pain of the muscle cramp but can also release the energy of the original emotional experience. Even though not all massage techniques are based on the bodywork principle, it is common knowledge that there is a close relationship between tight muscles and stress arousal. Therefore, it follows that massage can be an effective relaxation and stress-management tool. If nothing else, the time out, self-indulgence, and quiet relaxing environment offers a respite from one's busy day. Although one may realize some results from gently massaging their own body parts or having a friend do the massage, best results can be achieved from visiting a trained professional. The following description of the most popularly available types of massage can be viewed somewhat as a consumer's guide to the type of massage that may be beneficial for stress management.

Traditional Massage

The massage most readily available to us is based on traditional concepts of anatomy, physiology, and soft-tissue manipulation. It includes soft-tissue manipulation tracing the outer contours of the body usually toward the heart. A very popular technique in the United States was imported from Sweden and is called *Swedish massage*. It uses a system of long gliding strokes, kneading, and friction techniques on the more superficial layers of muscles. It usually goes in the direction of blood flow toward the heart because it emphasizes stimulation of the blood circulation through the body's soft tissues. Swedish massage can be relatively vigorous with a great deal of joint movement included. Oil is usually used to facilitate the stroking and kneading of the body, thereby stimulating metabolism and circulation. Its active and passive movements of the joints promote general relaxation, improve circulation and range of motion, and can relieve muscle tension. Swedish massage is often given as a complete, full-body technique, though sometimes only a part of the body is worked.

More vigorous massage techniques based on the Swedish concept are also popular and generally available. These techniques include neuromuscular massage, deep-tissue massage, sports massage, and manual lymph drainage. The focus is also on relieving muscle tension and increasing circulation, but it has the potential for creating deeper states of relaxation, beneficial states of consciousness, and general well-being.

Neuromuscular massage is a form of deep massage that applies concentrated finger pressure specifically to individual muscles. This is a very detailed approach, used to increase blood flow and to release *trigger points*, intense knots of muscle tension that refer pain to other parts of the body (they become trigger points when they seem to trigger a pain pattern). This form of massage helps to break the cycle of spasm and pain and is often used in pain control. Trigger-point massage and myotherapy are varieties of neuromuscular massage.

Moving toward a deeper, more clinical practice, the next level is *deep-tissue massage*. This approach is used to release chronic patterns of muscular tension using slow strokes, direct pressure, or friction. Often the movements are directed across the grain of the muscles (cross-fiber) using the fingers, thumbs, or elbows. This is applied with greater pressure and at deeper layers of the muscle than Swedish massage.

A type of deep-muscle massage known as *sports massage* is a deep-tissue massage more specifically adapted to deal with the needs of athletes and the effects of athletic performance on the body. Sports massage is used before or after events, as part of an athlete's training regimen, and to promote healing from injuries.

Structural/Functional/Movement Integration

These approaches organize and integrate the body in relationship to gravity through manipulating the soft tissues and/or through correcting inappropriate patterns of movement. These are methods that bring about more balanced use of the body and nervous system, creating greater integration and more ease of movement. This category of approaches is interesting in that some do not even involve the practitioner touching the client. There is no clear line of demarcation between where the bodywork therapies end and the movement therapies begin. Furthermore, many practitioners use multiple techniques that integrate massage, deeper-tissue work, and movement, all in the same session with a client.

There are numerous techniques that work on the body structure and how it moves. Remember that chronically stressed muscles can alter their shape, structure, and function. At this point the very act of moving creates pain and heightened stress-response feedback. Relief must include a *restructuring*, often called a reorganization of the tissue. The most common approaches include Rolfing, Hellerwork, the Rosen method, the Trager approach, the Feldenkrais method, the Alexander technique, and Ortho-Bionomy.

Rolfing is perhaps the mostly widely known of these deep tissue approaches. It is used for reordering the body to bring its major segments—head, shoulder, thorax, pelvis, and legs—into a finer vertical alignment. The technique loosens or releases adhesions in the *fascia*, the flexible tissue that envelops our muscles and muscle groups. The fascia is supposed to move easily and allow easy *articulation*, or movement of muscles or muscle groups past each other. However, trauma such as injury or chronic stress can cause *stuck points*, or adhesions, in which the fascia is in a sense frozen, not allowing full freedom of movement.

The Rolfer works to restore this freedom of movement, resulting in a more balanced, vertical alignment of the body and often a lengthening or expansion of the body's trunk. Rolfing usually takes place over a series of ten organized sessions dealing with different areas of the body.

Another well-known technique is the Feldenkrais method. This approach was developed by Moshe Feldenkrais and uses physical movement to focus learning on the juncture of thought and action. It is known for its ability to improve posture and flexibility and alleviate muscular tension and pain. It works with the nervous system's capacity for change and learning new patterns for moving, feeling, and thinking. The method involves two applications: awareness through movement and functional integration. These consist of verbally directed, pleasurable, and effortless exercise lessons involving highly sophisticated movement sequences, the use of specific skilled touch and passive movement. It is known for its ability to address serious muscular and neurological problems and improve human functioning.

Even in the western world the Oriental methods are quiet popular. These are based on the principles of Chinese medicine and the flow of energy, or *chi*, through the meridians. The geography of the acupuncture meridians is relied upon to determine points of applying the techniques, and the ultimate goal is restoration of harmony or balance in the flow of chi. These forms may also be used in concert with herbs and acupuncture.

Pressure is applied by finger or thumb tips to predetermined points rather than by the sweeping broad strokes of Western-style massage. Strong pressure or very light pressure may be applied. There are over a dozen varieties of oriental massage and bodywork therapy, but the most common forms in this country are acupressure, shiatsu, jin shin jyutsu, and jin shin do.

Acupressure and *shiatsu* are similar varieties of finger-pressure massage. They are both based on applying pressure to a pattern of specific points that correspond with the acupuncture points. Pressure is applied with the thumb, finger, and palm rather than needles. The goal is the efficient and balanced flow of chi through the meridians. It is believed that where there is tension being held in the musculature, the flow of chi is impaired through those areas, which can lead to chronic problems not only in the musculature but also in the associated organs. Stretching and movement are also sometimes used.

Acupressure is the more generic term used for this approach, and shiatsu is the Japanese version. Jin shin jyutsu comes from an ancient Japanese healing tradition that uses touch to restore the internal flow of energy through the body by releasing energetic blockages. A session lasts about an hour, and the client is fully clothed, lying on a table. The practitioner uses pulse diagnosis to identify energy blocks and then gently holds or touches a specific combination of two of twenty-six acupuncture points to allow release of the blockage. As practiced in the United States, the holding uses less pressure than other forms of acupressure or shiatsu, and there is no application of massage like movements to specific points. Rather, the touch is very light and works to balance the flow of energy.

The Oriental methods just described are also energetic methods in that they are working with energy according to principles of Chinese medicine and view the human being as an energy system. However, there are other energetic methods that are not based on Chinese principles. The most prominent of these are therapeutic touch, polarity therapy, and reiki.

Therapeutic touch is unique in that it was born and reached its maturation within the context of conventional Western medicine. It was developed in the 1970s by Dolores Krieger (Ph.D., R.N., and a professor at New York University) and Dora Kunz, a natural healer. A contemporary interpretation of several ancient healing traditions, it is based on the principle that the human energy field extends beyond the skin and the practitioner can use the hands as sensors to locate problems in it that correspond with problems in the physical body. Disease is seen as a condition of energy imbalance or blocked energy flow. Assessment is done by passing the hands over the body from head to toe about two to four inches above the surface.

The practitioner then serves as a conduit for universal energy, consciously and actively transferring energy into the recipient. The hands are used to direct and focus the energy, sometimes in rhythmical, sweeping motions. The method is initially taught "off body," meaning the practitioner's hands do not touch the physical body, though later with experience some physical touch may take place. Because it is not necessary to touch the physical body, this method can be applied in situations in which the client may not be able to tolerate contact. Sessions last up to thirty minutes and can be done sitting or lying down fully clothed. Therapeutic touch is currently taught in over eighty universities and thirty countries and is practiced by twenty to thirty thousand health care professionals.

Polarity therapy is a form of energy work that was developed by Randolph Stone, a chiropractor, osteopath, and naturopath in the mid-1920s. The practitioner uses subtle touch or holding of specific points to harmonize the flow of energy through the body and also to enhance the body's structural balance. It is based on the principle that every cell has both negative and positive poles and the body is gently manipulated to enhance the energy flow. Emotional tension or physical pain are released as the flow of energy becomes more properly balanced. Polarity therapy is often given in a series of four sessions and may be accompanied by guidelines for diet and exercise.

Reiki is the Japanese word for "universal life force energy." It is an ancient approach in which the practitioner is a kind of healer in the sense that he or she serves as a conduit for healing energy coming from the universe. The reiki energy enters the practitioner through the top of the head and exits through the hands, being directed into the recipient's body or energy field. Reiki is another very subtle form of healing and may be done through clothing and without any physical contact between practitioner and client.

There are other approaches and combinations of approaches that do not fit neatly into categories. Many massage therapists and body workers use combinations of approaches that could be called integrative massage or integrative bodywork.

Reflexology involves the manual stimulation of reflex points on the ears, hands, and feet. Similar methods resembling shiatsu and acupressure have also been practiced in China for thousands of years. Thumb pressure is applied to specific points that correspond somatotopically to specific areas or organs of the body. Reflexology was introduced to this country by William Fitzgerald, who termed it "zone therapy," in the early 1900s. One of the contemporary explanations for how it works is that compression by specific touch techniques affects a system of points and areas that are thought to "reflex" through neurological pathways to distant parts of the body. The pressure on these reflex points (also called "cutaneo-organ reflex points") is used to relieve stress and tension, to improve blood supply, to promote the unblocking of nerve impulses, and to help restore homeostasis or balance in the body.

Zero balancing is a painless, hands-on method of aligning body energy with body structure. It is done through clothes and involves the practitioner using gentle pressure at key areas of the skeleton in order to balance the energy body with the structural body. The theory holds that each of us has an unseen energy body that exists like a glove surrounding the physical body. When injury or trauma occurs, healing of these two bodies does not necessarily occur simultaneously. "Balancing" refers to balancing the relationship between energy and structure. Zero balancing seeks to bridge the gap between those methods that work with structure and those working with energy.

SOURCES CITED

American Holistic Health Association. (1997). *Complete guide to alternative medicine*. New York: Warner Books.

Bernstein, D. A., and Carlson, C. R. (1993). Progressive relaxation: Abbreviated methods. In *Principles and practices of stress management*, eds. P. M. Lehrer and R. L. Woolfolk. New York: Guilford Press.

Carlson, C. R., and Hoyle, R. H. (1993). *Efficacy of abbreviated progressive muscle relaxation training: A quantitative review of behavioral medicine research*. Journal of Consulting and Clinical Psychology, 61 (6), 1059.

Good, M. (1995). *Relaxation techniques for surgical patients*. American Journal of Nursing, 95 (5), 38.

Jacobsen, E. (1977). *The origins and development of progressive relaxation*. Journal of Behavioral Therapy and Experimental Psychiatry, 8.

Lehrer, P. M., Carr, R., Sargunaraj, D., and Woolfolk, R. (1994). *Stress management techniques: Are they all equivalent, or do they have specific effects?* Biofeedback and Self-Regulation, 19 (4), 353–96.

Lehrer, P. M., and Woolfolk, R. L., eds. (1999). *Principles and practices of stress management*. New York: Guilford Press.

Morse, D. R. (1994). *Related exercise*. International Journal of Psychosomatics, 41, 17–22.

Pert, C. (1998). *Molecules of emotion*. New York: Simon and Schuster.

CHAPTER

14 Autogenics and Visual Imagery

Autogenic Relaxation Training: Relaxation Recall

The term *autogenesis* (self-generation) describes almost every form of relaxation exercise; however, the word *autogenic* has become synonymous with a form of relaxation involving self-directed mental images of relaxed states. W. Linden (1999) presents an excellent review of the original technique and its effectiveness.

Although autogenic training has been found highly effective in treating a wide variety of stress-related disorders, most of the research has been done in Europe using what is known as the "full procedure." The abbreviated technique popular in the United States has been found effective as a relaxation and stress-management technique but has not been as well researched as a technique to treat specific stress disorders (Linden 1994).

This simple yet advanced technique centers on conditioned patterns of responses that become associated with particular thoughts. Recall those moments when you have allowed your mind to run away and conjure up a tragic event. Recall how thinking of yourself or your loved ones dying or being involved in a serious accident gives you chills or raises the hair on the back of your neck. This represents a conditioned physical response to that particular association. The opposite is just as true and produces an equally dramatic physical response. Imagine sitting on a quiet beach with the sun warming your body, and a relaxation response is triggered. Unfortunately, many of us have become more conditioned to negative thoughts than to positive ones; thus the technique of relaxation recall was developed to help condition relaxation.

Relaxation recall is actually a very advanced form of relaxation training; it is learned more rapidly when the individual already possesses some other relaxation skills. For example, it is difficult to concentrate or control the direction of your thoughts if your mind is being bombarded by arousal impulses from the body. The components of relaxation recall—concentration and relaxation—are facilitated by your ability to vividly imagine a scene or feeling state and by the ability to concentrate without arousal. Let's examine in detail one of the techniques included in the exercise plan.

It is known that one of the physical responses that accompanies relaxation is *vasodilation*, an expansion of the arteries in the skin of the extremities. This produces a warm, heavy sensation as blood flow increases in that area. Generally speaking, relaxed individuals tend to have warmer hands than anxious or stressed individuals. If one can imagine warmth, or on a feeling level can reproduce the heavy sensation, the body has the tendency to "relive" or reproduce that state. A shift in blood flow is impossible without a change in nervous-system tone; thus relaxation is facilitated. After a degree of proficiency has been obtained, we will add a more complex imagination process by utilizing personal visual imagery of a time and place that was particularly relaxing to you. If your "feeling memory" is pretty good and if you have developed some fairly good body control and concentration abilities, the memory of the beautiful times in your life can be one of the keys to controlling stress and tension.

We have said that stress arousal is a mind-body response to a particular event. Each situation produces an immediate stress response but also leaves a residual amount of tension in the body. Response to subsequent stressors is augmented by the residual from previous responses. As the day wears on, response overactivity results from the inability to dissipate residual tension. The physical relaxation produced by relaxation exercises is an immediate reaction, but the more the relaxation state is induced, the more the carryover to times more removed from the exercise time. Gradually you experience a decrease of residual tension. Thus each new stressful situation will produce a reaction sufficient to deal only with that particular situation without the added-on effect of previous stress arousal. The longer you practice the relaxation exercises, the more your general state of arousal resembles the relaxed state, and the more the ongoing tensions most detrimental to the body are reduced. After a while, this relaxed state becomes a stable part of your behavior. The overactive, rushed individual can become a slowed, cooler-reacting person having the ability to respond with the intensity demanded of each situation as an isolated incident.

Chronically stressed and anxious people do not perceive internal states of arousal and do not associate physical states with emotional arousal. As in a positive feedback system, the physical arousal causes anxious feelings, which further cause physical arousal. Relaxation not only diminishes physical arousal but also promotes stress desensitization by allowing individuals to experience previously stressful situations in a relaxed state, gradually diminishing the stressful experience in their lives and reducing anxiety.

One essential ingredient of mental health—happiness—can be thought of as the ability to live each current situation in reality without the effect of adding imaginary consequences of what could or should happen. Perhaps the primary therapeutic benefit of this relaxation program is the development of the ability to concentrate attention on the present, to quiet the imagination, and to distinguish reality from fantasy. You can develop the ability to direct thoughts away from the ego self, the primary source of stress, and direct them to the problem at hand. You can become more problem centered and less ego centered. As you become less stressed, you automatically become more efficient; they go hand in hand. The exercises that are presented in the remainder of this chapter are time-honored, well-practiced examples of the relaxation technique we call relaxation recall. Follow the instructions and practice these for a few days; the effects can be felt immediately, and the long-term benefits can be substantial.

Legs Heavy and Warm

The exercises in this group are quiet concentration activities that can be done either sitting or lying down. The object is to tell yourself to reproduce feelings of heaviness and warmth in the legs. If you are successful, a heavy, warm sensation will occur as blood flow increases in that area. The body will "relive" or reproduce that state, and, as we have said, such a shift is impossible without a change in the nervous-system tone. Thus relaxation is facilitated. You must be quiet and undistracted, and you must concentrate.

Start by taking three deep breaths. Repeat the following phrases quietly to yourself: "I am relaxed. I am calm. I am quiet." Go slowly; allow time between each phrase to feel these sensations:

My right leg is heavy.
My right leg is heavy and warm.
My right leg is warm and relaxed.
I am calm and quite relaxed.
My left leg is heavy.
My left leg is heavy and warm.
My left leg is warm and relaxed.
I am calm and quite relaxed.
I am quiet and at peace.
I am relaxed.

This activity should take about five minutes. When you are done, remain quiet for a few minutes.

Center of Warmth

The exercises in this group are quiet concentration activities that may be done while sitting or lying down. You will need quiet, intense concentration on the trunk area of the body. You are going to try to imagine warmth being emitted from the nerve plexus lying behind the stomach and right above the navel. Focus your attention on what you feel is the exact center of your body. The nerves there form a plexus called the *solar plexus*. Softly, slowly, and quietly say to yourself:

I am relaxed.
I am calm.
I am quiet.
My solar plexus is warm.
I can feel the heat radiating throughout my entire body.
My body is warm and relaxed.
I am quiet and at peace.
I am relaxed.

This activity should take about five minutes. When you are finished, remain quiet for a few minutes.

Arms Heavy and Warm

By now you should be familiar with the procedure for this exercise. It will include quiet concentration of heaviness and warmth in the arms and hands. If you had any success with the two previous exercises, you will do very well here. If you had difficulty with those exercises, this one should provide you with a breakthrough because you have better control over hands and arms than over legs and trunk, more nerves innervating fewer muscles, and just more practice in using the upper extremities. You may sit or lie down. Start with a few deep breaths. Center yourself. Close your eyes and concentrate on your hands and arms. Your statements are as follows; repeat them to yourself slowly and quietly:

> I am relaxed.
> I am calm.
> I am quiet.
> My right arm is heavy.
> My right arm is heavy and warm.
> My right arm is warm.
> My right arm is warm and relaxed.
> I am calm and quite relaxed.
> My left arm is heavy.
> My left arm is heavy and warm.
> My left arm is warm.
> My left arm is warm and relaxed.
> I am calm and quite relaxed.
> My body is warm and relaxed.
> I am quiet and at peace.
> I am relaxed.

This activity should take about five minutes. When you are finished, remain quiet for a few minutes.

Freedom Posturing

Another form of autogenic or relaxation-recall type of relaxation is what we call *freedom posturing*. This exercise is designed to change thoughts and behaviors that continually fuel the stress response. The basic premise of freedom posturing lies in the interaction between mind and body—arousing thoughts produce a tense body, and a tense body stimulates central nervous-system arousal. The cycle can be broken by changing either the body position or thought process. In addition, this technique seeks to promote self-awareness and reduce stressful behavior, especially as it relates to dealing with the expectations others have of us.

After you learn some of these powerful relaxation techniques, you must then refine your use of them so that you are able to relax at will. Once you have developed the ability to relax at will, you can (1) practice and gradually condition your system to be more tranquil and relaxed and (2) use your ability to relax for immediate relief when you feel stressed. The catch in Item 2 is that we must be able to recognize stress as it builds and before it pushes us into unproductive emotional states and physical disability.

If you are working with another person, just sit back and have that person read the directions. If you are working by yourself, read the situation, get the idea of what you are being asked to do; then sit back, close your eyes, and work through it. Either way, always close your eyes because it greatly increases your power of concentration.

Situation 1

Close your eyes, but in your mind's eye see a tense person. It may be someone you know well or just someone you have seen once. What does this person look like when stressed? How is that person sitting? What is he or she doing with his or her legs, arms, and face? Concentrate on the person's breathing. Is it fast or slow; deep or shallow; through nose or mouth? What sounds is the person making?

Concentrate on the legs. Are they moving or still; crossed or open? Are the feet flat on the floor? Do they seem to be digging into the floor as if to resist movement; or just the opposite, to provide a firm base from which to spring? Are the legs generally taut, ready for action?

Concentrate on the midsection of the person's body. Is this person hunched over from the shoulders? Bent in the abdomen? Is the back arched? Is the back being pushed into the chair?

Concentrate on the hands and arms. Are they moving or still? Are the hands clenched into a fist, or are they open? Are they pushed down onto the arms of the chair? Are they gripping? Are they crossed in front of the body? Are they tensely straight?

Concentrate on the head, neck, and face. Are the eyes wide open or squinted? Is the head pulled down, and are the shoulders up? Is the forehead wrinkled? Are the jaws tightly clenched? Are the neck muscles tightly drawn?

Now assume that position yourself. Tense your muscles as the person you saw in your mind's eye tensed his or her muscles. See yourself in that position. Feel yourself in that position. Where are you? Who are you with? What message (verbal or nonverbal, explicit or implied) is that person giving you? What is he or she expecting from you? Are you feeling pushed to do something you do not want to do? Or are you feeling held back from doing something you want to do? Now leave those thoughts and rest for a moment.

Situation 2

Close your eyes and switch your mind's eye to a person you see as very relaxed. How is this person sitting? Concentrate on this person's arms, hands, breathing, legs, trunk, and face as you did in the previous exercise. How are they different from those of the tense person? Assume the relaxed position yourself. Where are you? Who are you with? Do you feel free to do what you want to do? In the absence of expectations, this is how your body feels. You can help yourself demand your personal freedom by telling your body to position itself in this fashion. Now slowly open your eyes, and reorient yourself to the world around you. Feel the energy flowing through your system vitalize your sense of commitment to your purpose and to yourself. When you feel someone is pushing you or holding you back, assume this freedom posture and be aware of how you are more willing to demand your personal freedom.

Your Special Place

Recall a time in your life when you felt very relaxed, peaceful, and tranquil. It may help to close your eyes, relax, and let the images come to you.
Describe the place in the following terms.

1. When was it? _____

2. Who was with you? _____
   Note: Even though you might have traveled with another person, do not list anyone else unless that person's image is vividly associated with the relaxation feeling.

3. Where was it? Look around; describe what you see; describe your feelings and sensations:

   _____
   _____
   _____
   _____
   _____
   _____
   _____
   _____

Note: Feelings and sensations are more important than exact topographical descriptions. Here is an example of Item 3, somewhat overdone to drive home the point that the location must have feeling.

> See a lonely stretch of beach with the waves forcefully pounding the rocks and teasing the sand. With each wave the sand feels cool, solid, and resisting, then warm and accepting, caressing my feet. The gentle breeze massages my skin, and my hair resembles the grass, bending in response to the wind's gentle persuasion. The sun seductively bathes my skin with warmth, which is then cooled by the breeze. The gulls, precocious and curious, clamor for attention as they proclaim the ecstasy and freedom of flight. My spirit soars with their flight, and as I ride the wind I feel free, open, part of the wind, the sun, the sea, the universe.

Take this a step further into the realm of fantasy. See yourself gently floating on a raft, drifting deeply into relaxation. Your raft may have the ability to float not only on water but also in the air. Feel the wind pick up your raft and gently and safely carry it off the ground as high as you wish it to go, closer to the warmth of the sun. You can fly as high and as far as you wish, looking down on your surroundings, relaxed and calm, as you look at the activities of people and events below. Perhaps you wish to visit a special place and view from your gently floating raft the activities of a special event, knowing that you are above it all, relaxed and calm, gently floating on the wind, leaving all your worries on the ground. Continue your travel for a few minutes, and enjoy this special place and experience. As you return from your trip, know that you can return anytime you wish just by closing your eyes, taking a deep breath, and seeing yourself floating on your special raft.

Visual Imagery

Aristotle wrote, "The soul never thinks without a picture." It is well documented that the pictures in our minds are closely related to physical arousal and the stress reaction. We now know that what works against us can be turned around to work for us—if we can control the pictures in our mind. The basic premise is that imagery is an experience and can be regarded in many important aspects as equivalent to an actual experience with a concomitant elevation of stress arousal or relaxation response (Ganim and Fox 1999, Sheikh and Sheikh 1996, Thomas 1997).

This exercise is only one type in the broad spectrum of visual imagery that is rapidly becoming perhaps the most widely used and researched area in stress management and healing. A guided imagery or fantasy is one in which an individual, by describing an experience, helps another individual form internal visual images. This differs slightly from what we will use here in that you will be working alone, using a story based on your own experience to elicit internal images that will produce a relaxation response. Construct a guided fantasy illustration to help stimulate your personal imagery that, although based on your personal experience, goes beyond that experience to a relaxation fantasy. Create your own imagined relaxation place and use it in the following exercise:

1. In a quiet room and in a comfortable chair, assume a restful position and a quiet, passive attitude. Take four deep breaths. Make each one deeper than the one before. Hold the first inhalation for four seconds, the second one for five seconds, the third one for six seconds, and the fourth one for seven seconds. Pull the tension from all parts of your body into your lungs, and exhale it with each expiration. Feel more relaxed with each breath.

2. Count backward from ten to zero. Breathe naturally, and with each exhalation count one number and feel more and more relaxed as you approach zero. With each count you descend a relaxation stairway and become more deeply relaxed until you are totally relaxed at zero.

3. Now go to the relaxation place outlined in the previous exercise. Stay there for four minutes. Try to vividly, but passively, recall the feelings of that place and time that were very relaxing.

4. Bring your attention back to yourself. Count from zero to ten. Energize your body. Feel the energy, vitality, and health flow through your system. Feel alert and eager to resume your activities. Open your eyes.

Lusk (1992), Naparstek (1995), and Schwartz (1995) provide imagery scripts for calming, centering, coping, and other aspects of staying well.

SOURCES CITED

Ganim, B. and Fox-Wood, S. (1999). *Visual journaling: Going deeper than words.* New York: Quest Books.

Linden, W. (1994). *Autogenic training: A narrative and quantitative review of clinical outcome.* Biofeedback and Self-regulation, 19 (3), 227.

Linden, W. (1999). The autogenic training method of J. H. Schultz. In *Principles and practice of stress management,* 2d ed., eds. P. M. Lehrer and R. L. Woolfolk. New York: Guilford Press.

Lusk, J. T. (1992). *Relaxation imagery and inner healing.* New York: Whole Person.

Naparstek, B. (1995). *Staying well with guided imagery.* New York: Time Warner.

Schwartz, A. E. (1995). *Guided imagery for groups.* New York: Whole Person.

Sheikh, A., and Sheikh, K. (1996). *Healing east and west.* New York: John Wiley and Sons.

Thomas, P. S., ed. (1997). *Image-guided pain management.* New York: Lippincott Williams and Wilkins.

CHAPTER

15 Yoga and Stretch-Relaxation

Yoga

The word *yoga* is derived from the Sanskrit word meaning "union" or "reunion" and is a method of physical, mental, and spiritual development based on the philosophies of Krishna. Knowledge of these philosophies was passed from enlightened master to student, generation after generation, for thousands of years before the first written record appeared around 200 B.C. in Patanjali's Sutras. Since then, thousands of books have been written describing the many types of yoga, called "paths," which have developed into spiritual schools, in many instances becoming distinctly separate schools in themselves. *Raja yoga*, or royal yoga, meaning the path to self-realization and enlightenment, is very similar to the meditative practice described in Chapter 16.

Yoga is a mental discipline that is not directly associated with any religion, although some religions encourage its use as a method to establish a relationship with the divine (Muni 1994). Yoga also has been reported to heal the body—strengthen immunity and breath, improve body alignment, open up blocked energy, and aid meditation (Weller 1995).

The most popular path in the Western world is *hatha yoga*, which uses positions and exercises to promote physical and mental harmony. Most yoga practice starts with hatha yoga because it is thought to provide the body with the health and endurance needed to learn more advanced forms of yoga.

Hatha yoga is practiced for its own rewards, which include strength, flexibility, and reduction of muscle tension, and is used as a technique to quiet the body in preparation for quiet mental states.

Stretch-Relaxation Exercises

The health benefits of stretch-relaxation techniques have been known for centuries; these exercises form the basis for hatha yoga programs, are an essential part of most calisthenics programs, and represent an innate pattern of movement. Notice your pet dog or cat especially on awakening but at other times during the day also. It never attempts to get up without first stretching. Humans also naturally go through a series of stretches before arising from sleep or after prolonged sitting. When tightness or tension is sensed, stretching is a natural reflex.

247

Our modern living patterns are directly responsible for a multitude of health problems, many of which have already been listed in earlier sections of the book. One of the most pervasive is shortened muscles, tendons, and ligaments. Our basic body structure and function have not changed since the days of prehistoric humans, yet our daily activities have changed drastically. Because the body is adaptive, continual sitting during work and leisure will eventually result in shortened muscles, tendons, and ligaments and eventually result in restricted movements. It is not unusual for adults in their midtwenties to be so restricted that touching their fingers to their toes while keeping the knees straight is impossible or at least very painful. The spine will condition itself to the state demanded by chronic sitting and lose its natural erect capabilities; the result will be a sitting-type posture while one is standing or walking. This posture naturally produces pain and tension because body parts are positioned unnaturally. Neck and facial muscles, tendons, and ligaments will pull unnaturally, producing pain in the sensitive tissue around the head, and thus causing headache. It is not at all unusual for the posture and tone of the muscles under the skin to resemble those of the very old. Age lines are not a natural process of aging and are surely not natural in the young or even in those in the middle years.

Chronically shortened muscles do not function properly; excess tension and internal viscosity prohibit normal functioning, and a vicious cycle of the tension reflex develops. Gradually, movements become inefficient and labored; more energy than necessary is required, and fatigue causes a chronic tired feeling even after adequate amounts of sleep. It has long been known that a muscle with proper stretch capabilities is stronger, more efficient, and more enduring than one that is chronically shortened. Moreover, such a muscle is more contractible, exhibits less residual tension, and can be relaxed more easily.

Again, one must realize that yoga masters come from a different culture in which both physical structure and physical activity patterns are significantly different from those of Western cultures. Thus, it is difficult for Westerners to completely master all of the positions. Nevertheless, positive results can be derived from yoga, especially if the exercises are chosen for specific outcomes in specific groups of people. For relaxation, we have developed some exercises and postures derived from principles of hatha yoga. These carefully developed exercises have been shown to yield maximal results in the shortest period of time in groups of individuals with no prior experience or special physical conditioning. This program is sequenced to condition natural readiness. Do not go beyond your point of pain, or you will tear the tissue and retard your progress. You have spent many years conditioning this state, and you cannot reverse it overnight. Do not set goals too high too fast. These are powerful exercises with the capability of restoring the natural structure and function to your tissue. Use them as directed until you have reconditioned your body.

Toe Raise, Knee Stretch, Toe Touch

Even though muscles will contract during these positions, the emphasis is on stretch of muscles and joints. The first exercise is a simple toe raise (Figure 15.1). In a standing position with hands on hips or raised in front of you, balance yourself as high on the tips of your toes as possible. Hold for a count of ten and relax. Repeat this exercise five times and relax.

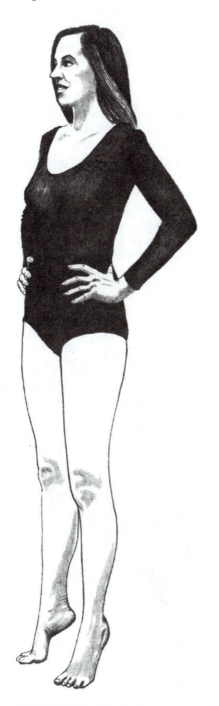

FIGURE 15.1   Toe Raise

The second exercise is the knee stretch (Figure 15.2). Sit with your legs folded under you so that your buttocks are resting on your ankles. Your toes should be pointed backward. Place your hands on the floor outside and behind your feet. Straighten your body with head raised high. Hold for a count of ten; relax and repeat five times.

The third exercise, the toe touch (Figure 15.3), stretches the muscles in the back of the leg in three positions. In a standing position with the heels together, toes angled slightly outward and legs straight, bend forward from the waist and place your hands on your knees. Hold for a count of ten, and return to standing. If this produced no pain, the second repetition should find you reaching for your ankles. If pain was experienced, repeat the position to your knees. Don't force it; your body will tell you when it is ready to go lower. Hold for a count of ten, and return to standing. On the third repetition, place the tips of your fingers on the floor, but assume this position only if no pain was experienced during the last one. Hold for ten and return to standing. The final position, assuming no pain to this point, is to place your palms flat on the floor. Keep your legs straight, bend at the waist, and hold for a count of ten. You will do four repetitions whether you reach the floor or not. Remember, go slowly; your body will tell you when to go on to the next position.

Back Stretch Forward and Reverse, Standing Trunk Bend

Here again, the emphasis is on the stretch of the muscle, the recoil, and the sense of relaxation that follows. Concentrate on the "afterfeeling" of extreme relaxation. The stretch relieves the partial contraction and allows the muscle to relax fully.

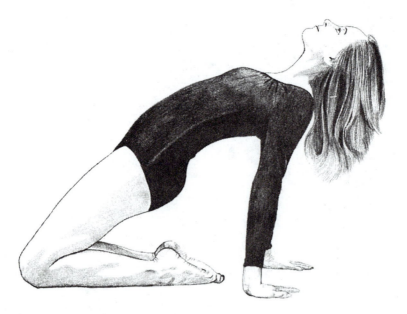

FIGURE 15.2   Knee Stretch

The first exercise is the back stretch forward (Figure 15.4). As its name implies, you will feel the stretch in different parts of your back as the exercise advances. Lie on the floor. Slowly tensing your stomach muscles, raise your trunk through the sitting position to a point where your head is as close to your knees as possible. Once there, place your hands on your knees, thumb on the inside of your leg, and elbow held as high as possible. Hold for ten counts and return to the lying position. Move very slowly. Feel the stomach muscles contract as they raise and lower your upper body. Feel the stretch in the lower back.

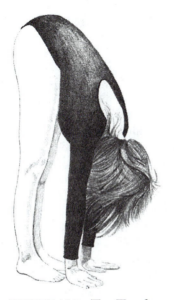

FIGURE 15.3   Toe Touch

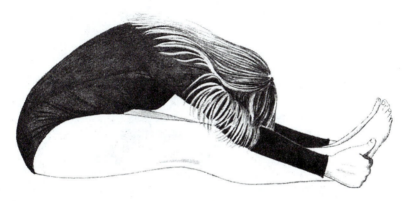

FIGURE 15.4   Back Stretch Forward

On the second repetition, place your hands halfway between your knees and ankles. Try to get your head to your knees; however, go only as far as your flexibility allows. Don't force it—you will get there one day soon. Hold for a count of ten, and relax back to the lying position. Feel the stretch and subsequent relaxation in the back slightly higher than in the first repetition.

On the third repetition, try for your ankles. Go slowly; feel the stretch a little higher on the back. Try to get your head on your knees. Hold for a count of ten and relax. For the fourth repetition, try to hold your hands on the bottoms of your feet. Draw the trunk toward your legs. Allow your elbows to rest on the floor. Hold for a count of ten, and slowly return to the lying position. Relax, feeling the tension release.

For the second exercise, the trunk stretch reverse (Figure 15.5), you will need to lie down on your stomach. This exercise will stretch the back in the opposite direction. You will feel the muscles in both the back and stomach stretch. Place your hands, palms down on the floor, one on each side of your face. Slowly raise your upper body until you can rest your elbows on the floor. Hold in this position for a count of ten. If this produces no pain, arch your back slowly, moving your head high and back. Hold this position for a count of ten and rest. If this produces no pain, place your palms on the floor and continue to raise your upper body until your arms are straight. Go very slowly, and if you feel pain, return to the last position. Hold for a count of ten, and return to the floor and relax. Feel the tension release in your back and stomach. Relax and breathe softly. Repeat the entire sequence five times.

The third exercise is the standing trunk bend (Figures 15.6 to 15.8). Stand with your feet together, legs straight. The first motion will be a side bend. Stretch your arms over your head. Bend your trunk to the right. Go as far as possible. Try to achieve a right angle to your lower body. Go only as far as you can, and, when there, hold for a count of ten, and return to an erect position. Now repeat to the left. Hold for ten and return. The final move is forward. Bend to a right angle, hold for ten, and return. Move very slowly, feeling the stretch and the contraction. When you have done all three moves, bring your arms down to your side and relax. Sense the feeling of relaxation. Repeat the entire sequence five times.

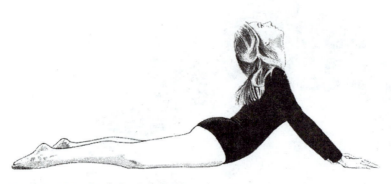

FIGURE 15.5   Back Stretch Reverse

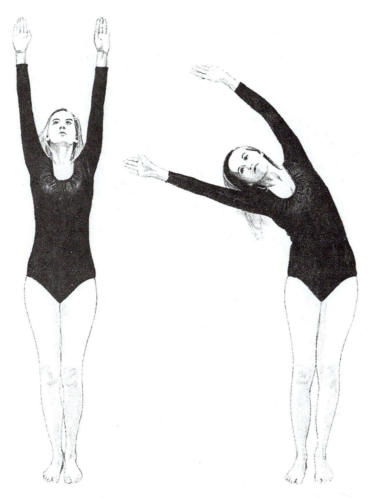

FIGURE 15.6   Standing Trunk Bend (first part)

Wall Reach, Sky Reach, Shoulder Roll, Back Reach, Shoulder Elevation

Chances are that you have noticed in yourself or others that, after hours of writing or other deskwork, the natural tendency is to try to stretch out those cramped fingers, elbows, and shoulders. It is a natural reaction, but most people start too late. First of all, they should have prepared themselves better, and second, they should have stopped more frequently and stretched before cramps developed. That is the purpose of this set of exercises. The emphasis is on the relaxation that follows the recoil of the stretch. Sense it, and sense the difference between that feeling and muscle tension.

The first exercise in this group is the wall reach (Figure 15.9), which is done in the standing position. Stand in front of a wall so that

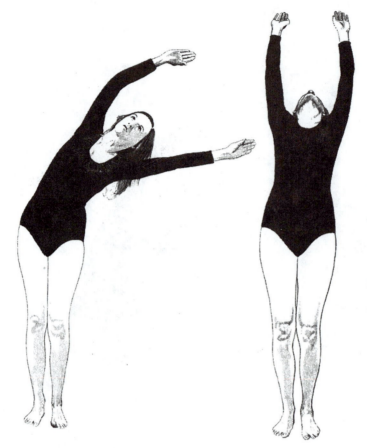

FIGURE 15.7   Standing Trunk Bend (second part)

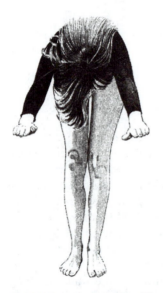

FIGURE 15.8   Standing Trunk Bend (final part)

254

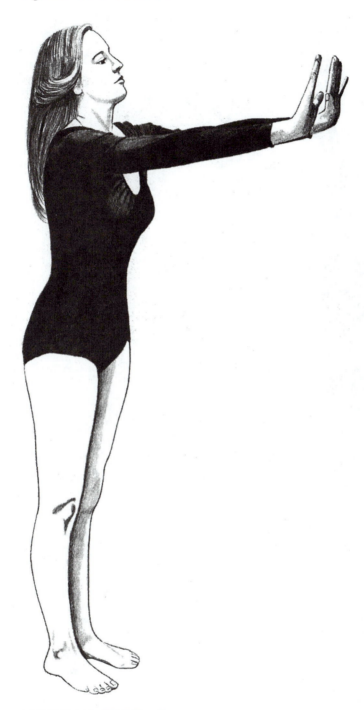

FIGURE 15.9   Wall Reach

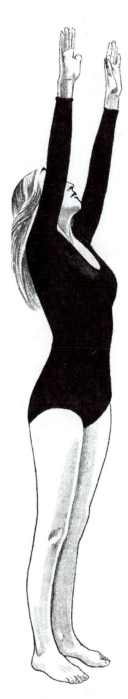

FIGURE 15.10   Sky Reach

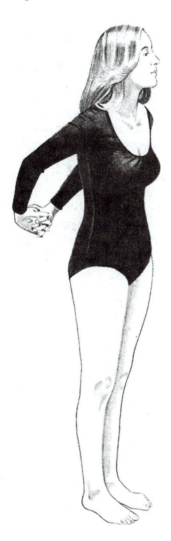

FIGURE 15.11 Shoulder Roll

your outstretched arms just reach the wall. Place the palms of your hands against the wall. Now step back about six inches. Extending your arms primarily from the shoulder, reach for the wall. At the same time spread your fingers and extend them backward. When you make contact with the wall, your shoulder, elbow, wrist, and finger joints should be at full extension and stretch. Hold the stretch for a count of five and return. Repeat five times.

The next one, the sky reach (Figure 15.10), is very similar except that your arms are outstretched over your head. At full reach pause, then with shoulder movement reach a few inches farther, almost as if you were taking something from a shelf just inches out of your reach or as if you were reaching for the sky. The movement is in the shoulder, so be sure not to rise onto your toes. At maximal extension, hold for a count of five and return to rest. Repeat five times.

While you are standing, do the third exercise, the shoulder roll (Figure 15.11). Clasp your hands behind your back. The objective is to roll your shoulders by first dropping them to the lowest possible point, rolling them back, then up in a shoulder shrug, and then forward before they are lowered once again. Complete five circles and return to rest.

The next exercise, the back reach (Figure 15.12), can be done while standing or while sitting if the back of the chair is not high. Raise your arms above your head and clasp your hands together. Then bend your arms back so that your hands touch the back of your neck. Pause and then stretch so that your hands touch a point farther down your back. Hold the extreme position for a count of five, then rest. Repeat five times.

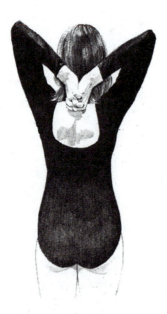

FIGURE 15.12   Back Reach

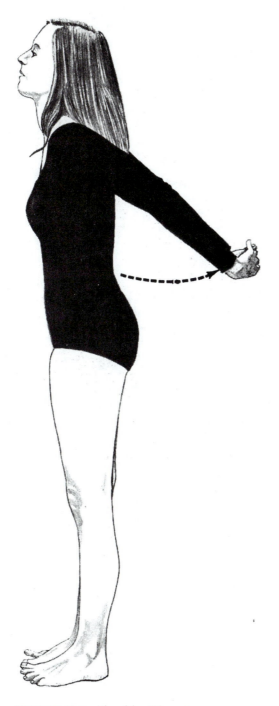

FIGURE 15.3 Shoulder Elevation

The last exercise, shoulder elevation (Figure 15.13), is done while either sitting on the floor or standing. Clasp your hands behind your back, allowing them to rest comfortably against your buttocks. Keeping your back straight, raise your arms as high as possible. Hold in the extreme position for a count of five and return to the resting position, but do not unclasp hands. Feel the stretch in shoulders, elbows, and wrists. Feel the relaxation as you return to rest. Repeat five times.

SOURCES CITED

Muni, S. R. (1994). *Awakening life force*. St. Paul, MN: Llewellyn.
Weller, S. (1995). *Yoga therapy*. London: Thorsons.

CHAPTER

16 Meditation

One of the most important components of a program of stress management is the conditioning of the mind to reduce internal arousal. Meditation is a time-honored technique for going within and moving beyond thoughts and habits to a quiet centeredness.

Meditation teaches us to let go of the past, let go of the future, and just "be" in the present. Our childhood enculturation conditions us to be "human doings"; we are rewarded for doing things to please others. Rarely do we learn to tap into the deep essence of our personal being. It is as though we are hyperactive children reacting to all stimuli coming in, without the ability to damp out unimportant messages. Like the hyperactive child, the undisciplined mind jumps from worries about yesterday to fears of tomorrow, from desires to demands to planning, all the while judging, complaining, and comparing. Meditation disciplines the mind to tune out the tensions and pressures from others and from ourselves. It tunes us in to our own centeredness, which is the basis of our physical, mental, emotional, and spiritual health.

One of the main benefits of meditation is an increase in one's resistance to negativity, which results in a reduction of one's reactivity to former stressors. Practiced meditators learn to eliminate the surface chatter of the mind, the constant thinking, planning, remembering, and fantasizing that occupy the mind's every waking second and keep the mind firmly implanted in the physical matters of living. As mind chatter diminishes, so do one's acquired defenses of physical and psychological survival. Anxiety is reduced, and thus arousal is reduced as both the body and mind achieve the quiet and peace natural to a self-transcendent state of consciousness. Westerners come to meditation for many multilayered reasons such as to cultivate ideals such as wisdom and love; to slow down restless minds; to handle problems that have mental or emotional components; to reconnect the body and spirit; to control a mind filled with uncontrollable fear or anger; to better understand behaviors; to meet fellow seekers; to open the heart and awaken the mind; to realize God; and to become enlightened (Lama Surya Das 1999).

The art of meditation is the ability to maintain a state of passive concentration in which alertness and control are maintained but tension is not produced. The meditator is in complete control of the experience.

Brain Waves

In the meditative state, one is aware of subtle thoughts, energy, and creative intelligence. It is an intended process that takes thought, preparation, and practice. The meditator is thus left with feelings of creativity and accomplishment and a generally positive feeling about the activity. Because there is a marked reduction in the activity of most bodily systems governed by the autonomic nervous system, the meditator usually feels a heaviness or numbness in the extremities and an extreme sense of relaxation and calm. Electroencephalographic (EEG) studies of experienced students of transcendental meditation (TM) show that brain waves are slowed during meditation, suggesting that the meditative state and a low-brain-wave state are synonymous. The increase in popularity of yoga and meditation, coupled with our reverence for time- and energy-saving machines, gave rise to the popularity of using biofeedback as an instrument to control and condition brain wave states. Many people were convinced that the presence of the alpha (8-to-13-cycles-per-second) brain waves resulted in instant mind control. Intuition, accelerated healing, control over pain, higher IQ, improved sleep, and even weight loss have been attributed to control over alpha brain waves. The alpha-theta brain-wave instrument, which roughly resembles the electroencephalograph (EEG), measures the brain's electrical activity in a manner similar to the way the EMG measures muscle activity. There are some important differences, however, in that nerve cells, unlike muscle cells, are always in action and do not stop generating electrical activity until they die. The nerve-cell membrane potentials (the electric differential between the inside and outside of the cell) are not fixed but oscillate continuously near the threshold level. Electrical potentials in any part of the nerve cell create an open field of current flow that can be detected at the surface of the scalp. This continuous variation and accompanying impulse discharge produce a spontaneous and often rhythmical flow of current.

As one might expect, with millions of cells simultaneously performing thousands of functions, it is impossible for the entire brain to be producing activity at any one frequency at any given time. Thus, the EEG shows a complex pattern of mixed waveforms occurring at varying frequencies. However, at any given point, there appears to be a dominant frequency emitted from a specific section of the brain, and the analysis of this dominant frequency has become an important area of study as researchers have begun to associate brain-wave patterns with cognitive functioning, emotion, and states of consciousness (see Figure 16.1).

The third slowest brain wave is called the *alpha wave*. There is nothing mystical or magical about alpha, however. It is a slow, synchronized wave, which means that it occurs in rhythmical, stepwise fashion indicative of a predictable, nonfluctuating, nonprocessing state. Everyone has alpha waves. When you close your eyes, alpha bursts begin to appear with greater frequency. It is more difficult to remain in alpha for any length of time than to produce it in spurts, but one can be trained to do so.

Subjective reports of the feelings that accompany the alpha state indicate that it is an awake, alert, but a calm, restful, and peaceful state, often described as idyllic. It is often difficult to validate such subjective accounts because most people hold preconceived opinions regarding what alpha is supposed to be like. However, most (but cer-

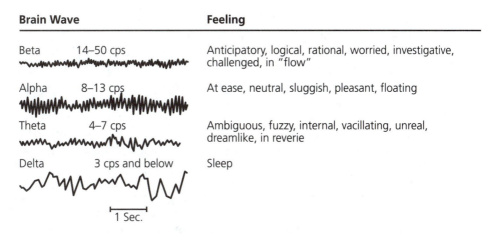

Brain Wave	Feeling
Beta 14–50 cps	Anticipatory, logical, rational, worried, investigative, challenged, in "flow"
Alpha 8–13 cps	At ease, neutral, sluggish, pleasant, floating
Theta 4–7 cps	Ambiguous, fuzzy, internal, vacillating, unreal, dreamlike, in reverie
Delta 3 cps and below	Sleep

1 Sec.

FIGURE 16.1   Brain-Wave States and Associated Feelings

tainly not all) authorities in the field agree that alpha waves characterize a state of consciousness free from ongoing personality-involved thought processes. This relative absence of sustained thought pattern is responsible for the relaxed feeling. As has been mentioned many times, a large part of stress is triggered or augmented by personality-involved arousal thoughts; these thoughts are not present during the typical alpha state. Feeding information back to an individual about the general activity of the brain promotes the ability to decrease potentially stress-producing thought patterns.

Perhaps more intriguing than alpha states are the *theta states*. The dreamlike reverie associated with the production of slowed theta waves has been likened to an advanced meditation experience. This state has been described as being highly creative, producing integrative mental pictures and a low-stress inner-awareness dissociated from the outside world. High-quality instrumentation capable of sophisticated brainwave feedback is expensive and not readily available, thus, although fascinating, it is for most of us academic. Meditation on the other hand, is available to everyone.

Types of Meditation

Perhaps the greatest source of our stress problems is our extreme attachment to our senses, thoughts, and imagination. Peace can best be attained when we free ourselves from these attachments, directing our awareness inward, transcending the incessant bombardment of the consciousness in order to experience a quiet body, a subtle mind, and a unified spirit.

These are the simple goals of meditation, which have motivated millions of seekers for hundreds of years. Although the goals are simple, the fundamentals of meditation are often misunderstood, for meditation itself is difficult to define. Meditation is not a physiological state, nor is it a specific psychological state. Meditation is not East as opposed to West; it is not now as opposed to then, it is not the domain of any organized religion or prayer. It is a practice universal to all who wish to connect to their quiet mind and their spirit. Meditation is so basic that it has transcended time, culture, races, religions, and ideologies. It is so simple that millions have used it, yet so advanced that it represents the highest state of being—the living condition that most closely approximates the tranquil, spiritual state.

Meditation can be best understood as a state of mind, of consciousness, or of spirit. But it is most often defined in terms of an act or a technique. There are numerous meditation techniques embodied in different philosophies. Although meditation is intended to be a central component in one complete style of living, a few of its techniques have been successfully extrapolated for the purposes of relaxation and tension reduction.

The philosophical goals of meditation cannot be achieved without training. The great number of meditation groups that have arisen throughout the world are the result of differences in techniques and ways of mastering techniques rather than of different philosophies (Carrington 1999).

Concentration

Common to all forms of meditation are concentration and the closely related techniques of contemplation and mental repetition. Concentration here implies attention to one subject and thus control of the mind's usual habit of flipping from one subject to another. Mind control through selective attention reduces ego consciousness, and nondirected attention heightens awareness and, in some disciplines, is thought to release energy. Concentrating on physical processes, such as the rhythm of one's breathing, or internal sensations, such as the mystical "third eye," is used in several disciplines. One type of yoga, *Kundalini yoga*, theorizes potential energy coiled up in the nervous system that can be awakened by concentrating on the energy centers that progress up the spine. Visual imagery is used in many practices, including focusing the mind's eye on a thousand-petaled lotus. Another popular practice is to concentrate on breathing by counting breaths while working to eliminate all other thoughts and feelings. When ten breaths are counted without losing the count, the mind is more ready to contemplate. Whatever the technique, to the masters, concentration of the mind away from the worries and cares of the personality is the only real freedom a person will ever experience (Dalai Lama and Cuther 1999, Goldstein 1993, Surya Das 1999).

A time-honored vehicle for concentrative meditation is the verbal or mental repetition of a word or sound called a *mantra*, meaning "hymn" or "calming sound." A mantra can be a single word, such as "mu" or "om"; a phrase from holy scripture; a name for a god, or specially selected words thought to be calming because of their resonance qualities. Using such words is the practice in popular transcendental meditation (TM).

Words with "meaning" tend to elicit many associations. Although the Sanskrit mantras are meaningless for Westerners, most have deep meaning for eastern practitioners. For example, "Om" ("I am one, we are one") is known in Eastern cultures as the universal mantra that is believed to give cosmic power. In the meditative traditions of Judaism, Christianity, and Islam, the repetition of God's name has mystical meaning. For Westerners, although the Sanskrit mantras may not be understood literally, they can still have meaning.

Benson (1992) chose the word "one" as the mantra for his "relaxation response" because it is basically neutral and low in association value, but as a connotation of "Om," it can be meaningful for some people.

The "emotionality" of words used for meditation can induce either stress or relaxation depending upon the word's associations and the effects on the involved individuals. In a physiological and psychological study, on a group given a choice of emotional or unemotional mantras for meditation, most subjects preferred the emotional words (such as *happy, garden, sail,* or *love*) to the neutral words (*om, one*) (Morse 1995). (Mantras will be discussed further in the section "How to Meditate.")

Contemplation

Contemplation is closely related to concentration, the primary difference being that the object of contemplation (usually an external object, or *mandala*) is symbolic, and it is the significance rather than the object that becomes the focus. The Zen Buddhist *koan*, a question puzzle or riddle such as "What is the sound of one hand clapping?" has no answer. Rather, it is an artificial instrument to force an open mind and develop in students the Zen consciousness.

The same is true for Christian meditation that uses objects such as the crucifix, a picture or statue of a religious figure, or spiritual passages and prayers as a focus for contemplation as a means to consciousness of Christ. One of the more complete systems of Christian or religious meditation has been outlined by the Association for Research and Enlightenment, made up of the followers of the "Sleeping Prophet," Edgar Cayce. Cayce was adamant in his belief that contemplation should be only a means and not an end, and he quoted Jesus' warning in the Parable of the Displaced Demon, in which the evil spirits that were cast out of an empty mind quickly returned with other devils, leaving the man worse off than before. To Cayce, meditation was attuning the mental and physical body to its spiritual source, seeking to know the relationship to the Maker. There is no emptying in the mind-void sense, only emptying of that which hinders the creative forces from rising along the natural channels or centers. An example of these natural channels are the seven spiritual centers, or *chakras*, also recognized as being related to the endocrine glands, which in this case provide energy for psychic and religious experiences. Cayce additionally defined meditation as a prayer from within the inner self and made a distinction between prayer and meditation: Prayer was external attunement, a pleading, a petition to the Holy Spirit; meditation was an internal attunement, a seeking to know one's relationship with God, an inpouring from the Holy Spirit. Cayce's form of meditation uses the Lord's Prayer as a focus for contemplation.

The contemplation techniques of Christian meditation are similar to those of other types in that they are employed to transcend one's daily cares and worries. The primary difference is in the focus of the contemplation. Contemplative meditation is for the purpose of contemplating what you desire to experience. You become relaxed and think of the spiritual state to which you aspire (Maharishi Mahesh Yogi 1995). Whatever the technique, though, the desired outcome is control of consciousness and direction of mind.

Meditation and the Reduction of Stress Arousal

The primary purpose of meditation—peace, enlightenment, and spiritual growth— cannot be obtained as long as the mind is in turmoil and the body is aroused. Thus, most meditative techniques have seemingly elaborate preparatory procedures designed to induce physical relaxation, and meditation itself quiets the mind. Relaxation, an indirect product of meditation, can be therapeutic in the treatment or prevention of stress-related disorders.

Even though meditation is thousands of years old and the physiological feats of meditation masters are legend, the "scientific" study of the body-mind processes of meditation is still quite new. Meditation became scientific when Wallace (1970) published the results of a study showing that the body significantly decreases its consumption of oxygen during meditation, thus producing a hypometabolic state (a slowing down of the body processes). Wallace also found that the skin showed an increased resistance to the passage of an electrical current, which indicates decreased arousal of the autonomic nervous system. Additional findings from this study were a decrease in the lactate/ion concentration, another measure of decreased metabolism; a decrease in heart rate and cardiac output (quantity of blood pumped by the heart per minute), indicating a reduction in the heart's workload; a decrease in respiration rate; and an increase in the amount of time the brain emits slowed brain waves, indicating a more restful state. This restful state physiologically resembled sleep in many ways but was significantly different from it. The meditator was found to be in a restful state but was awake and alert and exhibited increased reaction time, improved coordination, and improved efficiency of perception and auditory ability.

Later research both supported and refuted, at least in degree, Wallace's early findings. This only points out the difficulty of such research, which is largely the result of subject variability and differences in meditation techniques. For example, variations in the length of the meditative session and experience of the meditator are extremely important. Obviously, the more one meditates, the greater should be one's ability to change psychophysiological states. EEG records of meditation masters show a predominance of alpha and theta brain waves during meditation, which become more marked with years of practice; beginning meditators, on the other hand, show only slight changes in brain-wave patterns.

Another difficulty in research is the difference in the meditative state itself. As mentioned, meditation is not a unitary phenomenon but a series of states including quiet sitting, passive concentration, mental deautomatization or desynchronization, a neutral or mind-void stage, and, especially in accomplished meditators, a brain-directed state.

As we have seen, stress arousal is a mind and body response to a particular psychosocial or environmental situation. Each situation produces an immediate stress response but may also leave a residual amount of tension in the body. Response to subsequent stressors is augmented by this leftover tension. As the day wears on, response overactivity results from the inability to dissipate residual tension. The physiological relaxation experienced by the meditator is a short-term phenomenon, but the more the relaxation state is induced, the more carryover there is to the nonmeditative state. Meditation helps dissolve tension by quieting the mind's tendency toward "afterthoughts," which prolong the stress response and at least temporarily reduce the physical arousal of the organs. Thus each new stressful situation will produce a reaction sufficient to deal with that particular situation without the added effect of previous stress arousal. The longer one meditates, the more one's general state of arousal resembles the meditative state, and the more ongoing tensions most detrimental to the body are reduced. The accomplished meditator develops the ability to direct thoughts away from physical, mental, and emotional defense, the primary source of stress. The meditator experiences temporary transcendence, but just as the physiological state gradually becomes a stable trait, so can an individual learn to live a life of increased transcendence (Patel 1999).

A review of literature covering 25 years, 500 scientific studies from 210 different universities in 35 countries in summary shows that meditation reduced stress, increased creativity, improved memory, increased energy, increased inner calm, reduced insomnia, increased happiness and self-esteem, reduced anxiety and depression, improved interpersonal relations, improved breathing, and promoted younger biological age (Roth 1994).

How to Meditate

There are many types of meditation, each representing a variation in purpose and technique. The type presented in this section is thought to be the best suited for stress reduction, the easiest to learn, and the one most void of cultic, religious, and spiritual overtones. The technique is complete for the purpose of meditation; however, it can also serve as an introduction to more specific types because they all have at least this technique as their core experience. What follows is both explicit instruction and clarifying explanation.

1. The first essential element is a quiet environment—both external and internal. A quiet room away from others who are not also meditating is essential, especially while you are learning. Put out the dog, cat, or whatever. Unplug the phone or find a room without one. Generally, do whatever you can do to reduce external noise. If you cannot completely eliminate the noise, as is often the case in busy households or in college dorms, use earplugs, play a record or tape of soft instrumental sounds, or use any of the numerous environmental sounds that have been commercially recorded. Many enterprising people take their tape recorders to the woods to record the sound of the wind singing in the trees, a mountain stream, or just the birds at dawn. The sounds of the waves at the seashore also make an excellent background for meditation. In addition to blocking out noise, such sounds help promote relaxation as they usually bring back memories of pleasant feelings.

2. Next, work on quieting your internal environment. One way is to reduce muscle tension. Remember that it is practically impossible to induce a meditative state while the reticular activating system is bombarding the cortex with sensory signals emitted from the muscles. Muscle tension represents one of the largest obstacles to successful meditation. Spend some time, no more than five minutes, relaxing your muscles. You may want to choose one or several of the relaxation exercises from Chapters 12 through 15 and work on the area that is most troublesome for you.

One way to reduce excess muscle tension is to sit comfortably. You may not feel like real meditators unless you use the cross-legged position; if you desire this position, sit on the floor with a pillow under your buttocks. In this position the legs are crossed so that the left foot rests on the right thigh and the right foot rests on the left thigh. Unless you have practiced this position or are naturally flexible, you will find this uncomfortable, however. A simple tailor's position will suffice, if you really want to sit on the floor. If you don't mind being too Western, sit in a straight-backed, comfortable chair, feet on the floor, legs not crossed, hands resting on the thighs, fingers slightly open, not interlocked.

You should sit still, but remember meditation is not a trance; if you are uncomfortable or feel too much pressure on any one spot, move. If you itch, scratch. Do not assume a tight, inflexible position or attitude. Relax. Do not lie down or support your head or you will tend to fall asleep. Keep your head, neck, and spine in a straight vertical line. A small but significant amount of muscular effort is needed to maintain this posture, and this effort helps prevent sleep from occurring.

If shoes, belt, bra, tie, or collar are too tight, loosen them. The goal is to diminish sensory input to the central nervous system. Most people like to have a clock where it can be seen at a glance to reduce the anxiety that arises from the feeling that more time is being spent than was anticipated. Twenty to thirty minutes is the standard amount of time spent per session, although five minutes is better than none. Although not recommended for the first few sessions, occasionally interspersing a one-hour session has been reported to be most profound and relaxing.

3. Before you start, relax and stretch your neck muscles. Move your chin toward your chest, then back in place. Repeat this three times. Move your head toward your back. Do this three times. Rotate your head clockwise three complete rotations. Repeat this counterclockwise three times. Now relax your neck. Allow your head to drop slightly forward. This is more comfortable than slightly backward.

Sit quietly. Close your eyes. Notice immediately how that simple movement quiets the environment. Most of our sensory input enters through the eyes; the simple act of closing the eyes does much to quiet the mind. The ambient noise is reduced, the eyes are closed, muscle tension is reduced, and tactile sensory stimulation is at a minimum. The external and physical environment of the body should now be quiet. Now concentrate on quieting the mind. Foremost in this effort is developing a tranquil or passive attitude. Even if meditation is done for a specific reason, such as to reduce hypertension, cut down on smoking, or increase self-assuredness, you must not dwell on the outcome of meditation or even on how well that particular meditation is proceeding. Such thoughts represent an ongoing competitive type of thought process that the meditation is trying to suppress. The body's external physical environment should now be quiet.

4. Spend ten minutes in "neutral," a period of not controlling or focusing your thoughts. Concentrate on quieting the mind. Foremost in this effort is developing a tranquil or passive attitude. Flow with whatever you may feel, and stay calm with relaxed interest. Touch with your thoughts whatever comes to your mind, and then let it go.

Direct your thoughts away from self, away from the parts you play in the stories of your mind. If you have music or environmental sounds playing, direct your attention to the sound. Float with the sound like a cloud, white and fluffy against blue sky . . . like a leaf floating down a stream, floating, and twirling around the rocks, over a waterfall. You may notice some warmth or heaviness in your arms or legs. This is an indication of muscles in those areas beginning to relax. You might also notice your head dropping with the relaxation of your neck muscles. Your breathing is probably slower and a bit deeper.

For a moment, concentrate on your breathing. As you breathe in, think "in," let the air out and think "out." You should breathe in through your nose, think "in," and breathe out through your mouth, think "out," but do not force the expiration . . . just open your mouth and let the air out. Think in . . . out . . . in . . . out. . . . Now each time you breathe out, count the breath. Count ten consecutive breaths without missing a count. If you happen to miss one, start over. When you get to ten, start at one again. Concentrate, anticipate the breath, and block all other thoughts from your mind. Concentrating on breathing is a means of focusing attention inward away from the self in relation to the external world. It is an example of a mental device.

Most meditative techniques utilize some form of mental device to direct consciousness away from logical, cause-and-effect, goal-directed thought processes. The device may be spiritual contemplation, the contemplation of geometric designs, concentration on a body process such as breathing, an internal light, or an external light, as in a biofeedback display, but most often the device is a mantra.

The mantra is used to quiet the mind. Think of the mind as a lake, choppy on the top but calm below. Just as the choppy waters of a lake are caused by the external environment, so too are reflective thoughts churning around the cortex (top layer of the brain) in response to external stimulation of your senses, your memory, and your thought habits. Concentrating on the mantra directs your attention toward it. But because the word has no denotative or connotative meaning, stories are not formed, memory and imagination are not stimulated, and arousal does not occur. Automatization of brain function breaks down, and you drift into an altered state of consciousness. As in the quiet depths of the lake, the quiet, subtler state of mind emerges into consciousness. Gradually, the concentration on the mantra will also disappear and you will remain in a neutral state until a new thought pops into your consciousness, as sporadic thoughts often do. At that point, you can consciously void the thought just by telling yourself, "No, I do not want to think about it," or you can go back to the mantra, or you can direct the thought to a pattern of nonstressful thinking consistent with the particular type of meditation you are practicing.

5. During the concentration part of your meditation period, you may wish to repeat a word, idea, or phrase that depicts peace, beauty, or a spiritual ideal for you. "Om" is the universal mantra. More than just spoken, it is softly chanted aloud on each exhilaration (as "aaaaaaooooommmmm") at your individual pitch and tonality. Also during the concentration part of your meditation, you may wish to use a visual focus rather than using sound. A candle flame, a picture that produces serenity for you, or a mandala may be a good eyes-open focus. Whatever visual focus you use, be sure that it does not offer your left hemisphere food for thought, or it will be busy analyzing, planning, and evaluating. A mandala (a simple geometric pattern) is used for meditation because the left hemisphere quickly tires of the simple pattern while the rest of the mind continues to focus on it. A circle with a dot in the center, an equilateral triangle, and a square have been used for centuries as meditation aids. Some meditators use visual imagery (eyes closed) as their concentrative focus.

In all cases, you are teaching your mind not to think about or form stories around sporadic thoughts. You are eliminating a bad habit acquired over the course of your life. This method is a form of reeducation of the mind and the central nervous system. We can make an analogy between this practice and dieting. Dieting can help you lose weight, and, you hope, the practice of dieting may help you to develop new eating habits to lessen the chance of becoming overweight again. Similarly, meditation will help make you calm, and the practice of meditation can help develop new thought habits that should diminish stress arousal in the future.

Breathe softly, but now do not concentrate on your breathing. Repeat one of the mantras aloud. Say it over and over. Each time say it more softly until it becomes just a mental thought with no muscular action involved. Pace yourself, gradually lengthening the interval between thoughts of the mantra. Allow the mantra to repeat itself in your mind. Do not force it; just let it flow. Gradually the mantra will fade, and your mind will remain quiet. The quiet will occasionally be broken by sporadic thoughts. Let them come, experience them, go with them until you feel that you are controlling them. At that point they become daydreams and usually involve ego arousal. When this happens, stop the thought process and go back to the mantra.

Remember that meditation is a feeling, a state of mind. It is not simply a technique; it is not saying the mantra. Sit quietly for ten to fifteen minutes and meditate. Keep your movements to a minimum, but if you are uncomfortable, move; if you are worried about time, look at a clock, or the discomfort and anxiety will prevent your full attainment of the meditative state.

6. When you finish meditating, do not be in too much of a hurry to get up. Open your eyes, and stretch a little. Contract your muscles and reactivate yourself slowly. Having at least temporarily altered your emotional reactivity, continue your day with renewed inner capacity for meeting the day's challenges.

One of the greatest obstacles preventing the full attainment of the meditative state is usually the lack of physical and/or mental quietness. Physical quietness is the easier of the two to surmount. A quiet room, dim lights, closing the eyes, working to relax the muscles, sitting comfortably, and loosening clothes all tend to diminish sensory stimulation. You should also eliminate the stimulation that can come from too much food and drugs (including caffeine and nicotine) by abstaining from either before meditating. Meditation is a discipline that necessitates having faculties at full command; drugs have no place in the practice.

Mental quietness is more difficult to attain, especially at first. But do not be discouraged. It took many years to develop your current thought processes, and they will not change overnight. Many people are uncomfortable with quietness. They have been so bombarded with stimulation every waking minute since the cradle that they have not learned how to sit still by themselves and simply think of nothing. When one finally does sit down and seek quiet, the mind is filled with: "The car needs a tune-up," "What time will Dick be home? . . . I hope he remembers our anniversary," "Should I buy that new computer?" But as you learn to disregard these thoughts, they will gradually diminish and finally disappear.

Mindfulness and Insight Meditation

The previous meditation exercise is an example of the technique popularized by transcendental meditation and utilizes concentration or similar practices as a point of focus to stabilize the mind, reduce distractions, and maintain nonstressful attention in an attempt to promote the relaxation response (Benson 1992).

Another school of meditation practice is called *mindfulness*, or insight meditation. In the practice of mindfulness, you begin by utilizing the concentration meditation to produce calmness and stability, and then you introducing an observing focus as well. When thoughts or feelings come up in your mind, you don't ignore or suppress them, nor do you analyze or judge their content. Rather, you simply note any thoughts as they occur as best you can and observe them intentionally but nonjudgmentally, moment by moment, as events in the field of your awareness. (Kabat-Zinn 1993)

Deeply buried in the mind lies a mental mechanism that accepts what the mind perceives as beautiful and pleasant experiences and rejects those experiences that are perceived as painful. This mechanism gives rise to states of mind that cause stress (what we have previously described as sufferings, emotional states such as fear, anger, greed, envy, lust, hatred, aversion, and jealousy). We choose to avoid these hindrances not because they are evil in the normal sense of the word but because they are compulsive and because, once attention is focused on them, it tends to remain fixated in feedback loops that never lead to problem solving, only to stress arousal. Conscious thought has the habit of adding to our experience and of loading us down with concepts and ideas, plans and worries, fears and fantasies. Mindfulness teaches us to see things as they really are. It adds nothing to perception and it subtracts nothing. It distorts nothing. It is bare attention and just looks at whatever comes up.

Paradoxically noting of thoughts that come and go in your mind can lead you to feel less caught up in them and give you a deeper perspective on your reaction to everyday stress and pressures. By observing your thoughts and emotions as if you had taken a step back from them, you can see much more clearly what is actually on your mind and how you react emotionally to those thoughts.

The key to mindfulness meditation is not so much what you choose to focus on but the quality of the awareness that you bring to each moment. It is very important that it be nonjudgmental—more of a silent witnessing, a detached observing. Observing without judging, moment by moment, helps you see what is on your mind without editing or censoring it, without intellectualizing it or getting lost in your own incessant thinking. The goal of mindfulness is for you to be more aware, more in touch with life and with whatever is happening in your own body and mind at the time it is happening—that is, in the present

The goal is to resist the impulse to try to escape the unpleasantness; instead, you attempt to see it clearly as it is and accept it because it is already present in this moment. It is psychologically impossible for us to objectively observe what is going on within us if we do not at the same time accept the occurrence of our various states of mind. This is especially true with unpleasant states of mind. In order to observe our own fear, we must accept the fact that we are afraid. We can't examine our own depression without accepting it fully. The same is true for irritation and agitation, frustration, and all those other uncomfortable emotional states. You can't examine something fully if you are busy rejecting its existence. Whatever experience we may be having, mindfulness just accepts it. It is simply another of life's occurrences, just another thing to be aware of. Without judging it there is no pride, no shame, and no self-deprecation, nothing personal at stake—what is there, is there.

With this explanation in mind, sit comfortably and quietly. Close your eyes and allow your mind to be quiet, yet alert. As thoughts arise in your consciousness, accept them and concentrate on how your body is responding to the thoughts. Concentrate but don't manipulate the thoughts. Just be aware of your thoughts, your feelings, and your body's reaction. Resist the temptation to judge the experience as pleasant or unpleasant, worthwhile or worthless. Gradually the experience loses its emotional valence, and you begin to break the bond between the thought and the emotion. The training or conditioning has started. Continued practice can result in this detachment becoming your automatic choice for experiencing both the ups and downs of life with a more even keel.

The Need for Practice

Meditation is a skill you must practice if you are to enjoy its benefits. Meditation is not difficult to learn. However, many people are hindered by lack of confidence in their ability to meet their expectation of what meditation is and can do for them. Meditation is not so simple that mere ritual will overcome the hyperactivity of a mind planning, scheming, thinking about, and reacting to the distractions to which we are all subjected. One cannot go full steam one minute and be tranquil the next. Preparation for quietness is an essential step.

Meditation must be practiced, but one cannot labor at it. You cannot force yourself into transcendence. The key phrase in learning meditation is "let go." Some may be tempted to withdraw from life through meditation. The purpose of meditation, however, is to enhance the experience of life, not to be a vehicle for withdrawing from it. Meditative tranquility trains the mind to allow active participation in an active life without unnecessary stress. Meditation is not a substitute for living.

SOURCES CITED

Benson, H. (1992). *The relaxation response.* New York: Avon.

Carrington, P. (1999). Modern forms of meditation. In *Principles and practice of stress management,* eds. P. M. Lehrer and R. L. Woolfolk. New York: Guilford.

Dalai Lama, and Cutler, H. (1999). *The art of happiness.* NY: Riverhead.

Goldstein, J. (1993). *Insight meditation.* Boston: Shambala.

Kabat-Zinn, H. G. J. (1993). *Mindfulness in plain English.* Mind/Body Medicine.

Morse, R., (1995). *Love and hate: Their many guises and stressful effects.* Stress Medicine, 11, 177–97.

Patel, C. (1999). Yoga-based therapy. In *Principles and practice of stress management,* eds. P. M. Lehrer and R. L. Woolfolk. New York: Guilford.

Roth, R. (1994). *Transcendental meditation.* New York: Primus.

Surya, D. (1999). *Awakening to the sacred.* New York: Broadway Books.

Wallace, R. K. (1970). *Physiological effects of transcendental meditation.* Science, 167, 1751–54.

Yogi, M. M. (1995). *The science of being and the art of living: Transcendental meditation.* New York: Meridian Books.

CHAPTER
17 Stress Reduction through Physical Activity

This chapter presents a natural body-awareness technique that has proven itself again and again to all who love to lose themselves in physical activity—to revert to an original mind-body unity, to rediscover play. Physical activity is a natural way of putting mind and body back together. Movements such as dancing, running, hiking, and walking through the woods are natural and necessary for normal growth and development.

Under the influence of the dualistic philosophy, the mind became of great importance to humankind, and the body was demoted to a lesser role except when in ill health. The pendulum started to swing toward the mind when human beings found that the mind could accomplish more than the body through its use of written and stored information, the basis of technology. The body had been quite perfected by this time and lived in harmony with mind and nature. It was delicately balanced, with an innate drive to conserve energy. Thus, all species survived by becoming efficient, by reading the current and swimming only when necessary. We began to let the mind work while the body conserved its energy, and the mind began to think of ways of extending the body without expending human energy—enter the machine. Through use, the mind grew into the fantastic organ that even now we don't fully understand.

To that innate drive of energy conservation humankind added another drive—toward time efficiency. Reducing the time involved in one activity allows for completion of more activities. The mind is responsible for technological advances, so it is no wonder that development of the mind has taken precedence over development of the body in industrialized nations. But as we move away from a mere survival epoch to one of life quality, we have begun to ask the questions "Save energy for what?" "Save time to do what?" We have also begun to realize that physical inactivity results in degenerative disease and have found it increasingly difficult to cope with the mental overstimulation that accompanies rapid technological growth. Perhaps this is an epoch in which we will allow the body to catch up with the mind's giant strides.

The physical nature of human beings is beginning to take a more prominent position in our lives once again, but instead of casting off technology, people in developed countries have learned to live with it by replacing physical work with "artificial work" in the form of recreational activity. The difficulty in finding an open tennis court, the packed ski-area parking lots, and the boom in the athletic outfitting industry all attest to the fact that physical activity has become important. In conjunction with its recreational nature, physical activity is regaining recognition for its potential as a relaxation technique, which is in some ways similar to those already discussed but with several unique characteristics as well.

Relaxation techniques such as meditation, neuromuscular relaxation, or autogenic training are highly preventive in nature; however, they contribute little to alleviation of tension once the stress response has occurred. A primary contribution of physical activity, on the other hand, is the alleviation of stress-product buildup, with prevention being a secondary aspect. This being the case, we focus here on three aspects of physical activity: (1) using activity to dissipate or use up the stress products produced by fear, threat, or anger that has provoked the hormonal and nervous systems into defensive posture, (2) using exercise preventively to decrease one's reactivity to future stress, and (3) using physical activity to promote a feeling of well-being, tranquility, and transcendence.

Physical Activity as Treatment

Let us look at the treatment role of physical activity in stress management by focusing on a particular problem. Imagine yourself in your work or school situation being asked to give more time than you have and to do more work than you can possibly accomplish. Then imagine that your personal relations are strained because of this overload. An underlying state of tension is becoming a part of your life, and you begin to doubt your personal effectiveness. Then the crowning blow comes—you are berated in front of others, and you undergo a massive stress response. Anger, fear, indignation, and rage boil through your body. This is the response we have described many times before—the hormonal and nervous systems ready the body for fight or flight. Now is the time to do one of these actions and do it physically.

It is important to understand that the human stress response is intended to end in physical activity. The outpouring of sugar and fats into the blood is meant to feed the muscles and the brain so that they can actively contend with the provoking stressor. The dilation of pupils occurs to give better visual acuity and to visually take in apparent threats. The increased heart and respiration rates are to pump blood and oxygen to active muscles and stimulated control centers in the brain. This is not a time to sit and feel all of these sensations tearing away at the body's systems and eroding good health. This is the time to move, to use up the products, and to relieve the body of the destructive forces of stress on a sedentary system. Appropriate activity in this case would be total-body exercise such as swimming, running, dancing, biking, or any active sport that lasts at least one hour (assuming that you are in adequate physical condition to perform such a task). Such activities will use up the stress products that might otherwise be harmful and that are likely to play a part in a degenerative disease process such as cardiovascular disease or ulcers.

Research has definitively shown the benefits of exercise in cardiac rehabilitation for decades, and exercise is now a standard component of postcardiac treatment. Historically, the prevalence of heart attacks in men was greater; thus the data were generated on men. Even a short-term exercise program for only one week started as soon as possible after myocardial infarction was shown by Greif (1995) to have beneficial effects for male patients.

It has been shown that women realize the same benefits. After a cardiac rehabilitation exercise program, women showed significant improvements in percentage of body fat, exercise capacity, and most components of behavior and quality of life (Lavie and Milani 1995). In addition to the use of exercise for the cardiovascular health of both men and women, it is used for treatment in many other diseases as well (Leutholtz and Ripoll 1999).

We have mentioned that during the stress response the two hormones of the adrenal medulla, epinephrine and norepinephrine, are pumped into the system to prepare the body for fight or flight. In laboratory experiments, when norepinephrine is injected into the body, it causes a feeling of underlying anxiety until a social situation triggers a known emotion. For example, if an individual is injected with norepinephrine and is then annoyed by someone, the reported feeling is anger; if intimidated by someone or a situation, the feeling reported is fear. As norepinephrine is a product of the stress response, it makes the individual highly volatile and vulnerable to adverse emotions if it is not used for its intended purpose—physical activity. The mental and emotional implications here should be apparent. How many times under stress do you "fly off the handle" at very little provocation?

A picture should be forming that the stress response evolved to be nothing more than preparation for physical activity. Thus, a natural release, which is also socially acceptable for everyone, is physical activity. It is also a treatment everyone can afford.

Such treatment was notably used by two professional coaches. After football games a former football coach would run to wear off the stress products and bring himself down. The other, a basketball coach, had four piles of dirt in his backyard and moved dirt pile A to spot B and so on until his stress level subsided. To some extent all of us are coaches of a sort—we watch the game (both literally and metaphorically) being played, we get emotionally involved, and then we suffer the consequences of not being able to interact physically. The key factor for all of us is to recognize when we're stressed and act physically on that response soon after.

Physical Activity in the Prevention of Disease

The second nature of physical activity is that of prophylaxis—preventive treatment. The value of physical activity in preventing the untoward effects of stress are such that if they could be bottled and sold for people to take a dose a day, the bottler and sales agents would be rich beyond compare, so effective is the product.

Deep within most of us we fear abnormality of the heart; if it beats too fast or too loudly or "skips a beat," we become anxious because we are this muscular organ—when it expires, we expire! The heart, just like other muscles, is the epitome of syntropy—it becomes stronger as we use it appropriately. Exercise is a stressor, so it forces the body to adapt to the stressor. The heart gains in muscular strength during exercise, and that strength carries into the resting state. When it is strong, fewer beats are required to supply the body with blood, so the heart gets more rest and relaxation time (Wilmore and Costell 1999).

The respiratory system reacts to exercise in the same syntropic manner, increasing its capacity to take in air and exchange oxygen for carbon dioxide at the capillary level. This respiratory efficiency also carries over into the resting state.

The working muscles, the hormonal system, metabolic reactions, the responsiveness of the central nervous system—all the body's systems—react in a like manner to physical activity, strengthening one's ability to cope (Berger 1994, Bird, Smith, and Gibbins 1998, Viru and Smirnova 1995).

The unifying feature of physical exercise is that (1) during activity the body reacts in an ergotropic manner, that is, all systems are stimulated for action, and (2) after physical activity, the systems are slowed down in a trophotropic manner, dominated by the parasympathetic nervous system, causing tranquillity. About ninety minutes after a good physical bout of exercise, one usually feels deeply relaxed. If you are a consistent exerciser, you know that feeling and perhaps are aware of its lasting effects throughout the day. The relaxation that comes after exercise brings with it a certain imperturbability, a lowered resting reactivity to the environment, which helps the regular exerciser react more appropriately to stimuli. Your step is a little lighter, your attitude more positive, and it takes more to make you upset (Crocker and Grozelle 1991).

In using activity as a preventive agent, you should use up stress products daily rather than wait for a stressor to trigger the system. This calls for a regular exercise regime. In a preventive exercise program your motivation is of a higher level than the urge to run or hit a ball against a wall when angry or upset. Because of this difference in intensity of purpose, a regular pattern of exercise must somehow be rewarded in its initial stages until it becomes a reward in itself. Exercising with a partner, joining a club, or making certain to engage in an enjoyable activity is helpful for this purpose.

Exercise for Well-Being and Tranquility

The highest purpose of physical exercise is to gain a sense of well-being—you participate because it feels right (and conversely, feels wrong when you don't), because it enhances positive feelings toward yourself that bounce off others as positive energy, and because it helps make your life complete. The tranquility state, the oneness, the internal calm experienced by those who really become involved in their activity make the prospect of a regular exercise program intriguing.

Exercise is a natural form of expression. We were made to move. And when we do, if social sanctions do not prevent our psychological acceptance of the activity, we rediscover the original unifying thread of mind and body. It makes us feel naturally healthy, just as we feel when we know that we're eating the right foods and dealing with social problems in a self-enhancing manner. But we cannot achieve this feeling unless we enter into activity in a noncompetitive way.

Beyond Competition

As we have discussed at length, physical activity can significantly reduce the immediate stress arousal; however, playing a highly competitive game of golf and wrapping a putter around a tree are not relaxing activities. Nor is a game of tennis when your self-esteem is on the line. This is one reason that singular activities such as running, biking, or skiing often have greater relaxation rewards than competitive sports, in which winning is more important than playing your best.

We are competitive people with a competitive heritage. We compete for money, jobs, space, and glorification of the self. It may seem odd that our leisure and recreation activities, intended as diversions from competition, are themselves competitive. We become conditioned to seek self-esteem enhancement from beating others, and there is no reason to believe we can stop competing just because we are not on the job or in school—the drive to win carries over into all aspects of life. Most of us measure ourselves by comparing ourselves to others. As was mentioned, exercise will burn off much of the stress arousal products, but competition often creates more stress in the form of lingering self-doubt, anger, and embarrassment. Think about your recreational activities. How transcendental are they? Do you lose your sense of time, do the hours seem like minutes? Or do you lose your temper and/or patience with yourself and others? Do you lose your sense of self? Or are you constantly "seeing yourself" and admonishing yourself for poor performance?

Research by Morse (1994) and DeGeus and colleagues (1993) added to this concept. In their projects subjects were asked to complete identical exercise tasks while in a "hateful" and then in a "loving" emotional state. During the "hateful thoughts" bout of exercise, subjects had elevated maximum heart rate and blood pressure when compared to the "loving thoughts" bout of exercise. These researchers concluded that although exercise has been touted as a beneficial means of getting rid of hostility, physical activity that is hostile in nature or is performed by individuals who have a hostile personality can be deleterious to an individual's health.

Competitive sports are not the only leisure activities that are the culprits here. Performance of singular activities (such as running or skiing) is no guarantee of self-transcendence. "Can I run three miles? Am I running as fast today as yesterday? What if I can't make it the entire distance? I really don't have it any more. Why can't I make a simple parallel turn?"

Some activities are not directly competitive, with a winner and loser in each event, but we can make them competitive by constantly rating our performance against our past performances or against the performances of others. More important, we allow the performance to influence our feelings about ourselves. This is the "terrible athlete, therefore terrible person" syndrome. This syndrome was given life in a touching biographic account by a forty-five-year-old health educator who was recovering from coronary bypass surgery. He was confused because he had none of the cardiovascular risk factors and had constantly monitored his physiological performance data. Upon reflection, he remembered his ever-improving times as he pedaled a rigorous mountain road, while in the back of his mind he heard, "You're not good enough. Do better." Only afterward did he realize he could not remember the beautiful scenery on his ride. Lucky to be alive, he does the same ride now, takes his time, enjoys the scenery, and constantly affirms that he is good enough at the things that really matter in life (Kearns 1995).

To remove the conscious, critical analyst, top performers go into a mindful state in which they "merely perform." In each of us is the inherent athlete who can perform without constant self-instruction; who can get lost in the joy of the movement, flow with the feeling of the activity, and correct movements through somatic and visual feedback, not through conscious criticism.

High-Risk Activity

Each year more people than ever take to what is called high-risk recreation. They try to exist in the wilderness for days with no food, tents, or weapons; climb high mountains; navigate wild rivers; sail around the world alone; and other dangerous activities. The reasons for the upsurge in the popularity of high-risk activities are numerous, but one that stands out is the pleasure and exhilaration the individual receives from success. Many of these situations are "dare not lose" (in the sense that to lose would mean death), so survival is winning. More important, survival is possible only if one totally concentrates on the activity. The innate survival instinct takes over and demands total attention. High-risk activity is used by many athletes to quiet their mind as they use the activity as a form of concentrative meditation.

Exercise Assessment

In the Activity Assessment (Table 17.1) on the following pages, if you score below 40 points, you are a very sedentary person and should consider engaging in an activity higher in the point system than the activities you usually engage in. If you score above 55, you are probably enjoying the benefits of physical activity. Everyone who is physically able should have some regular activity worth more than 5 points per hour. To be a "regular exerciser," you should perform that activity five times a week for at least half an hour per session.

Concerning the last four questions on the exercise, if you do not use physical activity to burn off stress products, try it. Choose an activity compatible to you and your lifestyle (Table 17.2 may be of help), and try it the next time you can't seem to calm down after a confrontation. Do it long enough for it to be physically effective—you'll need to walk longer than you would run to use up similar energy products. If you find you can tolerate this activity, try doing it regularly so you can keep a low stress profile. And if you really learn to love the activity, you will recognize the rewards and want to pass them on to others.

TABLE 17.1   Activity Assessment

The following self-assessment of your activity level lists activities that are part of many people's daily routine. In addition, a sample of other activities is given. If you engage in an activity other than that listed, try to approximate that activity with one given here, and use the points accorded to it. After completing the exercise, you will have twenty-four hours of activity listed. For each hour or partial hour, multiply the weighted score given for the activity, and then total the points. This is your physical-activity score.

After filling out the activity assessment, answer the four questions dealing with your motivational state and physical activity.

List the number of hours per day you spend

Sleeping	_____ hours	@ .85 points/hour	_____
Sitting		@ 1.5 points/hour	_____
Riding/driving	_____ hours		
Studying/deskwork	_____ hours		
Meals	_____ hours		
Watching TV	_____ hours		
Reading	_____ hours		
Other	_____ hours		
	_____ hours		
	_____ hours	(total sitting × 1.5) _____	
Standing		@ 2 points/hour	
Standing	_____ hours		
Dressing	_____ hours		
Showering	_____ hours		
Other	_____ hours		
	_____ hours		
	_____ hours	(total standing × 2) _____	
Walking			
Slow walk	_____ hours	@ 3 points/hour	_____
Moderate speed	_____ hours	@ 4 points/hour	_____
Very fast walk	_____ hours	@ 5 points/hour	_____
Occupational			
Housework and/ or light physical work	_____ hours	@ 3 points/hour	_____
Heavy physical labor	_____ hours	@ 4 points/hour	_____
Heavy total-body physical exertion			
Rapid calisthentics	_____ hours	@ 4 points/hour	_____
Slow run (jog)	_____ hours	@ 6 points/hour	_____
Fast run	_____ hours	@ 7 points/hour	_____
Recreational			
Racket sports	_____ hours	@ 8 points/hour	_____
Team sports (e.g., basketball)	_____ hours	@ 9–10 points/hour	_____
Stair climbing	_____ hours	@ 8 points/hour	_____
Total hours	24	*Total Points*	_____

Do you have an exercise outlet for stress buildup?	Yes _____	No _____
Do you use it?	Yes _____	No _____
Do you exercise regularly for its preventive rewards?	Yes _____	No _____
Have you discovered the transcendental nature of exercise?	Yes _____	No _____

TABLE 17.2 Activity Chart

Activity	Advantages	Possible Disadvantages*
Walking	No cost, no equipment, no special facilities. Everyone can participate. Year-round activity.	Time commitment, must walk fast for conditioning effect.
Jogging (less than 5 mph)	Promotes weight loss, leg strength, cardiovascular endurance. No special facilities.	May be hard on knees and other joints. Must have physical checkup, proper shoes.
Running (more than 5 mph) Stair climbing Step training	Promotes weight loss, cardiovascular conditioning, and well-being.	Must have physical checkup, good shoes. Can be hard on joints.
Dancing (folk, rock, aerobic, and other vigorous fast dances)	Promotes weight control, total-body conditioning, especially aerobic dancing (doing cardiovascular exercises to music). Year-round activity.	Must be brisk for conditioning. Requires coordination, rhythm for set dance patterns. May be hard on joints.
Biking	Good cardiovascular conditioning, promotes weight control, easier on joints than walking, jogging, running. Energy-saving transportation.	Danger from autos, cost of bike, requires learned skill.
Alpine skiing	Promotes total body-conditioning, especially legs. Enjoyable, apt to promote well-being.	Requires learned skill, expensive equipment. Can be dangerous (especially if not in condition) from falls, cold weather, and altitude. Seasonal.
Cross-country skiing	Excellent for cardiovascular conditioning, total-body fitness. Little jarring to body joints. Apt to promote well-being.	Requires some learned skill, special equipment. Cold and altitude may be a negative factor. Seasonal.
Swimming	Excellent for cardiovascular conditioning and muscle toning. No jarring to joints.	Requires some skill, pool, minimum cost of swimsuit.
Racket sports (tennis, squash, racketball)	Excellent total-body conditioner if fast game is played. Promotes weight loss.	Requires learned skill, special equipment, and facilities. Must play at high level for conditioning effect.
Golf (walk, carry own clubs)	Enjoyable and relaxing if not self-critical. Some of the same benefits of walking.	Requires learned skill, special equipment. Walking briskly without intermittent stops is a better conditioner.
Bowling	Relaxing and enjoyable if not self-critical. Better than just sitting.	Almost no conditioning effect. Requires learned skill and special equipment. Not recommended as treatment or preventive relaxation technique.
Slow, low-impact aerobic dance	Brisk, total-body exercises have conditioning value, especially muscle toning. No cost, little or no equipment. Year-round activity.	May exacerbate existing muscle problems. Tendency to overdo initially.
Weight lifting	Increases strength, improves physique, and may improve self-image. Can improve cardiovascular efficiency by lifting lighter weights for greater repetitions or by circuit training.	Requires special equipment. Some risk of muscular injury unless properly trained and prudently utilized.

*A possible disadvantage in most of these activities is high-level ego-involved competition.

Exercise Program Benefits and Guidelines

The benefits of regular exercise are worth the effort it may take to overcome inertia and begin an exercise program. In addition to the stress-management benefits that have been outlined in this chapter, there are other benefits that we have not yet mentioned and that may help to explain why a fitness program contributes to stress management.

Stronger Heart and Better "Tuning" of the Heartbeat

The heart is a muscle that, with use, increases in size and strength. It is the prime mover of the blood, which provides the tissues with oxygen and nutrients. Regular aerobic activity puts overload demands on the myocardial tissue, which responds by becoming stronger. As the heart becomes stronger, it can pump out more blood per beat, resulting in a slower resting heart rate. Aerobic training also changes the timing of the heart so that it spends less time in contraction and more time at rest. During the rest portion of the heart cycle, blood flows into the emptied cavities and also through the coronary arteries (the arteries that feed the heart muscle itself). This leaves more time for unrestricted blood flow to the myocardium, which in turn allows better nutrient flow and removal of wastes.

Increased Muscle Strength and Endurance

Exercise involving the large muscle groups helps develop the size and fluid capacity of the muscles through greater capillarization, increased muscle-fiber mass, and greater efficiency of contraction (Shephard and Astrand 2000). Because muscles act as pumps to help blood return to the heart, they develop a positive feedback cycle; they send more blood back to the heart, which pumps out more nutrients and oxygen to the muscles. Without the help of the muscles to send blood back to the heart, the heart takes on the full load of pumping blood throughout the system. This is why it is physiologically correct to cool down slowly rather than to just stop after vigorous activity.

Increased Lung Capacity

Just as in other deep-breathing relaxation exercises, vigorous aerobic activity demands that the lungs expand and the diaphragm drop, which helps squeeze blood from the trunk back to the heart. In addition, intercostal muscles are strengthened, and greater oxygenation of the blood occurs (Morris and Froelicher 1993).

Stronger Bones

When the body's bones are stressed with exercise, they respond by becoming denser (thus stronger). Weight-bearing exercise has been shown to prevent osteoporosis at any age (Shephard 1997).

Improved Serum-Cholesterol Level and HDL/LDL Ratio

Chronic aerobic exercisers have higher high-density lipoprotein (HDL) as opposed to low-density lipoprotein (LDL) levels than nonexercisers. HDLs are blood constituents that carry cholesterol to storage, getting it out of the blood stream so that it is not as likely to be involved in atherosclerotic plaquing of the smooth arterial walls (Wilmore and Costell 1999).

Improved Body Composition

As an individual becomes involved in an aerobic program, the body begins to use up fat stored in adipose tissue and develop more muscle tissue. Fat pads diminish, and muscular curves develop and become more apparent. An aerobic exercise program is a must for weight management (Lavie and Milani 1995).

Increased Range of Motion

As a safety measure, part of every exercise program involves stretching exercises. Without this kind of exercise, the muscles become organized at the semicontracted length and may create muscle cramps, soreness, and chronic pain. The exerciser should be able to enjoy a full range of motion in all muscles. As discussed in Chapter 15, stretching exercises also stimulate the relaxation response (Shephard 1997).

Greater Efficiency, Attention, and Economy of Movement

Another safety factor and stress-management benefit of a regular physical activity program is that the body becomes more efficient, cutting down on useless expenditure of energy. It is the difference between the beginning swimmer who thrashes around in the pool, expending great amounts of energy, and the trained swimmer who uses only the energy necessary to get from one end of the pool to the other. Because an activity program contributes to the alleviation of fatigue and anxiety, less meaningless activity is generated in this way.

Greater Alertness

Aerobic fitness improves nerve transactions throughout the body. All electrochemical transactions become more efficient, resulting in greater overall alertness and awareness.

Diminished Effects of Aging

Many of the characteristics that we attribute to the aging process are those that characterize the unfit individual. If we were to state the opposing side of each of the nine items just listed, we would get a picture of a debilitating process: inflexibility, low endurance, brittle bones, low respiratory capacity, creeping obesity, less alertness and awareness, and so on. When comparing our senior citizens, those who have been more physically active throughout their lives and continue to engage in vigorous activity appear to be younger and healthier than their nonactive counterparts (Blumenthal, Emery, and Madden 1991, Jette 1999, Shephard 1997).

The benefits outlined here, along with the specific stress-management benefits discussed earlier, are compelling evidence that everyone should conduct a personal exercise program. The latter part of this chapter describes how to set up such a program.

Preprogram Guidelines and Principles

Before starting an exercise program, consider the three following principles and guidelines to help you understand and enjoy exercise and the physical conditioning you will see and feel in yourself.

Regularity

The most beneficial exercise is regular exercise. Set up specific days and hours for exercise, and stick to this schedule. Most colleges offer regular exercise programs either in physical education classes or in intramural sports. Most cities also have recreation programs that offer a variety of physical activities.

If you are planning your own program, set aside three to five hours a week for vigorous exercise. If you take a formal exercise class, complement it with an independent program on weekends. Three to five one-hour periods of activity per week should provide a good exercise program.

Variety

A total fitness program includes stretching, muscle-strengthening exercises, and aerobic activity. A mixture of these will keep your fitness program interesting and beneficial.

The Overload Principle

In order to increase physical strength and endurance, you must push yourself beyond what you can easily do. For example, if you can walk at a brisk pace without being out of breath, you must move faster—at a jog or run—in order to improve your aerobic capacity. If you can easily lift and use a ten-pound weight, a heavier one is necessary to develop your arm muscles beyond their present state. Throughout a fitness program, work with greater resistance until it feels comfortable, and then increase the resistance again. When you get to the level of fitness at which you are aiming, level off with a maintenance program (that is, one designed to help you maintain a strength and endurance level).

In order for exercise to contribute to a stress-management program, it is not necessary to strive for marathon endurance or the strength of an Olympic weight lifter.

However, the greatest benefits to all-around health demand that the program increases your fitness level rather than just giving you sporadic exercise (McArdle 1999).

Aerobics Program

Most of the benefits of physical fitness come from a program of aerobic exercise, that is, activities that are vigorous, rhythmic, and involve the large muscle groups of the body. Cardiorespiratory fitness is effectively enhanced when an individual works at 60 percent of maximum capacity or more (capacity being measured according to heart rate).

Heart Rate

Your heart rate tells you two important things about aerobic exercise: (1) how vigorous the activity must be for you to benefit from the exercise and (2) how your system is responding to the exercise program, as reflected by your resting heart rate.

To find out how strenuous your workouts should be, you must have several items of information. One is your resting heart rate. Take your pulse for sixty seconds while lying in bed after just waking up. Your pulse is located on the thumb side of your wrist, on the outer side of the tendon that goes down to your hand. It is also located at your temples and other pressure points on your body, including the neck. However, when pressure is applied to the neck to find a pulse rate, the heart responds to the pressure, and you might not obtain a true reading.

Take your pulse several mornings in a row, and average the three readings. Enter your resting heart rate here:

Date _____ Resting heart rate _____

A second item of information you need to have is your maximal heart rate. The formula to determine this is 226 (for females) or 220 (for males) minus your age. Your maximal heart rate tells you how fast your heart can beat under a strenuous workload. The figures for men and women are slightly different because women apparently have a slightly higher maximal capacity (Althoff, Svoboda, and Girdano 1996). Enter your maximal heart rate here:

Women: 226 – _____ (age) = _____
(beats per minute)
Men: 220 – _____ (age) = _____
(beats per minute)

When you begin an aerobic or a maintenance program, you must determine your starting abilities. If you are minimally fit (that is, if even minor exertion is exhausting for you), you should begin your aerobic program at 50 to 60 percent of your maximal capacity. As your program gets easier for you, you can increase the load to 60 to 70 percent and higher. If you already engage in vigorous activity, begin your program at 70 to 80 percent maximal. If you are highly trained and very physically fit, you will want to use a range of 80 to 90 percent.

The last item of information that you must have is how to calculate your training heart rate. To do this, take 60, 70, 80, and 90 percent of your maximal heart rate. For example, a twenty-year-old male would have a maximal heart rate of 200. Sixty percent of that is 120 beats per minute. Seventy percent of 200 is 140. If this individual is beginning a program at a 60 to 70 percent range of maximal, he should keep his heart rate between 120 and 140 beats per minute during his workout. As he becomes conditioned during his program, he will move up to a 70 to 80 percent range, which then demands that he keep his heart rate between 140 and 160 beats per minute.

When you are doing aerobic exercise, it is important to keep moving slowly as you take your heart rate so that you do not let blood pool in the lower extremities with only the heart beat to pump the blood back up the body. When you move, your legs work as muscle pumps to continually squeeze blood back up to the heart. For this reason, rather than take the pulse for sixty seconds, you should take it for six seconds and multiply by ten.

To easily determine whether you are working within your target range, divide the top and bottom figures of the range by ten to identify what a six-second reading should be. In the previous example, when working at a 60 to 70 percent range, this man's six-second pulse should be between 12 and 14. When taking a six-second pulse, always count the first pulse as zero in case you just missed a beat. It is better to err on the low side than on the high side.

To determine how intensely you must exercise to get to your training heart rate range, you must experiment. Begin walking at a slow pace for two minutes, and then take your six-second pulse. If your heart rate is too slow, pick up the pace and repeat. Repeat this process until you find an intensity that will lift you into your range and keep you there. Take your pulse immediately after you exercise because your heart rate starts to slow down as soon as you slow down. It is extremely important that you adhere to your beginning heart-rate range to avoid burnout. Many people who start an exercise program are so highly motivated that they try to get all the benefits in just one day. They exercise too strenuously for too long a time, ending up with aching muscles, joints, and bones, and decide that exercise is not for them.

Intensity and Duration

An aerobic program will not maximally benefit you unless its intensity is at your training heart rate and its duration is at least fifteen minutes. However, there is an inverse relationship between intensity and duration that enables you to gain training effects at lower intensity levels if the duration is longer. This means that even a low-intensity walking program will give you training effects if you walk for a long period of time. Performing an exercise for three hours at a heart rate of 110 beats per minute will give you the same training effect as performing one for twenty minutes at a rate of 140 beats per minute (Cooper 1994).

The American College of Sports Medicine and the Centers for Disease Control and Prevention recommend that every U.S. adult should accumulate thirty minutes or more of moderate-intensity exercise (comparable to a brisk walk) on most, preferably all, days of the week (American College of Sports Medicine 1995).

When beginning a program, the duration of exercise should be low, perhaps as little as five to ten minutes per day (especially if fitness level is very low). Duration should then increase progressively.

For developing and maintaining cardiorespiratory fitness, perform large-muscle, rhythmic exercise three to five days a week, fifteen to sixty minutes per workout at 60 to 90 percent of your maximal heart rate.

When you choose an activity, keep your interests, abilities, and objectives in mind. Make sure the activities you choose are compatible with your lifestyle.

Set realistic short- and long-term goals for yourself, and chart your progress. This helps with motivation and adherence to the program.

Get assistance in starting your program if you need more information or even for motivation. It may be helpful to work out with others.

Always warm up and cool down.

Aerobic exercises include running, jogging, walking, cycling, rowing, cross-country skiing, aerobic dance, rope skipping, hiking, swimming, and stair climbing. Depending on how they are played, many games, such as handball, racquetball, soccer, tennis, and basketball, may be aerobic.

Intermittent activity or activity of low energy output has some effect on increasing cardiovascular fitness, but more vigorous exercise gives greater increase in fitness.

Flexibility Program

Stretching exercises are essential to any fitness program. Exercises such as the ones discussed in Chapter 15 should be performed for your relaxation program as well as a part of your aerobic activity. The key to safe, effective stretching is slow, constant pressure. Do not bounce—it may cause harm.

Muscular Strength and Endurance Programs

Two kinds of programs to develop muscular strength and endurance are available. One is a weightlifting program in which dumbbells, barbells, or machines are used for resistance. These programs are becoming very popular with both men and women and are available in schools, recreation centers, and workout studios. The second program involves using yourself as the resistance. The exercises in this kind of program are often called *calisthenics*. Whichever program you choose, follow the safety guidelines that apply to the kinds of exercises you will be doing. One does not have to be a stock-market analyst to realize that one of the fastest-growing industries in the world is recreation. People are beginning to recognize that it is very difficult to remain healthy while performing only sedentary tasks. So while some are driven to physical activity to counter boredom, others are trying to prevent degenerative diseases, and still others are driven to activity because the activity itself is "right" and feels good. Now add stress management as an additional motivating factor, perhaps the most compelling motivation of all. To many, physical activity is the only transcending experience they have ever had, so they seek to reproduce the feeling and search for more active leisure-time pursuits.

Unfortunately, modern men and women (at least in the industrialized world) are obsessed with recreation and pursue it with the same diligence and competition with which they pursue work. In fact, for many the only difference between work and recreation is that one may be done behind a desk, and the other is done on a basketball court. Everything else is the same. Critical analysis is present, as are competition and ego defense, so the participant is often left with self-doubt and extended worry over performance and its reflection on personality and character. In order for you to use a physical activity as a relaxation technique, it must be void of competition and ego involvement. Otherwise it is a mere diversion of your time.

SOURCES CITED

Althoff, S. A., Svoboda, M., and Girdano, D. A. (1996). *Choices in health and fitness.* Scottsdale, AZ: Gorsuch and Scarisbrick.

American College of Sports Medicine. (1995). *Recommendations from the Centers for Disease Control and Prevention and the American College of Sports Medicine.* Journal of the American Medical Association, 273, 402–7.

Berger, B. G. (1994). *Coping with stress: The effectiveness of exercise and other techniques.* Quest, 46 (1), 100.

Bird, S., Smith, A., and Gibbins, K. (1998). *Exercise benefits and prescription.* New York: Stanley Thomas.

Blumenthal, J. A., Emery, C. F., and Madden, D. J. (1991). *Effects of exercise training in men and women over 60 years of age.* The American Journal of Cardiology, 67 (7), 633.

Cooper, K. H. (1994). *The antioxidant revolution.* Nashville: Nelson.

Crocker, P. R. E., and Grozelle, C. (1991). *Reducing induced state anxiety: Effects of acute aerobic exercise and autogenic relaxation.* Journal of Sports Medicine and Physical Fitness, 31 (2), 277.

DeGeus, E. J. C., Lorenz, J. P., Van Doormen, L. J. P., and Orlebeke, J. F. (1993). *Regular exercise and aerobic fitness in relation to psychological make-up and physiologic stress reactivity.* Psychosomatic Medicine, 55, 347–63.

Greif, M. A. (1995). *The effects of short-term exercise on the cognitive orientation for health and adjustment in myocardial infarction patients.* Behavioral Medicine, 21 (2), 75–85.

Jette, A. (1999). *Benefits of home exercise in the elderly.* American Journal of Public Health, 89, 66–72.

Kearns, L. E. (1995). *The transformation of Lee Edward.* Journal of Health Education, 26 (3), 186–87.

Lavie, C. J., and Milani, R. V. (1995). *The effects of cardiac rehabilitation and exercise training on exercise capacity, coronary risk factors, behavioral characteristics, and quality of life in women.* The American Journal of Cardiology, 75 (5), 340.

Leutholtz, B., and Ripoll, I. (1999). *Exercise and disease management.* Boca Raton, FL: CRC Press.

McArdle, W. D. (1999). *Essentials of exercise physiology.* Philadelphia: Lea and Febiger.

Morris, C. K., and Froelicher, V. F. (1993). *Cardiovascular benefits of improved exercise capacity.* Sports Medicine: An International Journal, 16 (4), 225–36.

Morse, D. R. (1994). *Related exercise.* International Journal of Psychosomatics, 41, 17–22.

Shephard, R. J. (1997). *Aging, physical activity and health.* Champaign, IL: Human Kinetics.

Shephard, R., and Astrand, P.-O., eds. (2000). *Endurance in sport.* Champaign, IL: Human Kinetics.

Viru, A., and Smirnova, T. (1995). *Health promotion and exercise training.* Sports Medicine, 19 (2), 123–36.

Wilmore, J., and Costell, D. (1999). *Physiology of sport and exercise.* Champaign, IL: Human Kinetics.

CHAPTER

18 Your Personal Stress-Management Plan

Up to this point we have discussed what stress is and what can be done to avoid excessive stress and burnout. However, knowing educational theory alone is usually insufficient for initiating a lasting behavior change. Most people require a plan of attack. This chapter is designed to help you develop an individualized plan for personal stress management. This approach to developing a plan involves some introspection and some diligence in record keeping. Many people do not want to bother with the specifics; they would just rather deal in generalities and try a few comfortable exercises. That is understandable because there are a lot more fun and pressing things to do with your time. However, it is well to remember that in the behavior change research literature, the highest predictor of failure in smoking-cessation programs was unwillingness to fill in the forms about smoking habits. Likewise in weight management, the highest predictor of failure was unwillingness to fill out diet recall forms and track calories. Stress-management research yields the same results; failure is associated with noncompliance with doing the exercises. Pure and simple, compliance signifies commitment and motivation equals success.

In an overwhelming majority of cases, people experience stress because they have a stressful lifestyle and have learned through years of conditioning to react in a stressful manner. With regard to health and illness, a stressed person is one who exhibits physical arousal in response to social-emotional conditions. This exaggerated arousal is usually unnecessary for dealing effectively with the situation. A vicious cycle develops until minor happenings are met with major arousal, and the individual never really relaxes.

The stressed person experiences what can be termed mind-body arousal because both psychological and physiological systems are activated. Usually various physical, mental, and emotional arousals occur together, but the precise way that individuals manifest the stress reaction varies greatly. Because stress reactions are so complex and varied, it follows that no two individuals will react in exactly the same manner to a similar stressor. The type of stimulus that causes the stress response in individuals is highly variable; what causes one person excessive stress may cause less stress or even no stress for another individual. This is because stress is a reaction based on an individual's perception of the circumstances or situation, and it is safe to say that no two individuals perceive any given stimulus in exactly the same manner.

By understanding the concepts and nature of stress, it becomes evident that the management of stress is best achieved by an intervention plan that is custom made for an individual. You will recall from an earlier section of this volume that personal stress management is best when holistic, that is,

- individualized
- practically designed to suit personal preferences
- multidimensional
- flexible

Developing the Plan

A good starting point is to address your stress reaction. Summarize what you feel are your serious or obvious symptoms of stress. Give them serious thought. Try this visualization exercise.

Step 1. What Do You Want to Accomplish?

Exercise 1: Goals.   Find a comfortable sitting position. Kick off your shoes, lean back, and relax. Sit quietly. Tell yourself that you are going to use the next five minutes to focus on yourself and to relax. Gently close your eyes. As you inhale, feel the air filling and expanding your chest, your stomach area, and your abdomen. When your lungs feel full, hold the breath for five seconds, and then begin to slowly exhale, controlling the air as your abdomen begins to contract. Push all of the air out of your body at the end of your exhalation. Repeat three times.

After practicing the full breathing part of the exercise, shift your attention to your body. Scan your face, shoulders, upper back, lower back, abdomen, legs, knees, and ankles. Ask yourself, "How do I experience the stress in my life?" "Which sections of my body are affected when I am stressed?" "What happens to those body parts?" Scan your body, becoming more and more aware of it as you go inside yourself to gather this information. Remember this information for further use. Focus on your breathing again, and, when you are ready, open your eyes. Slowly stretch your hands, feet, arms, and legs as you become active again. The preceding exercise is an opportunity to get in touch with yourself and to discover the ways in which you internalize stress. Use the following lines to write what you felt during this first body-scanning exercise.

Exercise 1: Report

_____

_____

_____

_____

To further your insights about how stress affects you and to begin developing that awareness, complete Exercise 2. Your responses to this exercise may indicate which systems in your body are likely to be subjected to stress arousal and become weakened. This exercise lists some of the potential arousal signs in three major categories. Check the symptoms you usually experience, and then describe (on the lines provided) additional symptoms you may also experience.

Exercise 2: Signs and Symptoms.
Check the items that you often experience.

Musculoskeletal Signs
_____ stiffness in neck

_____ fingers and hands tremble or shake

_____ twitch in muscles (specific muscle: _____)

_____ difficulty standing still or sitting quietly

_____ stuttering or stammering speech

_____ frequent headaches (location on head: _____)

_____ muscle tension (specific muscles: _____)

_____ voice quivers

_____ nervous mannerisms; for example, biting nails, twisting hair, tapping feet, and so on.

_____ other

Visceral Signs
_____ heart pounding

_____ feeling light-headed or faint

_____ cold chills

_____ cold hands

_____ cold feet

_____ dry mouth

_____ profuse sweating (location: _____)

_____ upset stomach

_____ sinking feeling in stomach

_____ frequent digestive disturbance

_____ moist or sweaty palms

_____ flushed or hot face

_____ other

Mood and Disposition
_____ preoccupied

_____ frequent insomnia

_____ uneasy or uncomfortable

_____ nervous or shaky

_____ confused

_____ forgetful

_____ insecure

_____ overexcited

_____ angry

_____ irritated

_____ worried

_____ anxious

_____ exhausted

_____ other

Exercise 3: Stress and Stressors.   After you get a picture of your stress reaction, next concentrate on your usual triggers of the stress reaction. For this exercise, close your eyes to let visualization help you picture your stress and stressors. Think about each question, and then open your eyes and write your thoughts in the space provided.

1. Close your eyes, but in your mind picture a tense person. Scan your picture of this stressed person. What does the person look like when stressed? What is the person doing with his or her legs . . . arms . . . face? How is this person sitting or standing? Also picture the people and activities surrounding this individual in the stressful situation.

2. How are you like the image of the stressed person? How are you different?

3. Can you recall a stressful environment or situation in your life? How is this environment like your image, and how is it different?

Generally, what are the major ongoing stressors in your life? To better understand these stressors and to add to your picture of your stress reaction, do the following exercise.

1. Go to your stressor profile (Appendix A), and examine each of the stressor self-assessments.
2. Identify the stressors to which you feel vulnerable. Your self-assessment scores will reveal your current degree of stress for each stressor.

3. List your top three stressors in descending order.
   My most significant stressors are
   a. (score: _____)
   b. (score: _____)
   c. (score: _____)
   Pick one of these three to work on first and write it here:

   _____

   Write a short statement about why you have chosen this stressor over the other possibilities.

   _____

   _____

   Have you ever taken steps to reduce this stressor before?
   _____ Yes _____ No

   If yes, what were the results? _____

   If no, why not? _____
   Write a brief but specific outcome statement.

   I want to _____

   _____

   Rate on a scale of 1 to 10 how ready you are to alleviate this stressor.
   1 - - - - - - - - - -10
   Low   High

   Rate your ability to do it now.
   1 - - - - - - - - - -10
   Low   High

If you did not give yourself at least an "8" on both scales, your chances of success will be decreased. In that case you may wish to reconsider your other major stressors and focus on your second choice.

Step 2. How Will Things Be Different or Better in Your Life?

This question is often overlooked in stress-management programs. It is the motivation question. Everyone is committed to some degree, and everyone undertaking a stress-management program would like to be more in control, but only the very committed will finish the program and change the behaviors necessary to be successful. The committed will be able to visualize the new behavior and clearly see how life will be different or better than it was with the old behavior. To strengthen that picture in your mind try the following visualization exercise.

Outcome Visualization

Outcome visualization is used for programming or imprinting a new thought about behavior or belief about oneself. The technique involves seeing, hearing, and feeling yourself doing the new behavior. By mentally practicing the desired new behavior, a potentially stressful situation that would have previously triggered the old behavior instead triggers the new behavior because it has been rehearsed in the mind. Try this now.

Exercise 4: Visualization.   Close your eyes, and visualize yourself having accomplished the new behavior. Visualize yourself without the stressor or as a more relaxed person in the old stressful situation.

If you have difficulty in this exercise, it may mean that you are ambivalent about giving up the stressful behavior because, on some level, that behavior has served a very useful purpose, possibly for many years. Sometimes individuals cling to stressful behaviors because of some conscious or subconscious gain or benefit. Most stress behaviors are done for a positive reason, regardless of whether that purpose is consciously known. When an individual experiences difficulty in or ambiguity about giving up an old behavior, it is time to explore the cause of this reluctance. The phenomenon of continuing a negative behavior because it fulfills some need is called *secondary gain,* and the exact nature of the secondary gain is often not realized on a conscious level. For example, some commonly observed secondary gains accompanying stress are the following:

1. Maintaining control of life—many people fear becoming lazy and feel that keeping their "nose to the grindstone" protects them.
2. A strong need to please others and gain recognition often pushes people to take on more than they can handle. Again it provides external motivation for those who cannot do it for themselves.
3. Control of others through manipulation or to give oneself permission to rest or quit—this occurs when people overwork themselves to the point of fatigue, illness, or accident.

Step 3. How Do You Know When You Have Achieved an Outcome?

What Will You Accept as Proof?   As with Step 2, this critical phase of the program is often forgotten or omitted. It is easy to accept vague statements such as "I will feel better," "I will look better," or "I will have more energy." However, you must have definite, measurable proofs. How will you know that you feel better, look better, or have more energy? What will you accept as proof of these outcomes? The important word in this step is *measurable.* If your outcome is being more relaxed, how will you measure that outcome?

If you are having difficulty setting behavioral proofs, think of how you would observe this behavior in someone else. For example, how would you know a person was energetic; what behavior would be proof or evidence of that to you? You might make a list of the behaviors and apply them to your situation. If you are still experiencing difficulty, choose a personal friend or someone in the movies or on TV who exhibits the behavior you desire. What would you accept as proof or evidence that the other person has the behavior? Can you make a similar observation in your life? If the answer is yes, it can be accepted as proof, and the process continues.

One of our students who was working on a stress-management program with an outcome of self-confidence had difficulty with Step 3 until he identified the character Luke from the movie *Cool Hand Luke* as the model for his behavior. *Cool Hand Luke* not only provided him with a model for his targeted behavior, but the name also became a reminder or "anchor" of a time when he was self-confident.

Write a short list of ways you can prove to yourself that you have achieved your stated outcome.

These are proofs:

_____

_____

_____

Step 4. What Are Your Useful Resources?

This is an enjoyable part of the program because it helps build self-esteem by recalling resources and successes. When you feel confident about your ability to succeed in obtaining your outcomes, almost nothing will hold you back. Resources are both internal (personal characteristics) and external (environmental, social, or economic). Examples of internal resources are integrity, tenacity, willpower, energy, a sense of humor, self-love, and other self-concept issues. External resources may be the money to buy a good set of running shoes, the availability of certain facilities, or a devoted partner who will give support during the program. Resources may be general (as the suggestions given earlier) or specific to a situation (such as the *Cool Hand Luke* example). Both are very useful, but the best resources are those that use a specific skill that has been programmed in a certain situation.

Finding a Resource State

The intent of finding a resource state is to give you access to positive feeling states within yourself. The process itself builds self-esteem, promotes good feelings about the person at the time, and can be "anchored" into the mind and body for retrieval of these positive feelings at later times.

Exercise 5: Resources.   Scan through your experiences and choose a time when you felt very fulfilled, confident, joyful, or peaceful—a state that felt very good to you. There have probably been many, many experiences in the past that would be appropriate, but choose one specific time and experience.

The resource-state exercise gives the very best results when you can take yourself back to relive a specific experience. Generalities do not work as well because they are not as powerful as a singularly wonderful experience or feeling state. When finding a resource state, you should be able to vividly recall that experience. You can almost smell the flowers and look down and re-create all the details from the color of your shoes to the things you were saying to yourself and command the very same feeling you felt at the time of the original experience. Get back into the original experience, create a detailed picture, "hear" all the sounds in the experience, and re-create the feeling you had at the time. You might want to select a colorful name that will have special meaning and help you recall the feeling. Some of the effective names people have chosen have been Strawberry Blond, Cool Hand Luke, Smart Lady, Eagle Wings, and Hot Shot. Others have come up with words such as "confident" or "strong," which describe their resource state, or words such as "rock" or "soaring," which depict location or action at the time. The colorful and specific names elicit greater response than the generic names, perhaps because words such as "strong," "confident," or "rock" can conjure up many other meanings for many people.

Exercise 6: Coping Skills*

_____ 1. Give yourself 10 points if you feel that you have a supportive family.

_____ 2. Give yourself 10 points if you actively pursue a hobby.

_____ 3. Give yourself 10 points if you belong to a social or activity group that meets at least once a month (other than your family).

_____ 4. Give yourself 15 points if you are within five pounds of your "ideal" body weight, considering your height and bone structure.

_____ 5. Give yourself 15 points if you practice some form of deep relaxation at least three times a week. Deep-relaxation exercises include meditation, imagery, yoga, and so forth.

_____ 6. Give yourself 5 points for each time you exercise thirty minutes or longer during the course of an average week.

_____ 7. Give yourself 5 points for each nutritionally balanced and wholesome meal you consume in an average day.

_____ 8. Give yourself 5 points for each time you do something that you really enjoy, "just for yourself," in an average week.

_____ 9. Give yourself 10 points if you have some place in your home that you can go to relax and/or be by yourself.

_____10. Give yourself 10 points if you practice time management in your daily life.

_____11. Subtract 10 points for each pack of cigarettes you smoke in an average day.

_____12. Subtract 5 points for each evening during the course of an average week that you take any form of medication or chemical substance (including alcohol) to help you sleep.

_____13. Subtract 10 points for each day in an average week that you consume any form of medication or chemical substance (including alcohol) to reduce your anxiety or just calm you down.

_____14. Subtract 5 points for each evening during the course of an average week that you bring work home; if work that was meant to be done at your place of employment.

_____   Total Score

If you have not calculated your total score, do so now. A "perfect" score would be 115 points. If you scored in the 50 to 60 range, you probably have an adequate collection of coping strategies for most common sources of stress. However, you should keep in mind that the higher your score, the greater your ability to cope with stress in an effective and healthful manner. Also pay particular attention to the adaptive-versus-maladaptive coping dichotomy. Items 1–10 are all adaptive health-promoting coping tools, but items 11–14 are all maladaptive, health-eroding ways of coping with stress. How did you do? Ideally, you would limit your coping strategies to only adaptive techniques.

How do you cope with stress? What techniques do you employ to give yourself a sense of mastery (or self-efficacy) over the environment, and how do you handle the stress it can elicit? Exercise 6 was designed to help you see how you cope with the stress in your life. Coping can be defined as action-oriented and intrapsychic efforts to manage external and internal demands that tax or exceed a person's resources. Coping can occur prior to a stressful confrontation, in which case it is called *anticipatory coping*, as well as in reaction to a present or past confrontation. As was discussed earlier, coping behavior may be considered adaptive or maladaptive. Adaptive coping tactics are those that can be successfully employed to reduce stress and promote long-term health.

1. Look at your coping assessment. Items 1–10 help you manage stress and avoid burnout when practiced on a consistent basis. Items 11–14 may help you cope with stress in the short run, but they can erode your health in the long run.
2. List your three most commonly practiced coping tactics.
   My most commonly used coping techniques are as follows:
   a. _____
   b. _____
   c. _____
   (Are they adaptive, as in items 1–10? Or are they maladaptive, as in items 11–14?)

Write one or two statements describing a personal resource that will help you achieve your goal. Write them in the form of affirmative statements, as if you already have the resource—because you do. Example: "I am organized and I always obtain my goals."
   Affirmation 1. _____
   _____
   Affirmation 2._____
   _____

Everyone possesses the skills for achievement of outcomes—they usually have not associated their positive resources with the problem situations or have blocked their use for some reason. The following is an outline of the procedure used for maximizing the use of resources in obtaining outcomes.

1. List your resources.
2. If each resource is valid, you will feel good about it and be excited to use it.
3. Decide what you will accept as proof that you have use of the resource. Look for measurable behaviors.

4. You should be able to create a resource state. Going to your resource state should make you feel better.
5. Think of specific ways to recall and use each resource in getting your desired outcome.
6. If the resource is one of high energy, but you remain "down," either the resource is not a positive, well-anchored one, or you are choosing to be "down." When you choose to remain in the problem state, it is time to suspect a secondary gain, which, as mentioned, is a hidden benefit of being "down."
7. You should be seeking support in your environment for the use and reinforcement of stated resources.

Step 5. What Are Your Blocks to Success?

Within each individual who has ambiguous feelings about behavior change, there is a part that would like to achieve the outcome, but there is another part that is afraid to try or to succeed. Feelings and actions that prevent a person from achieving his or her outcomes are called *blocks to success*. Blocks may be exaggerated parts of the stress problem itself (for example, excessive anxiety; lack of skills such as assertiveness; behaviors such as excessive anger; or secondary gains, including fear of failure or fear of success).

Fear of Failure

If a person with stressful behavior fails to adopt the new outcome behavior or fails to change the problem behavior, conditions are no better or no worse. The negative behavior has simply been kept a while longer (which would have happened if the person had not attempted the program in the first place). Many people see this as no harm done. Others see that some harm has been done because failure at an attempted program diminishes self-esteem and self-efficacy. Individuals who "fail" at a program are likely to think less of themselves, and more important, the program is associated with negative feelings. It will take more motivation to try again. An individual may say, "I tried that once and it didn't work, so why bother?" Many people would rather not try than risk failure, so they simply do not go beyond finding out what the problem is, or they rationalize the situation away. If the activities in Step 2 did not result in a clear picture of how life will be better, you will need to work on activities to increase the probability of program success.

Fear of Success

Fear of success is the reason most people fail to change health behaviors. Health behaviors are developed to fulfill a need; they all have a positive intention behind them. Unfortunately sometimes the behavior turns out to be unhealthy. Nevertheless, it did something positive, or it would have spontaneously extinguished itself. When a certain behavior is eliminated (for example, a stressful lifestyle), the need for that behavior (recognition or sympathy from others for being a hard worker) will go unfulfilled unless a substitute behavior is adopted to fulfill the old need, or the old need is eliminated. Fear of success occurs when a person finds that the thought of being without that behavior or lifestyle is often too much to face, so the person "fails" to change. If you are not making progress at the expected rate, or if you are not practicing relaxation techniques or completing homework assignments, chances are that you are not ready to give up the old behavior.

Step 6. Devise an Action Plan

Exercise 7: Techniques and Times. Review the earlier chapters that presented stress-management techniques. As you do, your task will be to identify two or three of the techniques discussed there that you are not currently using. As you review the numerous options, remember to consider your personal preferences and be practical.

Write down some techniques or action plans that would help you accomplish your outcomes.

_____

_____

_____

_____

Set a timetable for achieving this goal.

1. Break the total time into smaller intervals (for example, one month into four weeks).
2. Make a calendar of specific day-to-day activities, and place it where you can see it. An example is provided. Specific exercises and techniques are abbreviated. A blank calendar is also provided to get you started. A large month-by-month appointment calendar is preferable for your ongoing program.

For each week write outcome and resource statements.
This week's outcomes:

_____

_____

_____

This week's resource statements:

_____

_____

_____

Establish a program of activities. Get help from a health professional if needed. Design a practical plan in order to implement the new stress-management techniques you've just selected. In the space that follows, describe how you will integrate these new techniques into your daily and/or weekly habits. Use the contract method that follows. Many participants have found it an effective method for organizing their activities and for helping with their motivation. For example:

Technique 1.

Yoga

How I will use it:

Every morning before breakfast when I feel excessive tightness in muscles

Stress-Management Activities Contract

On this day   _____   _____   _____

                (month)   (day)   (year)

I have decided to begin to use the following new stress-management techniques:

Technique 1

_____

How I will use it:

_____

_____

Technique 2

_____

How I will use it:

_____

_____

Technique 3

_____

How I will use it:

_____

_____

_____

_____   _____

          (signed)   (date)

_____

        (witnessed)

Remember, stay flexible, reevaluate your plan in two to four weeks, and if you need to change this personal plan, do so.

Step 7. Devise a Revised Plan

Technique 1

_____

How I will use it:

_____

_____

Technique 2.

_____

How I will use it:

_____

_____

Technique 3.

_____

How I will use it:

_____

_____

List these tools:

> Daily Feeling Diary
> Daily Stress-Response Diary
> Monthly Stress-Management Calendar

Using Chapters 12 through 17, choose one or more exercises provided in those chapters to create a monthly stress-management plan as shown on the Example of Monthly Stress-Management Calendar. Also, complete the two daily diaries, and record their completion with a check mark each day.

A Sample Practice Plan

A total plan is more than just a promise to use certain techniques. It includes keeping a list of carefully selected techniques, records of the times used, feedback on your progress, and evaluation of success. Here is a sample plan.

A. Techniques
  1. Breathing and centering
  2. Resource statements
  3. Technique 1: Goal Path Model or other cognitive activity
  4. Technique 2: Muscle relaxation
  5. Technique 3: Meditation
B. Practice Plan
  1. Practice each daily sequence twice a day.
  2. Ponder or repeat the resource statements you have made.
C. Record Keeping
  1. Record times and make some notes about your experience with the practice.
  2. Complete the daily diary as a monitor of your progress.

Most athletic coaches agree that good practice leads to good performance on game day. The same philosophy applies to stress management. Good practice of relaxation

TABLE 18.1

SUNDAY	MONDAY	TUESDAY	WEDNESDAY	THURSDAY	FRIDAY	SATURDAY
		31	**1** D.D. ✓✓	**2** AM Breathing exercise PM Breathing exercise D.D. ✓✓	**3** AM Breathing exercise PM Breathing exercise D.D. ✓✓	**4** AM Breathing exercise PM Breathing exercise Physical activity D.D. ✓✓
5 AM Breathing exercise PM Meditation D.D. ✓✓	**6** AM Breathing exercise PM Muscle relaxation D.D. ✓✓	**7** AM Breathing exercise PM Visual imagery D.D. ✓✓	**8** AM Breathing exercise Resource statement PM Stretch relaxation D.D. ✓✓	**9** AM Breathing exercise Resource statement PM Physical activity D.D. ✓	**10** AM Muscle relaxation Resource statement PM Muscle relaxation D.D. ✓	**11** AM Stretch relaxation Resource statement PM Physical activity D.D. ✓
12 NEW Resource statmt. AM Visual imagery PM Muscle relaxation Resource statement D.D. ✓✓	**13** AM Stretch relaxation Resource statement PM Meditation Resource statement D.D. ✓✓	**14** AM Breathing exercise Resource statement PM Physical activity D.D. ✓✓	**15** AM Breathing exercise PM Meditation D.D. ✓✓	**16** AM Breathing exercise Resource statement PM Breathing exercise Resource statement Physical activity D.D. ___	**17** AM Breathing medita. Resource statement PM Breathing exercise Stretch relaxation Resource statement D.D. ✓✓	**18** AM Your choice PM Your choice D.D. ✓
19 NEW Resource statmt. Meditation Resource statement D.D. ✓	**20** AM Your choice PM Physical activity D.D. ___	**21** AM Visual imagery Resource statement PM Resource statement Stretch relaxation D.D. ✓✓	**22** AM Meditation PM Physical activity Resource statement D.D. ___	**23** AM Visual imagery Resource statement PM Muscle relaxation D.D. ✓	**24** AM Meditation Resource statement PM Your choice D.D. ✓✓	**25** AM Physical activity Resource statement PM Your choice D.D. ✓✓
26 AM Meditation Resource statement PM Stretch relaxation D.D. ✓✓	**27** AM Your choice PM Breathing exercise Resource statement D.D. ✓	**28** AM Visual imagery PM Physical activity D.D. ___	**29** AM Your choice PM Relaxation Recall + Resource statement D.D. ✓✓	**30** AM Relaxation Recall + Resource statement D.D. ___		You are on your own. PEACE

302

TABLE 18.2

SUNDAY	MONDAY	TUESDAY	WEDNESDAY	THURSDAY	FRIDAY	SATURDAY

TABLE 18.3 Daily Stress-Response Diary

STRESS How felt in the body	STRESSOR Cause or situation	Underlying content or root cause	Your action	Potential ways of alleviating STRESS or STRESSOR

Complete one row for each stressful situation you experience daily.

TABLE 18.4   Daily Feeling Diary

Choose two different times of the day, and fill in the following information on how you feel. Try to do this at the same times each day.

Dull	1	2	3	4	5	6	7	Alert
Sluggish	1	2	3	4	5	6	7	Energetic
Sad	1	2	3	4	5	6	7	Happy
Doubtful	1	2	3	4	5	6	7	Self-assured
Anxious	1	2	3	4	5	6	7	Tranquil
Withdrawn	1	2	3	4	5	6	7	Outgoing
Depressed	1	2	3	4	5	6	7	Exhilarated
Hungry	1	2	3	4	5	6	7	Sated
Weather poor	1	2	3	4	5	6	7	Weather good
Concentration: Poor	1	2	3	4	5	6	7	Concentration: Good
Stress high	1	2	3	4	5	6	7	Stress low
No exercise	1	2	3	4	5	6	7	Good exercise
Poor quality of sleep	1	2	3	4	5	6	7	Good quality of sleep
Overall quality of day: Poor	1	2	3	4	5	6	7	Overall quality of day: Good

techniques will lead to good application of the skills when needed. Take time to fill out the practice feedback sheets. If your practice is not going well, do something about it now!

SOURCES CITED

Cohen, F., and Lazarus, R. (1979). Coping with the stresses of illness. In *Health psychology*, ed. G. Stone, E. Cohen, and N. Adler. San Francisco: Jossey-Bass, 217–54.

APPENDIX

Personal Stressor Profile Summary

This Appendix gives you a chance to get a total picture of your own stress vulnerability by transferring each of your scores from the eleven self-assessment exercises to the Personal Stressor Profile Sheet on the following page. After you have filled in your scores on each of the scales, connect all of the points. You have now plotted a graph of your stressor profile. Although there is no linear relationship between the self-assessment exercises, the line will help you visually assimilate your total profile and will be most helpful when you compare results from retests at some later date. Knowing the source of your stress is vital to managing that stress.

A final note: You may be quite vulnerable to stress from a specific determinant even though your score was low on the assessment test in which it occurred. The reason for this is simply that several of the exercises consisted of two or three aspects under the same general heading. For example, you may be a "catastrophizer" of the greatest magnitude, and this may cause your life to be a very stressful one. However, it is possible that your score on the anxiety scale was low because you didn't suffer from the other feedback mechanisms. Therefore, it is important that you carefully consider each question in which you score poorly and determine how significantly this aspect of stress affects your life.

On the other hand, remember that, although these eleven scales are extremely useful tools for beginning to assess the sources of stress in your life, they are not clinically validated psychological tests and should not be treated as such.

At some later dates you may want to come back and retake the self-assessment exercises, formulating a second, third, or fourth profile as a record of your progress. Using the same profile, simply use different colors to indicate different dates.

TABLE APPENDIX 1 Personal Stressor Profile Summary Sheet

Exercise	1 Emotion	2 Self-Perception	3 Type A Behavior	4 Anxiety	5 Control	6 Change	7 Frustration	8 Overload	9 Boredom, Loneliness	10 Nutrition	11 Occupational Stressors
Scores Indicative of:	45	40	40	40	40	400	40	40	40	40	40
High Vulnerability to Stressors	40, 35, 30	35, 30, 25	35, 30, 25	35, 30, 25	35, 30, 25	350, 300, 250	35, 30, 25	35, 30, 25	35, 30, 25	35, 30, 25	35, 30, 25
Moderate Vulnerability to Stressors	25	20	20	20	20	200	20	20	20	20	20
Low Vulnerability to Stressors	20, 15	15, 10	15, 10	15, 10	15, 10	150, 100	15, 10	15, 10	15, 10	15, 10	15, 10

This profile is an educational tool and was designed to promote basic health education. It is in no way designed to be a substitute for the diagnostic procedures used by physicans or psychologists. Any concerns about your physical or mental health should be directed to your family physican, your local medical society, or your local psychological society.

307

INDEX

Abuse, 54
Academic overload, 129
Acetylcholine, 15, 20
Acupressure, 236
Adaptation, 32, 33, 47, 109, 142, 144, 155, 157, 202
Adaptive stress, 109, 114
Adrenals, 57
Adrenal glands, 16, 17, 25, 26, 57
Adrenaline, 17
Aerobics, 285
Affirmations, 85
Aging, 283, 288
Alcohol, 150, 152, 158
Aldosterone, 27, 28
Alexander, Franz, 29, 49
Alternatives, 122
Altitude, 157
Ambiguity, 198
Amygdala, 50
Anger, 33, 34, 36, 38, 42, 50, 54, 56, 57, 58, 64, 65, 72, 76, 95, 106, 107
Anger management, 64
Anxiety, 72, 96, 97, 106, 144, 145, 146, 154, 156, 159, 167, 178, 185
Aristotle, 73
Aromatherapy, 218, 221
Arousal, 5
Arousal response, 16, 18, 25
Assertiveness, 86, 87, 89, 166, 167
Atherosclerosis, 27, 42
Attachment, 76, 96
Attitude, 61
Autogenic, 239, 242, 246
Autoimmune, 47
Autonomic nervous system, 16, 17, 18, 25, 53

Bandura, Albert, 100, 102, 106, 113, 139
Behavior, 80, 83, 105
Belief, 54, 61, 62, 63, 64, 65
Beliefs, 50, 54, 61, 62, 63, 65, 66, 91, 96, 122, 125, 133, 139

Biofeedback, 232, 233, 238
Blood pressure, 142, 144, 146, 153, 155, 156, 158
Body temperature, 142
Bodywork, 73, 234
Bonding, 51
Boredom, 108, 136, 138, 139, 200, 201
Bradshaw, John, 8
Brain, 15, 16, 17, 18, 19, 20, 21, 22, 23, 24, 25, 27, 28, 30, 34, 35, 36, 39, 40, 42, 46
Brainstem, 16, 19, 22, 25
Brain Waves, 262
Breath counting, 218
Breathing, 213
Buddha, 68
Bureaucracy, 119
Burnout, 119, 120

Caffeine, 144, 158
Cannon, Walter, 2, 14, 50
Cardiovascular, 40
Cardiovascular system, 213
Catastrophize, 66
Central nervous system, 16, 18, 20, 27
Cerebellum, 18
Cerebral cortex, 21, 16
Challenge, 113
Change, 76, 108, 109, 111, 112, 113, 114, 115, 122, 125, 133, 134, 140
Choices, 11, 15
Cholesterol, 42, 148, 283
Chopra, Deepak, 68, 56, 63, 66
Cigarettes, 154
Climate, 157
Coffee, 144
Cognitive restructuring, 104
Collective unconscious, 74
Commitment, 52, 57, 113, 289
Communication, 51, 52, 166
Compassion, 9, 10, 74, 75, 82, 83
Competition, 278
Concentration, 95, 264
Confiding, 71

Conflict, 2, 169
Confrontation, 51
Conscious, 20, 22, 23, 25, 148, 151, 154
Conscious mind, 61
Consciousness, 73
Contemplation, 265
Control, 100, 113
Coping, 8, 22, 33, 34, 49, 185, 296, 297
Corpus callosum, 52
Cortex, 30, 32, 35, 36, 42, 46, 51, 52, 53
Cortisol, 15, 27
Crisis, 178
Crowding, 116, 118, 129, 140

Dating, 165
Deadlines, 128
Decision-making, 10, 196
Demands, 108
Depression, 50, 56, 57, 76
Diaphragmatic breathing, 60
Diet, 154, 158
Discrimination, 118
Disasters, 179, 185
Disease, 1, 2, 4, 5, 6, 9, 16, 23, 26, 27, 28, 29, 30, 32, 33, 38, 40, 42, 43, 45, 46, 47, 48, 49, 84, 276, 286, 288
Diseases of arousal, 47
Distress, 3, 4
Dopamine, 17, 22, 27
Dogma, 68, 69
Domestic overload, 129
Drugs, 150, 151, 158
Dubos, Rene, 4, 14
Dysfunctional families, 58

Eating and drinking habits, 144
Ego, 3, 7, 8
Egocentric, 68, 71
Ego defense, 61
Einstein, Albert, 72
Electroencephalographic, 262

Emotions, 34, 50, 51, 53, 56, 57, 58, 59, 60, 63, 64, 66, 67, 73
Emotional quotient, 56, 58
Empathy, 56
Endocrine system, 46
Endurance, 282, 287, 288
Endocrine system, 25
Endorphins, 39, 46
Environmental stressors, 201
Epinephrine, 190, 276
Erickson, 29
Ergotropic, 24, 28
Eustress, 3
Exercise, 275, 276, 277, 278, 279, 282, 283, 284, 285, 286, 287, 288
Exhaustion, 33
Expectations, 72, 108
Extrasensory, 73
Eye strain, 206

Fatty acids, 17, 27
Fear, 50, 51, 54, 56, 57, 58, 60, 64, 65, 66, 72, 76
Fear history, 65
Feldenkrais, 235, 236
Fight-or-flight, 12, 13, 17, 24, 25 33, 36
Fighting, 168
Financial, 193
Flexibility, 287
Forebrain, 50, 52
Forgiveness, 10, 83
Frontal cortex, 15, 52
Free will, 74
Friedman, M., 92, 93, 95, 102, 106
Fragrant oils, 219
Frustration, 108, 116, 118, 119, 121, 122, 125, 133, 198

Gas, 32
Gastrointestinal, 17, 18, 27, 36
Gellhorn, 24, 28
Glucocorticoid, 146
Gluconeogenesis, 27, 144
Goal alternative system, 122
Goals, 290
Goleman, 50, 56, 66
Guilt, 50, 56, 57, 58, 72, 77
Gurdjeiff, 73

Happiness, 54, 57, 58, 77, 163
Hatha yoga, 247
Heart rate, 285
Helplessness, 84, 102, 180, 184, 186
High-risk activity, 279

Hippocampus, 53
Holistic, 290
Holmes, 109, 111, 112, 140
Homeostasis, 51, 73, 109
Honor code, 77
Human environment interaction, 141
Human spirit, 74
Huxley, 71
Hyemeyohsts storm, 69
Hypothalamus, 16, 18, 19, 20, 22, 23, 25, 26, 27, 30, 36, 37, 53
Humor, 57
Hunger, 50, 63
Hypersensitivity, 183, 185, 186

Immune system, 16, 27, 44, 46, 57
Immunity, 44, 45, 48, 49
Immunotransmitters, 46, 47
Inactivity, 200, 201
Individuality, 73, 74, 77
Insight meditation, 271
Intent, 52
Interpersonal skills, 56

Jacobsen, 223, 234, 238
Jealousy, 50, 57, 76, 172, 173, 177
Jesus, 68, 79
Jet lag, 142, 144, 158, 205
Job complexity, 196
Job stress, 189
Journaling, 103
Joy, 50, 54, 57, 58, 77
Jung, 73

Karma, 78

Lao Tsu, 69
Laughter, 54, 57, 58, 66
Law enforcement officers, 180
Lazarus, R., 57
Left hemisphere, 52, 61
Lies, 78
Life events, 109, 111, 112, 140
Ligands, 73
Lighting, 206
Limbic system, 16, 19, 20, 22, 23, 25, 26, 30, 37, 50, 183
Living together, 165
Loneliness, 108, 136, 138, 139, 140, 174
Lonely, 60
Love, 50, 51, 54, 57, 58, 68, 71, 72, 75, 159

Maclean, Paul, 20, 28, 51, 67

Management of stress, 9, 11, 12
Maslow, Abraham, 11, 63, 67, 183
Massage, 234
Medicine wheel, 69, 70
Meditation, 14, 261, 263, 264, 266, 267, 271, 272, 273
Migraines, 42
Mind-body, 1, 4, 5, 16, 50, 51, 57
Mindbody medicine, 73
Mindfulness, 10, 11, 72, 75, 271, 273
Molecules of emotion, 50
Money, 72, 75, 172
Moods, 61
Motivation, 289, 293, 294, 298, 300
Muscles, 33, 34, 35, 36, 38, 39, 42, 222, 223, 232, 233, 248, 250, 251, 252
Muscle relaxation, 222, 223, 232
Muscle strength, 282
Muscle tension, 35, 36, 222, 223, 233, 234, 235
Musculoskeletal disorder, 225
Music, 156
Myss, C., 75, 79

Native Americans, 68, 69
Natural foods, 145
Neurohormones, 15, 20
Neuromuscular exercises, 223
Neuropeptide, 38, 39, 43, 46, 50, 53, 57, 73, 213, 214
Noise, 154, 155, 205
Norepinephrine, 15, 17, 20, 27, 190, 276

Occupational overload, 128
Occupational stress management, 209
Occupational stressors, 191
Opinion, 61
Organ system, 33, 34
Organizational stressors, 193
Ouspensky, 73
Outcome, 121, 122, 294
Overload, 108, 119, 126, 128, 129, 130, 131, 132, 133, 138, 194, 195, 196, 197, 198, 203, 210
Overspecialization, 194
Overwanting, 76

Pain, 50, 56, 62
Parasympathetic, 17, 18, 20, 24, 26
Pearce, Joseph, 51, 52, 54
Perception, 76, 108, 111, 112, 116, 119, 134, 136
Peptides, 15, 18, 20

Personality, 51, 62, 73, 74, 76
Pert, Candace, 5, 6, 7, 14, 15, 20, 25, 50, 52, 53, 57, 67
Philosophy, 2, 161, 162, 175, 274
Physical activity, 13, 274, 275, 276, 277, 278, 279, 283, 287, 288
Pineal gland, 141
Pituitary, 16, 20, 24, 25, 26, 27
Plan of action, 299
Plato, 73
Pleasure, 50, 54, 56
Polarity therapy, 237
Polypeptides, 20
Postcardiac treatment, 275
Posttraumatic stress, 178, 180, 181
Posttraumatic stress disorder, 179, 180
Prejudice, 118
Premature cognitive commitment, 63
Progoff, 104, 107
Pseudostressors, 27
Psychogenic, 43
Psychology, 2, 11
Psychoneuroimmunology, 46, 73

Quantum physics, 56, 72

Rage, 54
Rahe, R., 109, 111, 112, 140
Rationalization, 61
Receptors, 15
Reflexology, 238
Reiki, 237
Rejection, 72
Relationships, 51, 52, 56, 66, 71, 108, 119, 130, 159, 161, 162, 174, 176
Relaxation, 213, 238, 239, 240, 246, 247, 248, 250, 252, 253, 260
Relaxation technique, 64
Relaxation training, 185
Religion, 68, 72
Relocation, 202
Remorse, 77
Resistance, 32, 33, 34
Resources, 85, 295, 115, 121, 122, 128, 129, 135
Respiratory ailments, 214
Responsibility, 191, 197, 198, 202
Retirement, 204
Right action, 77
Right hemisphere, 52
Risk-taking, 71
Rosenman, R., 92, 93, 95, 106,
Role conflict, 198

Rolfing, 235, 236
Rossi, E., 29, 46, 48, 49

Selye, Hans, 3, 14, 32, 33, 34, 36, 47, 49
Self-awareness, 56, 82
Self-concept, 77, 80, 82, 83, 84, 85, 87, 89, 91, 95
Self-confidence, 83
Self-esteem, 83
Self-image, 62
Self-love, 82
Self-management, 56
Self-motivation, 56
Self-perception, 80, 84, 89
Self-respect, 83
Self-talk, 51, 58, 64, 90, 95
Self-worth, 82
Separation, 173
Sex, 166, 167, 169, 170
Sexual relations, 169
Shiftwork, 141, 205, 212
Signs and symptoms, 291
Simonton, 46, 48, 49
Skin, 43, 44, 45, 47
Smoking, 151, 153, 154
Social readjustment rating scale, 109, 111
Social support, 185, 186
Socrates, 73
Spinal cord, 16, 18, 22
Spiritual health, 261
Stress, 1, 3, 4, 5, 8, 9, 13, 14, 15
Stress arousal, 15, 29, 30, 33, 34, 38, 39, 42, 43, 47, 48
Stress and stressors, 292
Stress-management plan, 289
Stress products, 15
Stretch-relaxation, 247
Stress response, 1, 2, 3, 4, 12, 13, 15, 25, 29
Stress symptoms, 33, 34
Stressors, 1, 3, 30, 33, 34, 62, 80, 100, 102, 104, 105, 108, 144, 145, 148, 153, 154, 155, 180, 191, 198, 201, 202, 209, 212
Stressful events, 178
Subconscious 6, 7, 8, 12, 22, 25
Subpersonalities, 85, 107
Suffering, 76
Suicide, 179
Soul, 71, 72, 74, 76, 79
Symbolic threat, 30, 42

Sympathetic nervous system, 17, 24, 26
Sympathomimetic, 144
Symptoms, 4, 8

Tao, 69
Taoism, 69
Taoists, 68
Temperature, 208
Tension, 247, 248, 252, 253
Thalamus, 53
Therapeutic touch, 237
Thirst, 50
Thought stopping, 100
Thoughts, 50, 51, 56, 57, 60, 61, 62, 63, 65, 71, 73, 74, 76, 77
Threats, 30, 34, 37, 42
Time, 141, 195, 196, 197, 198, 203, 205
Time and body rhythms, 141
Time pressure, 128, 130, 195
Time urgency, 195
Tobacco, 150, 153, 154
Tonus, 36
Tranquility, 275, 277
Traumatic events, 184
Travel, 141, 142
Triglycerides, 42
Trophotropic, 24, 25, 28
Type A, 92, 93, 95, 96, 102, 106

Unconscious, 61, 62
Universal intelligence, 68
Universe, 69, 71, 72, 77, 78
Urban Time management, 131

Vasodilation 239
Victimization, 179
Violence, 178, 179, 187, 188, 203, 211
Visual imagery, 245
Visualization, 294
Vitamins, 144, 145, 157, 158

Weil, Andrew, 24,28
Well-being, 277
Withdrawal, 61
Work, 191, 194, 210
Workplace, 189, 203, 204, 205, 211

Yoga, 247, 260

Zero balancing, 238